Stem Cell Therapy and Tissue Engineering for Cardiovascular Repair

Nabil Dib, MD
Doris A. Taylor, PhD
Edward B. Diethrich, MD
(Editors)

Stem Cell Therapy and Tissue Engineering for Cardiovascular Repair

From Basic Research to Clinical Applications

With 91 Illustrations, 64 in Full Color

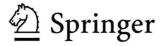 Springer

Nabil Dib, MD, MSc, FACC
Director of Cardiovascular Research
Arizona Heart Institute
2632 North 20th Street
Phoenix, AZ 85006
USA

Doris A. Taylor, PhD
Director
Center for Cardiovascular Repair
University of Minnesota
Minneapolis, MN
USA

Edward B. Diethrich, MD
Medical Director
Arizona Heart Institute
2632 North 20th Street
Phoenix, AZ 85006
USA

Library of Congress Control Number: 2005924728

ISBN-10: 0-387-25788-8   Printed on acid-free paper.
ISBN-13: 978-0387-25788-4

Printed in Singapore.   (SPI/KYO)

9 8 7 6 5 4 3 2 1

springeronline.com

Contributors

PETER ALTMAN, PH.D.
President
BioCardia Inc.
San Francisco, California

ELLEN AREMAN, M.S.
Biologist
United States Food and Drug Administration
Center for Biologics Evaluation and Research
Office of Cellular, Tissue and Gene Therapies
Division of Cellular and Gene Therapies
Cell Therapies Branch
Rockville, Maryland

FRANCISCO F. AVILESES, M.D., PH.D.
Professor of Cardiology
School of Medicine
University of Valladolid
Valladolid, Spain

KIMBERLY A. BENTON, PH.D.
Chief, Cell Therapies Branch
United States Food and Drug Administration
Center for Biologics Evaluation and Research
Office of Cellular, Tissue and Gene Therapies
Division of Cellular and Gene Therapies
Rockville, Maryland

RAVI K. BIRLA, PH.D.
Research Investigator
Section of Cardiac Surgery
University of Michigan
Ann Arbor, Michigan

MICHAEL BREHM, M.D.
Heinrich Heine University
Düsseldorf, Germany

DANIEL BURKHOFF, M.D., PH.D.
Adjunct Associate Professor of Medicine
Division of Cardiology
Columbia University
New York, New York

BLASÉ A. CARABELLO, M.D.
Professor of Medicine
Vice Chairman, Department of Medicine
Baylor College of Medicine
Michael E. DeBakey Veterans Affairs Medical Center
Houston, Texas

**NICOLAS A. F. CHRONOS, M.D., F.R.C.P.,
   F.A.C.C., F.E.S.C., F.A.H.A.**
Chief Medical and Scientific Officer
American Cardiovascular Research Institute
Atlanta, Georgia

NABIL DIB, M.D., M.Sc, F.A.C.C.
Director of Interventional Cardiology Research
Arizona Heart Institute and Heart Hospital
Phoenix, Arizona

MARCELO F. DI CARLI, M.D., F.A.C.C.
Associate Professor of Radiology
Harvard Medical School
Chief, Division of Nuclear Medicine/PET
Director, Nuclear Cardiology
Department of Radiology
Brigham and Women's Hospital
Boston, Massachusetts

EDWARD B. DIETHRICH, M.D.
Medical Director
Arizona Heart Institute and Heart Hospital
Phoenix, Arizona

SHARMILA DORBALA, M.D., F.AC.C.
Instructor in Radiology
Harvard Medical School
Associate Director, Nuclear Cardiology
Department of Radiology
Brigham and Women's Hospital
Boston, Massachusetts

EL MOSTAFA EL FAHIME, PH.D.
Associated Professor
Department of Anatomy/Physiology
Faculty of Medicine
Laval University
Quebec, Canada

STEPHEN G. ELLIS, M.D.
Professor of Medicine
The Ohio State University
Director, Sones Cardiac Catheterization Laboratories
Department of Cardiology
The Cleveland Clinic Foundation
Cleveland, Ohio
Columbus, Ohio

LUIS DE LA FUENTA, M.D.
School of Medicine
University of Valladolid
Valladolid, Spain

MANUEL GALIÑANES, M.D.
Professor of Cardiac Surgery
Cardiac Surgery Group
Department of Cardiovascular Sciences
University of Leicester
Leicester, United Kingdom

JAVIER GARCIA FRADE, M.D., PH.D.
Professor of Medicine
School of Medicine
University of Valladolid
Valladolid, Spain

JAVIER GARCIA-SANCHO, M.D., PH.D.
Professor of Physiology
School of Medicine
Institute of Biology and Molecular Genetics (IBGM)
University of Valladolid
Valladolid, Spain

MANUEL GÓMEZ BUENO, M.D.
School of Medicine
University of Valladolid
Valladolid, Spain

CAROLINA HERNÁNDEZ, M.D.
School of Medicine
University of Valladolid
Valladolid, Spain

STEFAN KLOTZ
Resident
Department of Thoracic and Cardiovascular Surgery
University Hospital Muenster
Muenster, Germany

HOWARD LEONHARDT
Chairman and CEO
BioHeart Inc.
Minneapolis, Minnesota

ATUL LIMAYE, M.D.
Clinical Fellow in Radiology
Harvard Medical School
Nuclear Cardiology Fellow
Division of Nuclear Medicine/PET
Department of Radiology
Brigham and Women's Hospital
Boston, Massachusetts

BRADLEY J. MARTIN, PH.D.
Associate Director
Cardiac Research
Osiris Therapeutics, Inc.
Baltimore, Maryland

MARK A. MARTIN, R.N., R.C.I.S.
Clinical Research Specialist
Clinical Research
Cordis Corporation
Warren, New Jersey

RICHARD MCFARLAND, M.D., PH.D.
Medical Officer
United States Food and Drug Administration
Center for Biologics Evaluation and Research
Office of Cellular, Tissue and Gene Therapies
Division of Clinical Evaluation and Pharmacology/Toxicology
Pharmacology/Toxicology Branch
Rockville, Maryland

PHILIPPE MENASCHE, M.D., PH.D.
Professor of Thoracic and Cardiovascular Surgery
Department of Cardiovascular Surgery
Hôpital Européen Georges Pompidou
Paris, France

SIMÓN MÉNDEZ-FERRER, PH.D
Postdoctoral Associate
Cardiovascular Research Institute
Department of Medicine
New York Medical College
Valhalla, New York

BERNARDO NADAL-GINARD, M.D., PH.D.
Professor
Cardiovascular Research Institute
Department of Medicine
New York Medical College
Valhalla, New York

HARALD OTT, PH.D.
Research Associate
Center for Cardiovascular Repair
University of Minnesota
Minneapolis, Minnesota

NICHOLAS PETERS, M.D., F.R.C.P.
Director of Electrophysiology Research
American Cardiovascular Research Institute
Atlanta, Georgia
Professor of Cardiology
Imperial College at St. Mary's Hospital
London, United Kingdom

MARK PITTENGER, PH.D.
Vice President, Research
Senior Research Scientist
Osiris Therapeutics, Inc.
Baltimore, Maryland

ROBERT RAPOZA
Senior Clinical Education Specialist
Clinical Affairs
Boston Scientific Corporation
Natick, Massachusetts

UCHECHUKWA SAMPSON, M.D., M.P.H., M.B.A.
Clinical Fellow in Radiology
Harvard Medical School
Nuclear Cardiology Fellow
Division of Nuclear Medicine/PET
Department of Radiology
Brigham and Women's Hospital
Boston, Massachusetts

ALBERTO SAN ROMÁN, M.D. PH.D.
School of Medicine
University of Valladolid
Valladolid, Spain

ANA SÁNCHEZ, M.D., PH.D.
Lecturer in Physiology
School of Medicine
Institute of Biology and Molecular Genetics (IBGM)
University of Valladolid
Valladolid, Spain

PEDRO L. SANCHEZ, M.D., PH.D.
School of Medicine
University of Valladolid
Valladolid, Spain

RICHARDO SANZ, M.D.
School of Medicine
University of Valladolid
Valladolid, Spain

DANIEL SKUK, M.D.
Associated Professor
Department of Anatomy/Physiology
Faculty of Medicine
Laval University
Quebec, Canada

BODO E. STRAUER, M.D.
Professor of Medicine
Heinrich Heine University
Düsseldorf, Germany

DORIS TAYLOR, PH.D.
Bakken Professor
Director, Center for Cardiovascular Repair
University of Minnesota
Minneapolis, Minnesota

FERNANDO TONDATO
Senior Scientist, Cardiac Electrophysiology
American Cardiovascular Research Institute
Atlanta, Georgia

JACQUES P. TREMBLAY, PH.D.
Professor, Department of Anatomy/Physiology
Laval University
Unit of Human Genetics
Quebec, Canada

OUSSAMA WAZNI, M.D.
Cardiology Fellow
Department of Cardiology
Cleveland Clinic Foundation
Cleveland, Ohio

TOBIAS ZEUS, M.D.
Heinrich Heine University
Düsseldorf, Germany

Preface

In the brief history of modern cardiovascular medicine, it has not been uncommon for scientists, researchers and clinicians to join forces in an effort to dramatically change the development and treatment of a specific pathology. The introduction of coronary arteriography, bypass surgery, angioplasty and, now, drug-eluting stents has positively influenced the care of patients suffering from lifestyle-limiting anginal symptoms due to obliterative coronary artery disease. In each of these and many other areas currently under study, the common denominator for success has been the ability to create a specific focal point where every available element of laboratory information is translated into a potential broad clinical application.

The publication of this inaugural text, *Stem Cell Therapy and Tissue Engineering for Cardiovascular Repair: From Basic Research to Clinical Applications*, is highly noteworthy and, more importantly, extremely timely in its focus on a disease of epidemic proportions. Statistics verify that myocardial infarction and congestive heart failure (CHF) are the most prevalent heart conditions not only in the United States (US) but also in other leading developed countries of the world. In US hospitals, myocardial infarction and CHF are the number one diagnoses in cardiovascular units today! This problem will not be solved with conventional procedures or enhancements of interventional devices. The answer will be found only in a better understanding and clinical application of gene, cell and tissue engineering.

The topics in this book, addressed by world-renowned authorities, were selected to cover the spectrum from basic development to clinical application. Pertinent information on cell isolation and expansion, both in animals and humans, is prevalent throughout, providing guidance for the clinical scientist interested in this area. There are detailed explanations of an FDA-accepted animal model for examining various cell lines, which hopefully will create some uniformity in experimental design. Regulatory authorities also discuss required cell manufacturing and pre-clinical pathways to eliminate the pre-clinical frustration of protocol deficiencies based on lack of requisite information and procedural mechanisms. This scenario is brilliantly illustrated in the description of the steps required for FDA approval of percutaneous myoblast transplantation.

The vital contents of this publication verify that which we have observed repeatedly from past experiences—great talent will assemble to conquer a great problem! It is not so much a question of which cell or process will ultimately be successful, but rather when and how it will come to fruition. Our hope is that the material presented here will speed us along that pathway, ultimately reining in yet another cause of human morbidity and mortality.

The Editors

Acknowledgments

I am privileged to have this opportunity to thank special people who affected me and my work throughout my life.

I would like to express my special appreciation to my mother, who cared, loved, educated and spent days and nights following my progress in my early childhood. To my father and brothers, who supported me endlessly.

To the wonderful teachers, I. Shatty, M. Joukhadar, and Dr. F. Sabbagh, who were examples of leadership and knowledge in my early days of schooling in Damascus University. To the ones who opened the doors for me at Boston University. To the special teachers, Drs. J. Isner, A. Ropper, J. Pastore, and D. Paydafar, who drew the first steps in research for me at Tufts University. To Dr. D. Schmidt who enhanced my career at the University of Wisconsin.

The unsurpassable education and attention at Harvard University gave me the skills for Interventional Cardiology with regards to procedure and technique, thanks to Drs. S. Shubrook, R. Nesto, D. Leeman, and S. Lewis. Special thanks to Dr. D. Baim for being an exemplary educator who built extreme self-confidence and a new horizon in my mind. To Drs. R. Kuntz and F. Cook, who supported me in the Harvard School of Public Health, where I truly learned the principles of research.

Without the support of Dr. E. Diethrich at the Arizona Heart Institute, the work on cell therapy and catheter based myoblast transplantation could not be possible. Special thanks to Ann Campbell, who helped me day and night to validate the catheter-based methodology for cell transplantation.

I am grateful to the authors for their contributions, Catherine Hamilton, for helping by coordinating and formatting this text, Sheila Ulrich, for corresponding with the authors, Springer, and VAS Communications, LLC who worked very hard despite limited time to make this text available.

Many thanks to my friend, Dr. Atileh for long and frequent conversations about the vision and the goal.

All my consideration and thanks to my wife Cheryl and daughter Lauren for understanding the time and hard work required to be where we are today.

Nabil

Contents

List of Contributors   v
Preface. xiii
Acknowledgements xv

Myocardial Remodeling

1. **Ventricular Remodeling in Ischemic Cardiomyopathy** **3**
   Stefan Klotz and Daniel Burkhoff

Myocardial Regeneration

2. **Myocardial Regeneration: Which Cell and Why** **25**
   Elmostafa El Fahime and Jacques Tremblay

Cardiac Stem Cells

3. **Cardiac Stem Cells for Myocardial Regeneration** **39**
   Bernardo Nadal-Ginard and Simón Méndez-Ferrer

Skeletal Myoblast

4. **A Historic Recapitulation of Myoblast Transplantation** **61**
   Daniel Skuk and Jacques Tremblay

5. **Myoblast Cell Transplantation Preclinical Studies** **81**
   Doris A. Taylor and Harald Ott

6. **Skeletal Myoblasts: The European Experience**   95
Philippe Menasche

7. **Skeletal Myoblasts: The U. S. Experience**   105
Edward B. Diethrich

Progenitor Cells

8. **Progenitor Cells for Cardiac Regeneration**   121
Ana Sánchez and Javier Garcia-Sancho

Bone Marrow

9. **Bone Marrow Derived Stem Cell for Myocardial Regeneration:
Preclinical Experience**   137
Bradley Martin and Mark Pittenger

10. **Bone Marrow Derived Stem Cell for Myocardial Regeneration:
Clinical Experience, Surgical Delivery**   159
Manuel Galiñanes

11. **Autologous Mononuclear Bone Marrow Cell Transplantation
for Myocardial Infarction: The German Experience**   169
Michael Brehm, Tobias Zeus and Bodo E. Strauer

12. **Autologous Mononuclear Bone Marrow Cell Transplantation
for Myocardial Infarction: The Spanish Experience**   187
*Francisco F. Avilés, Pedro Sanchez, Alberto San Román, Luis de la
Fuenta, Ricardo Sanz, Carolina Hernández, Manuel Gómez Bueno,
Ana Sánchez and Javier Garcia-Frade*

13. **Mobilizing Bone Marrow Stem Cells for Myocardial Repair
after Acute Myocardial Infarction**   203
Steve Ellis and Oussama Wazni

Percutanous Stem Cell Transplantation

14. **Percutaneous Myoblast Transplantation: Steps
in Translational Research**   213
Nabil Dib

15. **A Porcine Model of Myocardial Infarction for Evaluation
    of Cell Transplantation** 231
    *Nabil Dib, Edward B. Diethrich, Ann Campbell, Noreen Goodwin,
    Bark Robinson, James Gilbert, Dan W. Hobohm, and Doris A. Taylor*

Tissue Engineering

16. **Tissue Engineering for Myocardial Regeneration** 241
    Ravi K. Birla

**Functional and Electrophysiological Assessment
After Cell Transplantation**

17. **The Role of Pet Scan in Stem Cell Therapy** 257
    *Uchechukwu Sampson, Atul Limaye, Sharmila Dorbala,
    and Marcelo Di Carli*

18. **The Measurement of Systolic Function
    in the Mammalian Heart** 273
    Blasé Carabello

19. **Electrophysiological Aspects of Cell Transplantation** 289
    Nicholas S. Peters, Nicolas A.F. Chronos and Fernando Tondato

Regulatory Perspective

20. **Regulatory Considerations in Manufacturing, Product Testing,
    and Preclinical Development of Cellular Products for Cardiac
    Repair** 299
    Ellen Areman, Kim Benton and Richard McFarland

Appendix: Catheter Descriptions 315

Index 323

Myocardial Remodeling

1
Ventricular Remodeling In Ischemic Cardiomyopathy

STEFAN KLOTZ AND DANIEL BURKHOFF*

1. Introduction

Heart failure in the setting of reduced systolic pump function, if left untreated, is characterized by progressive ventricular dilation and dysfunction. Many of the major advances in pharmacologic treatments for heart failure achieved over the last two decades came with the recognition that this process, referred to as *ventricular remodeling*, results from abnormal mechanical stress on the myocardium (increased preload and afterload) and chronic neurohormonal activation (Figure 1). In the acute setting, loss of myocytes (as during infarction) or a defect of myocardial contraction (e.g., idiopathic cardiomyopathies) reduces overall ventricular pump function. This leads to reduced blood pressure and cardiac output, which activates autonomic reflexes that leads to increased circulating levels of neurohormones. It is believed, on a teleological basis, that these reflexes evolved in order to allow animals to cope with periods of increased energy demand (fight or flight) and to deal with acute blood loss.

In parallel with autonomic reflex activation, decreased systemic blood pressure and flow lead to renal hypoperfusion, which increases aldosterone, renin and angiotensin, I (which leads to angiotensin II) production. In the short term, these factors attempt to restore cardiac output and blood pressure via mechanisms that are considered adaptive. However, if sustained, neurohormonal activation and increased mechanical stresses conspire in a maladaptive process to drive cellular hypertrophy and elongation, global recapitulation of a fetal gene program, myocardial fibrosis, ventricular enlargement and dysfunction, apoptosis[1] and sets up a milieu for dyscoordinated myocardial contraction (e.g., conduction defects) and ventricular arrhythmias. A systemic inflammatory response also has been documented with increases of a multitude of cytokines which are also believed to contribute importantly to myocyte loss and disease progression.[2,3]

---

* Stefan Klotz and Daniel Burkhoff, Department of Medicine, Division of Cardiology, Columbia University Medical Center, New York, New York, 10032

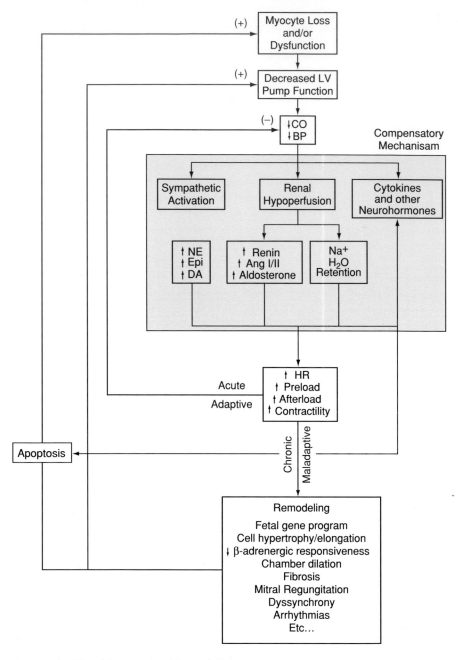

FIGURE 1. The vicious cycle of heart failure

It is now well known that ventricular remodeling involves molecular, biochemical, metabolic, cellular, extracellular matrix and ventricular structural characteristics as well as a multitude of effects on the peripheral circulation and viscera. Importantly, in the post infarct heart, the remodeling process affects not only regions of infarcted myocardium, but also normally perfused myocardium. Indeed, the previously normal myocardium is as affected by remodeling as the infarcted areas and changes in those regions assume a primary role in disease progression. The situation can be even further complicated in ischemic cardiomyopathy because noninfarcted regions can be supplied by stenosed coronary arteries so that active myocardial ischemia can be another factor influencing the remodeling process.

On a structural and functional basis, the remodeling process is readily represented on the ventricular pressure-volume diagram (Figure 2A). Within this framework, systolic and diastolic properties are represented by the end-systolic and end-diastolic pressure-volume relations, (ESPVR and EDPVR, respectively) which define the boundaries within which the normal pressure-volume loop resides (blue). An acute decrease in contractility, as with a myocardial infarction (MI), causes a downward shift of the ESPVR that results in a reduction in stroke volume and blood pressure (red solid line). The acute neurohormonal activation discussed above leads to increased heart rate, arterial and veno-constriction that increase arterial, venous and ventricular end-diastolic pressures (dashed purple line). With sustained neurohormonal activation and its consequences reviewed in Figure 1, the pressure-volume relations gradually shift towards larger volumes. Although stroke volume may be maintained to a large degree, ejection fraction is reduced because of the marked dilation of the left ventricle. In addition, marked myocardial hypertrophy occurs.

The goal of many heart failure treatments, be they pharmacologic, device- or cell-based, is to prevent, slow or reverse this process (Figure 2B). In particular the concept of *reverse remodeling* is an important principle for new treatments of heart failure.

Early experimental work on understanding the process of structural LV remodeling emerged from the studies of Pfeffer and Braunwald using a rat model of myocardial infarction.[4] Rats with induced large MIs underwent a substantially greater degree of chamber dilation over time compared to rats with a small MIs. In these early studies, the degree of chamber dilation was assessed by measurement of the *ex vivo* end-diastolic pressure-volume relationship (EDPVR). Through these studies, the term *ventricular remodeling* became synonymous with a rightward shift towards larger volumes of the EDPVR.

A graphic example of this remodeling process obtained from a canine model of heart failure is shown in Figure 3. A family of pressure-volume loops (obtained during a transient vena caval occlusion) from a normal dog chronically instrumented for measurement of left ventricular pressure (Konigsburg transducer) and ventricular volume (three orthogonally placed sonomicrometer crystals) is shown in Figure 3A. The loops delineate the

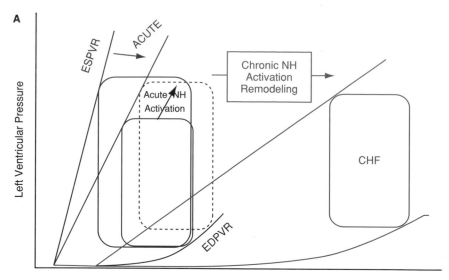

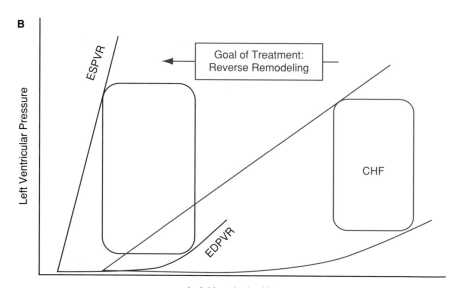

FIGURE 2. A. Changes in end-systolic and end-diastolic pressure-volume relations (ESPVR and EDPVR, respectively) and pressure volume loops with acute ventricular dysfunction (red solid line), with acute autonomic compensation (dashed purple line) and with chronic activation leading to structural ventricular remodeling (green). B. The goal of treatments is to reverse the remodeling process and restore more normal ventricular size, structure and function.

ESPVR and EDPVR. This same animal is then subjected to daily microembolisms via a chronically implanted left anterior descending coronary catheter.[5] Within about 6 to 8 weeks, this procedure induces a state of heart failure, which includes neurohormonal activation, fluid accumulation (ascites, pleural effusions), tachypnea, tachycardia and anorexia. On the pressure-volume plane (Figure 3B), the ESPVR shifts downward indicating reduced systolic performance. It is further seen that the EDPVR shift rightward towards larger volumes and the end-diastolic pressures is increased (arrow). Even after suspension of microembolization, the heart continues to remodel, characterized by further rightward shifts of both ESPVR and EDPVR (Figure 3C) and further elevations of end-diastolic pressure (arrow).

It is postulated that a similar course of events occurs in humans following a myocardial infarction. However, since serial measurements of pressure-volume relations require invasive techniques, it is not possible to delineate so clearly, the remodeling process in a given patient. However, significant insights about a multitude of aspects of ventricular remodeling in humans have been obtained through studies of hearts explanted from patients at the time of orthotopic heart transplant suffering from ischemic cardiomyopathy. Characteristics of these hearts are compared to those of normal human hearts not suitable for transplantation. In addition, studies of explanted hearts obtained from patients who required support with a left ventricular assist device (LVAD) prior to transplantation have provided important information about the extent to which the remodeling process can be reversed. The remainder of this chapter shall review results of these studies.

2.   Structural Remodeling in Ischemic Cardiomyopathy

There are several approaches available for studying the remodeling process in humans. Studies in our laboratory have employed the technique of measuring *ex vivo* passive pressure-volume relationships (EDPVRs) from hearts explanted at the time of orthotopic heart transplant; the following discussion will focus on results obtained from ischemic cardiomyopathic hearts. After explantation and preservation with 4°C cardioplegia solution, a compliant water-filled latex balloon is placed into the left ventricular chamber. While measuring pressure within the balloon, volume is varied from a volume adjusted for an intracavitary pressure of 0 mmHg to a volume yielding a pressure of at least 30 mmHg. The pressure-volume point at each volume step is then plotted, resulting in the passive pressure-volume relationship for that heart. Such curves have been obtained from non-failing hearts unsuitable for transplant, hearts explanted from patients with end-stage ischemic heart disease and from hearts that have undergone LVAD support prior to transplant.[7,8] Representative results are shown in Figure 4. Compared to normal hearts (crosses) the EDPVRs of ICM hearts (open circles) were shifted towards significantly larger volumes, a reflection of the gross dilation and

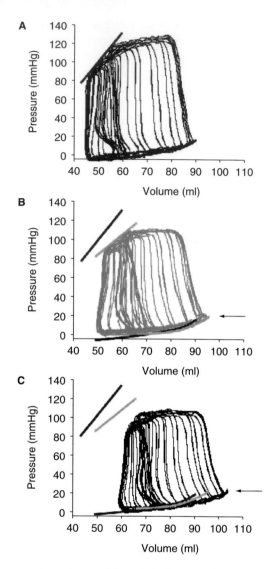

FIGURE 3. Pressure-volume loops obtained during transient vena caval occlusions in a normal dog (A), at the conclusion of an ~8 week period of daily coronary embolizations (B) and after an additional 10 weeks following suspension of embolizations (C). The ESPVR and EDPVR progressively shift towards larger volumes, indicative of remodeling. Once initiated, the remodeling process self propagates even without induction of additional myocardial injury.[6]

structural remodeling that is typical of end-stage cardiomyopathy. In addition, unitless chamber stiffness constant (k, obtained by curve fitting the data to $P=\beta e^{kV/Vw}$ where V_w is volume of the left ventricular wall[9]) is significantly reduced in end-stage ICM hearts compared to normal non-failing hearts.

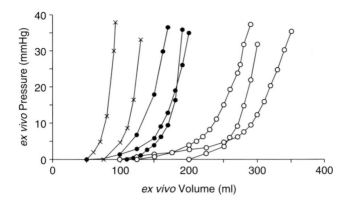

FIGURE 4. Representative left ventricular *ex vivo* pressure volume relationships (EDPVRs) for non-failing (*crosses*), end-stage ischemic heart failure (*open circles*) and LVAD supported ICM hearts (*filled circles*). The structural remodeling process in end-stage ICM leads to a rightward shift of the EDPVRs, but could be reversed following LVAD support.

At the root of these chamber structural changes is frank myocyte hypertrophy and cellular elongation with up to 70% increase in cell volume[10] (Figure 5A and B), increased collagen deposition and increased heart weight (Figure 5C). These changes, in turn, are due to the hemodynamic overload (increased preload and afterload stress) and neurohormonal activation present in these patients.

As late as the 1990's, it was generally believed that when such remodeling was longstanding and severe (such as observed in patients awaiting heart transplant) that these structural abnormalities would be irreversible. Soon after the introduction of LVADs, however, it was appreciated that these abnormalities were not permanent, but could be reversed, at least to some degree.

The primary action of LVADs is to improve cardiac output and blood pressure in terminally ill patients. However, there are several important indirect effects. First, along with normalization of the hemodynamic state comes normalization of the neurohormonal and cytokine milieu.[11] A second indirect benefit of LVADs derives from their anatomic position (withdrawing blood from the LV apex and returning it to the aorta) that results in profound pressure and volume unloading of the left ventricle.[12] Importantly, while the neurohormonal milieu is determined largely (though not entirely) by the blood perfusing the myocardium and is therefore common to the left and right ventricles, the hemodynamic benefits of LVADs are provided only to the left ventricle.[13] Consequently, comparisons of effects on the right and left ventricles further allowed for identification of whether the primary mechanism responsible for reverse remodeling relate to mechanical factors or neurohormonal factors.

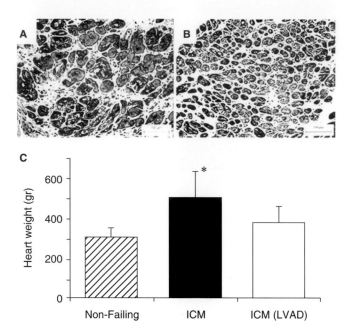

FIGURE 5. Sections of LV free wall demonstrating myocyte hypertrophy in end-stage ischemic cardiomyopathy (A) and following LVAD support (B). Original magnification 10α, Scale bar = 100 μm). (C) Average heart weights from ischemic cardiomyopathic hearts (ICM), ICM hearts following LVAD support, and non-failing heart not used for cardiac transplantation. In end-stage ischemic heart disease heart weight increases tremendously, but could be reverse to almost normal following LVAD support. $^{*}P<0.05$ vs. non-failing and LVAD.

As a consequence of the LVAD support, myocyte hypertrophy and heart mass are significantly reversed (Figure 4 and 5). Similar findings have been reported by Terracciano et al., who found a significant reduction in cell capacitance during LVAD support.[14] Zeifeiridis et al. examined isolated myocytes to evaluate changes in myocyte size and shape after LVAD support and observed a 60% regression of size.[15]

We found that associated with the reduction in cell size and ventricular mass, were significant leftward shifts towards normal of EDPVRs measured in LVAD-supported hearts (Figure 4, filled circles). This observation lead to the concept that the gross structural remodeling of end-stage failing heart could be reversed: *reverse remodeling*.

Interestingly, while the right ventricular EDPVR of patients with end-stage ischemic cardiomyopathy are also shifted towards higher than normal volumes, this relationship is not influenced by LVAD support.[13] This suggests that the primary mechanism of reverse structural remodeling is due to the hemodynamic unloading provided by LVADs, since the RV does not receive the same profound unloading experienced by the LV. Further support for this concept is derived from the fact that hearts supported by a right ventricular assist device (RVAD) do show RV EDPVR shifts towards lower volumes, similar to what is observed in the LV following LVAD support.[16]

3.   Molecular and Cellular Remodeling in Ischemic Cardiomyopathy

The anatomic changes of myocytes that accompanies increased pressure and volume within any heart chamber triggers a sequence of events, some of which are calcium-regulated,[17] that eventually leads to remodeling of individual cells. While physical stretch on the myocardium is believed to be a major regulator of this process, it also involves systemic neurohormones and intracardiac paracrine/autocrine mediators. These individual factors coalesce to produce a cascade of immediate and ultimately prolonged molecular and cellular events mediated in part by altered expression of a variety of genes within both myocytes and non-contractile elements of the myocardium.[18] One of the more widely studied genes is that encoding for the activity of the sarcoplasmic endoreticular calcium-ATPase subtype 2a (SERCA2a) which is known to be down regulated in heart failure. Down regulation of this gene has been linked with transformation of the myocardial force-frequency relationship (FFR). Normally, contractile force increases as contraction frequency is increased and this is referred to as a *positive* FFR. However, in heart failure, contractile force typically declines with increased contraction frequency and this is referred to as a *negative* FFR[19] (see chapter 5, Myocardial contractile performance following MI). In addition, alterations in the expression and/or function of SERCA2a,[20-23] the ryanodine-sensitive calcium release channel (RyR),[24,25] and the sarcolemmal sodium-calcium (Na^+/Ca^{2+}) exchanger[26,27] appear to be associated with various aspects of contractile dysfunction in severe heart failure, although there is some controversy, especially as it relates to changes in Na^+/Ca^{2+} exchanger gene expression. Some studies have indicated that with decreased SERCA2a function in heart failure, a compensatory increase in the activity of the Na^+/Ca^{2+} exchanger occurs as this sarcolemmal protein assumes a greater role in extruding Ca^{2+} during diastole.[19,26,28] Consistent with this process are data indicating up-regulated myocardial expression of Na^+/Ca^{2+} exchanger mRNA in human heart failure.[27] Recent data indicate that levels of Na^+/Ca^{2+} exchanger protein are not necessarily changed in severe human heart failure,[23] and animal studies have suggested that there can be decreased gene expression, and reduced Ca^{2+} flux through the Na^+/Ca^{2+} exchanger in the setting of cardiac failure.[29-31] Our own studies have suggested that Na^+/Ca^{2+} exchanger gene expression is reduced in the heart failure state.

   Just as LVAD support has been shown to induce *reverse structural remodeling*, such changes in gene expression associated with heart failure are shown to be reversed following LVAD support: *reverse molecular remodeling*. So, for example, LVAD support has been shown to reverse the abnormalities of

SERCA2a, Na^+/Ca^{2+} and RyR gene expression.[7] In addition, comparison of gene expression of LV and RV myocardial samples it was shown that only LV SERCA2a gene expression and protein content are improved following LVAD support.[13] This suggests that regulation of the expression of these genes is linked with the volume and pressure unloading provided by the LVAD and not with the normalization of neurohormonal milieu. Similar effects are observed in human tissue samples of patients undergoing β-blocker therapy.[32]

While much attention has been given to changes in gene expression, it is increasingly recognized that examination of protein content and function may be more reveling. For example, while it is known that SERCA2a expression is markedly reduced when examined by Northern blot analysis, functional assays of calcium sequestration rates of isolated sarcolemmal vesicles reveals ~75% retention of calcium sequestration capabilities in end-stage heart failure compared to normal controls.[33] Thus, gene expression does not reveal the entire picture. Additionally, post translational modifications of protein function also play a key role in abnormal cell function underlying the pathophysiologic mechanisms of contractile dysfunction. For example, the sarcoplasmic reticular RyR channel, which regulates Ca^{2+} release to the myofilaments, also play a pivotal role in the ability of the SR to store and rapidly release Ca^{2+}.[20] Hyperphosphorylation of RyR in failing human myocardium disrupts the normal coupled gating of neighboring receptors resulting in abnormal ensemble gating patterns, less coordinated SR Ca^{2+} release during excitation, and Ca^{2+} leak during diastole (Figure 6).[25] These abnormalities are reversed during LVAD support.

The abnormalities of cellular properties are too numerous to delineate in this brief review and only a few examples are provided above. It is noteworthy, however, that there are increasing number of reports showing that many molecular, biochemical and cellular abnormalities occurring in the end-stage heart failure can be reversed and/or normalized during LVAD support. The most notable of these include LVAD-induced normalization of β-adrenergic and endothelin-A receptors,[34,35] modulation of antiapoptotic genes,[36] deactivation of nuclear factor-kappaB,[37] normalization of mitochondrial ultrastructure,[38] and down-regulation of matrix metalloproteinases,[39] tumor necrosis factor-α,[40] β-tubulin,[41] and MEK/Erks and Akt/GSK-3.[42]

4.   Myocardial Contractile Performance in Ischemic Cardiomyopathy

The molecular, biochemical and cellular remodeling noted in prior sections underlie myocardial contractile dysfunction at rest and in response to different types of stimulation. To study such phenomena, isolated endocardial trabeculae were excised from freshly explanted non-failing and end-stage ischemic cardiomyopathic hearts with and without LVAD support and mounted in a muscle bath connected to a force transducer. Muscles were pro-

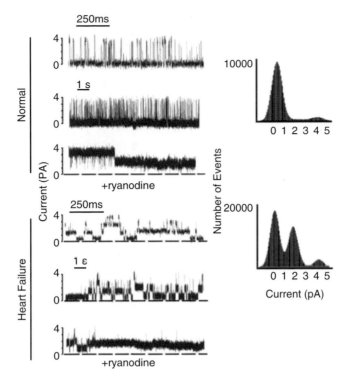

FIGURE 6. Single channel tracings of RyR2 from canine hearts in a non-failing state (top three tracings) and in ischemic cardiomyopathy (bottom three tracings). Corresponding amplitude histograms are at right. The bottom tracing in each set of three shows the characteristics modification of the RyR2 channels by ryanodine (1μM). Recording were at 0 mV.[25]

gressively stretched to the length of maximal force generation (L_{max}). Two separate experiments were performed. The first involved exploration of contractile response to increased rate of stimulation (the force-frequency relationship, FFR) and the second was a test of myocardial contractile response to β-adrenergic stimulation (isoproterenol, 1 μM).

For studies of FFR, stimulation frequency was initially set at 1 Hz and then increased at 0.5 Hz increments to a maximum of 3 Hz (Figure 7). At 1 Hz stimulation frequency, developed force generation of non-failing, ICM and LVAD supported hearts (normalized to cross-sectional area) were similar to each other. However, at higher rates of stimulation force increased in the normal myocardium (positive FFR) but declined in trabeculae from ICM hearts (negative FFR). As discussed above, this phenomenon is believed to be the result of the changes in expression and function of proteins involved with calcium cycling (e.g., SERCA2a).[7,13,26,43-45] In LVAD supported hearts, however, the positive FFR was restored. Interestingly, and paralleling the changes in

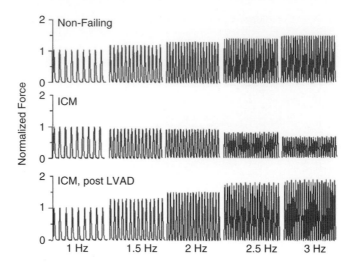

FIGURE 7. Representative force tracings from isometrically contracting trabeculae isolated from a non-failing and two ICM hearts with and without LVAD support. A positive FFR is evident following mechanical unloading. Bar=5 sec.

SERCA2a expression, FFR of the remodeled RV myocardium was also negative and did not revert to a positive FFR following LVAD support.[13]

Myocardial contractile force exhibited a blunted responsiveness to β-adrenergic stimulation in the failing, remodeling LV myocardium (Figure 8).[46] Concomitant with LVAD-induced normalization of β-adrenergic receptor density and phosphorylation of RyR calcium release channel, this response was significantly improved (Figure 8). In comparison to the FFR, however, β-adrenergic responsiveness is restored not only in the unloaded LV but also in the RV. This paralleled comparable recovery of β-adrenergic receptor density and RyR phosphorylation in both ventricles.[25]

5.   Pharmacologic Therapies and Other Devices also Induce Reverse Remodeling

With regard to reversal of remodeling, the present chapter focused on the effects of LVADs. It is clear that the degree and breadth of remodeling observed during LVAD support is far greater than with any other treatment investigated thus far, it is important to note that use of other devices and pharmacologic agents can also reverse remodel the failing heart, though to a lesser degree.

For example, experimental and clinical studies have clearly indicated that drugs such as angiotensin converting enzyme inhibitors and β-blockers can prevent or reverse structural and perhaps molecular remodeling in the setting

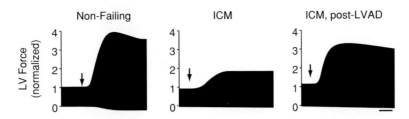

FIGURE 8. Representative continuous force tracings during exposure to isoproterenol (1 μM, arrow). The response from ICM is blunted, while LVAD supported hearts show a strong response similar to non-failing hearts. Scale bar=20 sec.

of heart failure.[47,48] Angiotensin converting enzyme inhibitors exert direct effects on ventricular preload and afterload as well as effects on the neuro-hormonal system and were shown to improve clinical outcome and LV function.[49,50] In addition, there are several potential mechanism of benefit from β-blockade in heart failure. At the tissue level experimental studies have provided insights into molecular and cellular mechanism contributing to prevention and/or reversal of remodeling by reducing apoptosis,[51] collagen deposition and myocyte hypertrophy.[52]

Similarly, devices such as a passive myocardial wrap[53] and cardiac resynchronization therapy[54] have also been associated with varying degrees of reversal of cardiac dilation and normalization of gene expression.

6.   The Challenge: Reverse Remodeling by Cell Therapy

There are three major problems with the use of LVADs to induce reverse remodeling. First is that in a vast majority of patients the degree of recovery, though on average vastly greater than achieved with pharmacologic agents, is insufficient to permit removal of the device.[55,56] Second, in cases when devices are removed, the reverse remodeling is not permanent, and the hearts remodel again once required to support the circulation.[55-57] Third, currently available LVADs are extremely invasive and associated with high morbidity and mortality.[58] Their use will therefore be limited to the vast minority of critically ill, end-stage heart failure patients. Thus, current LVADs provide proof of the concept that sufficient mechanical unloading and normalization of neurohormones and cytokines can improve LV function, but new technologies will be needed to optimize and take advantage of this remarkable property of the myocardium in order to more substantially help greater numbers of patients with debilitating symptoms.

Accordingly, many technologies are currently being investigated. One such class of technology is cell-based therapies such as the use of stem cells, progenitor cells and autologous myoblasts to repopulate infarcted regions of ischemic cardiomyopathic hearts.[59] There are many challenges that need to be overcome in order to arrive at a successful cell therapy for heart failure (Figure 9). The challenge begins with choosing a suitable cell to be used. Many different types are being investigated, each with its own theoretical advantages and disadvantages. Independent of type, sufficient quantities of the cell need to be made available. In patients with ischemic cardiomyopathy it is possible that as much as 40-50% of the original myocyte number is lost, which would amount to as myocardial masses in the range of 40 to 60 grams of tissue. Thus, even if the goal were to replace a relatively small fraction of lost myocardium there is a need to either develop means of producing and injecting large quantities of cells or to establish an environment that will allow proliferation of cells once they take up residence. In either case, the cells need to engraft, which may require disruption of the dense collagen scar present in infarcted areas. In order to ensure long-term survival, the cells need to be appropriately nourished so a vascular supply needs to be generated. The energetic cost of meaningful contraction is high and would need to be supported by aerobic metabolism. In order to most effectively contribute to contraction the engrafted cells need to be activated in synchrony with the native myocardium. This could be achieved either by formation of electrical connects between the graft and native myocardium (which would typically involve generation of gap junctions), by artificial pacing of the graft, or pos-

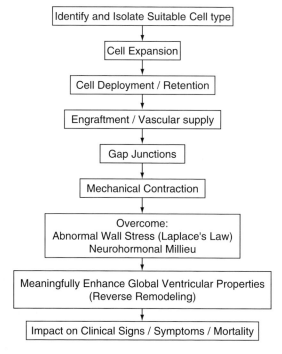

FIGURE 9. Summary of the milestones that need to be achieved in order to arrive at a successful cell therapy for heart failure. See text for details.

sibly via a mechanism whereby mechanical stretch created by the native myocardium could activate the engrafted cells. The engrafted cells would be then required to contract. For this, formation of myofilaments in an organized manner is required along with all necessary regulatory proteins (tropoinin, tropomyosin, etc) and control mechanisms for calcium handling. Due to the preexistent disease state, these cells are engrafted into a hostile environment. According to Laplace's Law (pressure is proportional to wall stress divided by radius of curvature: $P \propto \sigma/r$) the cells are placed at a mechanical disadvantage so that there is less efficient transformation of the force they generate into ventricular pressure. The high stress state may unfavorable affect the cells. Similarly, the neurohormonal milieu into which they are placed is in many ways cytotoxic and may induce undesirable effects on cellular function. Despite these factors, the cells must contract to a sufficient degree to meaningfully influence global ventricular performance. Ultimately, it must be demonstrated that these effects on function translate to beneficial effects on patient symptoms, quality of life and longevity.

The discussion above is predicated on the assumption that indeed the goal of cell-based therapies is to repopulate the infarcted heart with cells that contract and contribute to contraction. However, this assumption is not universally accepted as a requirement for a successful treatment. Some advocate that it would be sufficient that by as yet unspecified mechanisms, injected cells may favorably influence properties of the scar and induce beneficial effects on ventricular structure which in the long run may induce reverse remodeling of other aspects of myocardial structure and function. Our own preliminary studies in an animal model of ischemic cardiomyopathy suggest that autologous skeletal myoblasts injections, whether via a surgical procedure or during a catheter-based percutaneous procedure, are associated with reverse structural remodeling as evidenced by shifts of the end-systolic and end-diastolic pressure-volume relationships back towards lower, more normal volumes. This was observed even though we were unable to identify any significant regions of cell engraftment in the injection regions.

7.   Summary and Conclusions

Profound cardiac remodeling occurs in the setting of ischemic cardiomyopathy, which affects all regions of the heart, independent of whether a particular region is infracted, ischemic or normally perfused. The impact is broad, affecting molecular, biochemical, metabolic, cellular and structural aspects of the myocardium. This process is driven by increased mechanical stresses, in the form of increased preload and afterload, as well as abnormally elevated levels of cytokines and neurohormones. With respect to a majority of myocardial characteristics that undergo remodeling, the process appears to be similar in ischemic and non-ischemic cardiomyopathies, although in ischemic cardiomyopathic hearts there are the added factors of massive cell loss and regions of dense scar. Until the early 1990's it was commonly held that the end-stage failing heart was irreversibly dilated, hypertrophic and dysfunctional. Early clues from studies of pharmacologic neurohormonal blockade (specifically angiotensin II converting enzyme inhibitors and later β-blockers) indicated that the process could be slowed, halted and perhaps reversed. Following the introduction of LVADs, however, it because clear that almost every aspect of remodeling could be reversed. The only characteristic which does not seem to normalize during LVAD support relates to the extracellular matrix[39,60,61] which exhibits enhanced collagen turnover and interstitial fibrosis.

The precise mechanisms underlying the various aspects of remodeling and reverse remodeling remain to be determined. The mechanisms underlying hypertrophy and chamber remodeling in response to pressure and volume loading of the myocardium involve intricately orchestrated up- and down-regulations of a multitude of intracellular signaling cascades and post-translational modifications. Although having been investigated for over 40 years, these mechanisms are still not fully understood. It has been our working hypothesis that reverse remodeling involves the same mechanisms working in the opposite direction. Hopefully, future research will provide precise answers that will allow development of new treatments to achieve the same profound effects on reverse remodeling as LVADs. It is postulated that cell-based therapies may achieve this goal. The questions to be addressed broadly in this book are whether one or more cell types exist that can be injected into a heart with ischemic cardiomyopathy that can, by one mechanism or another, reverse remodel the grossly dilated heart and improve ventricular function to such a degree that will alleviate symptoms of heart failure and prolong life.

8.   References

1. Anversa P, Kajstura J, Olivetti G. Myocyte death in heart failure. Curr Opin Cardiol. May 1996;11(3):245–251.
2. Mann DL. Inflammatory mediators and the failing heart: past, present, and the foreseeable future. Circ Res. Nov 29 2002;91(11):988–998.
3. Mann DL. Stress-activated cytokines and the heart: from adaptation to maladaptation. Annu Rev Physiol. 2003;65:81–101.
4. Pfeffer MA, Braunwald E. Ventricular remodeling after myocardial infarction. Experimental observations and clinical implications. Circulation. Apr 1990;81(4):1161–1172.
5. Todaka K, Zhu S, Gu A, et al. Changes in left ventricular mechanics and energetics in canine microembolization model of heart failure. Journal of the American College of Cardiology. 1995;25:133A.
6. He KL, Dickstein M, Sabbah HN, et al. Mechanisms of heart failure with well preserved ejection fraction in dogs following limited coronary microembolization. Cardiovasc Res. Oct 1 2004;64(1):72–83.

7. Heerdt PM, Holmes JW, Cai B, et al. Chronic unloading by left ventricular assist device reverses contractile dysfunction and alters gene expression in end-stage heart failure. Circulation. Nov 28 2000;102(22):2713–2719.
8. Madigan JD, Barbone A, Choudhri AF, et al. Time course of reverse remodeling of the left ventricle during support with a left ventricular assist device. J Thorac Cardiovasc Surg. May 2001;121(5):902–908.
9. Mirsky I, Pasipoularides A. Clinical assessment of diastolic function. Prog Cardiovasc Dis. Jan-Feb 1990;32(4):291–318.
10. Anversa P, Beghi C, Kikkawa Y, et al. Myocardial response to infarction in the rat. Morphometric measurement of infarct size and myocyte cellular hypertrophy. Am J Pathol. Mar 1985;118(3):484–492.
11. McCarthy PM, Savage RM, Fraser CD, et al. Hemodynamic and physiologic changes during support with an implantable left ventricular assist device. J Thorac Cardiovasc Surg. Mar 1995;109(3):409–417; discussion 417–408.
12. Levin HR, Oz MC, Chen JM, et al. Reversal of chronic ventricular dilation in patients with end-stage cardiomyopathy by prolonged mechanical unloading. Circulation. Jun 1 1995;91(11):2717–2720.
13. Barbone A, Holmes JW, Heerdt PM, et al. Comparison of right and left ventricular responses to left ventricular assist device support in patients with severe heart failure: a primary role of mechanical unloading underlying reverse remodeling. Circulation. Aug 7 2001;104(6):670–675.
14. Terracciano CM, Hardy J, Birks EJ, et al. Clinical recovery from end-stage heart failure using left-ventricular assist device and pharmacological therapy correlates with increased sarcoplasmic reticulum calcium content but not with regression of cellular hypertrophy. Circulation. May 18 2004;109(19):2263–2265.
15. Zafeiridis A, Jeevanandam V, Houser SR, et al. Regression of cellular hypertrophy after left ventricular assist device support. Circulation. Aug 18 1998;98(7):656–662.
16. Klotz S, Naka Y, Oz M, et al. Biventricular Assist Device-Induced Right Ventricular Reverse Structural and Functional Remodeling. J Heart Lung Transplant. 2004;in press.
17. Calaghan SC, White E. The role of calcium in the response of cardiac muscle to stretch. Prog Biophys Mol Biol. 1999;71(1):59–90.
18. Swynghedauw B. Molecular mechanisms of myocardial remodeling. Physiol Rev. Jan 1999;79(1):215–262.
19. Houser SR, Piacentino V, 3rd, Weisser J. Abnormalities of calcium cycling in the hypertrophied and failing heart. J Mol Cell Cardiol. Sep 2000;32(9):1595–1607.
20. Arai M, Alpert NR, MacLennan DH, et al. Alterations in sarcoplasmic reticulum gene expression in human heart failure. A possible mechanism for alterations in systolic and diastolic properties of the failing myocardium. Circ Res. Feb 1993;72(2):463–469.
21. Linck B, Boknik P, Eschenhagen T, et al. Messenger RNA expression and immunological quantification of phospholamban and SR-Ca(2+)-ATPase in failing and nonfailing human hearts. Cardiovasc Res. Apr 1996;31(4):625–632.
22. Go LO, Moschella MC, Watras J, et al. Differential regulation of two types of intracellular calcium release channels during end-stage heart failure. J Clin Invest. Feb 1995;95(2):888–894.
23. Hasenfuss G, Reinecke H, Studer R, et al. Relation between myocardial function and expression of sarcoplasmic reticulum Ca(2+)-ATPase in failing and nonfailing human myocardium. Circ Res. Sep 1994;75(3):434–442.

24. Reiken S, Gaburjakova M, Guatimosim S, et al. Protein kinase A phosphorylation of the cardiac calcium release channel (ryanodine receptor) in normal and failing hearts. Role of phosphatases and response to isoproterenol. J Biol Chem. Jan 3 2003;278(1):444–453.

25. Marx SO, Reiken S, Hisamatsu Y, et al. PKA phosphorylation dissociates FKBP12.6 from the calcium release channel (ryanodine receptor): defective regulation in failing hearts. Cell. May 12 2000;101(4):365–376.

26. Hasenfuss G, Schillinger W, Lehnart SE, et al. Relationship between Na+-Ca2+-exchanger protein levels and diastolic function of failing human myocardium. Circulation. Feb 9 1999;99(5):641–648.

27. Studer R, Reinecke H, Bilger J, et al. Gene expression of the cardiac Na(+)-Ca2+ exchanger in end-stage human heart failure. Circ Res. Sep 1994;75(3):443–453.

28. Flesch M, Schwinger RH, Schiffer F, et al. Evidence for functional relevance of an enhanced expression of the Na(+)-Ca2+ exchanger in failing human myocardium. Circulation. Sep 1 1996;94(5):992–1002.

29. Yoshiyama M, Takeuchi K, Hanatani A, et al. Differences in expression of sarcoplasmic reticulum Ca2+-ATPase and Na+-Ca2+ exchanger genes between adjacent and remote noninfarcted myocardium after myocardial infarction. J Mol Cell Cardiol. Jan 1997;29(1):255–264.

30. Yao A, Su Z, Nonaka A, et al. Abnormal myocyte Ca2+ homeostasis in rabbits with pacing-induced heart failure. Am J Physiol. Oct 1998;275(4 Pt 2):H1441–1448.

31. Dixon IM, Hata T, Dhalla NS. Sarcolemmal calcium transport in congestive heart failure due to myocardial infarction in rats. Am J Physiol. May 1992;262(5 Pt 2):H1387–1394.

32. Lowes BD, Gilbert EM, Abraham WT, et al. Myocardial gene expression in dilated cardiomyopathy treated with beta-blocking agents. N Engl J Med. May 2 2002;346(18):1357–1365.

33. Heerdt PM, Burkhoff D. Reverse Molecular Remodeling of the Failing Human Heart Following Support with a Left Ventricular Assist Device. In: Dhalla NS, editor. Signal Transduction and Cardiac Hypertrophy. Boston: Kluwer Academic Publishers. 2002: 19–35.

34. Ogletree-Hughes ML, Stull LB, Sweet WE, et al. Mechanical unloading restores beta-adrenergic responsiveness and reverses receptor downregulation in the failing human heart. Circulation. Aug 21 2001;104(8):881–886.

35. Morawietz H, Szibor M, Goettsch W, et al. Deloading of the left ventricle by ventricular assist device normalizes increased expression of endothelin ET(A) receptors but not endothelin-converting enzyme-1 in patients with end-stage heart failure. Circulation. Nov 7 2000;102(19 Suppl 3):III188–193.

36. Bartling B, Milting H, Schumann H, et al. Myocardial gene expression of regulators of myocyte apoptosis and myocyte calcium homeostasis during hemodynamic unloading by ventricular assist devices in patients with end-stage heart failure. Circulation. Nov 9 1999;100(19 Suppl):II216–223.

37. Grabellus F, Levkau B, Sokoll A, et al. Reversible activation of nuclear factor-kappaB in human end-stage heart failure after left ventricular mechanical support. Cardiovasc Res. Jan 2002;53(1):124–130.

38. Heerdt PM, Schlame M, Jehle R, et al. Disease-specific remodeling of cardiac mitochondria after a left ventricular assist device. Ann Thorac Surg. Apr 2002; 73(4):1216–1221.

39. Li YY, Feng Y, McTiernan CF, et al. Downregulation of matrix metallopro-teinases and reduction in collagen damage in the failing human heart after support with left ventricular assist devices. Circulation. Sep 4 2001;104(10):1147–1152.

40. Razeghi P, Mukhopadhyay M, Myers TJ, et al. Myocardial tumor necrosis factor-alpha expression does not correlate with clinical indices of heart failure in patients on left ventricular assist device support. Ann Thorac Surg. Dec 2001;72(6):2044–2050.

41. Aquila-Pastir LA, McCarthy PM, Smedira NG, et al. Mechanical unloading decreases the expression of beta-tubulin in the failing human heart. J Heart Lung Transplant. Feb 2001;20(2):211.

42. Baba HA, Stypmann J, Grabellus F, et al. Dynamic regulation of MEK/Erks and Akt/GSK-3beta in human end-stage heart failure after left ventricular mechanical support: myocardial mechanotransduction-sensitivity as a possible molecular mechanism. Cardiovasc Res. Aug 1 2003;59(2):390–399.

43. Frank K, Bolck B, Bavendiek U, et al. Frequency dependent force generation cor-relates with sarcoplasmic calcium ATPase activity in human myocardium. Basic Res Cardiol. Oct 1998;93(5):405–411.

44. Holubarsch C, Ruf T, Goldstein DJ, et al. Existence of the Frank-Starling mech-anism in the failing human heart. Investigations on the organ, tissue, and sarcom-ere levels. Circulation. Aug 15 1996;94(4):683–689.

45. Mulieri LA, Hasenfuss G, Leavitt B, et al. Altered myocardial force-frequency relation in human heart failure. Circulation. May 1992;85(5):1743–1750.

46. Dipla K, Mattiello JA, Jeevanandam V, et al. Myocyte recovery after mechanical circulatory support in humans with end-stage heart failure. Circulation. Jun 16 1998;97(23):2316–2322.

47. Weber KT. Cardioreparation in hypertensive heart disease. Hypertension. Sep 2001;38(3 Pt 2):588–591.

48. Reiken S, Wehrens XH, Vest JA, et al. Beta-blockers restore calcium release chan-nel function and improve cardiac muscle performance in human heart failure. Cir-culation. May 20 2003;107(19):2459–2466.

49. Doughty RN, Whalley GA, Walsh HA, et al. Effects of carvedilol on left ventric-ular remodeling after acute myocardial infarction: the CAPRICORN Echo Sub-study. Circulation. Jan 20 2004;109(2):201–206.

50. Effect of enalapril on survival in patients with reduced left ventricular ejection fractions and congestive heart failure. The SOLVD Investigators. N Engl J Med. Aug 1 1991;325(5):293–302.

51. Yue TL, Ma XL, Wang X, et al. Possible involvement of stress-activated protein kinase signaling pathway and Fas receptor expression in prevention of ischemia/reperfusion-induced cardiomyocyte apoptosis by carvedilol. Circ Res. Feb 9 1998;82(2):166–174.

52. Wei S, Chow LT, Sanderson JE. Effect of carvedilol in comparison with metopro-lol on myocardial collagen postinfarction. J Am Coll Cardiol. Jul 2000;36(1):276–281.

53. Sabbah HN, Sharov VG, Chaudhry PA, et al. Chronic therapy with the acorn car-diac support device in dogs with chronic heart failure: three and six months hemo-dynamic, histologic and ultrastructural findings. J Heart Lung Transplant. Feb 2001;20(2):189.

54. St John Sutton MG, Plappert T, Abraham WT, et al. Effect of cardiac resynchro-nization therapy on left ventricular size and function in chronic heart failure. Cir-culation. Apr 22 2003;107(15):1985–1990.

55. Foray A, Williams D, Reemtsma K, et al. Assessment of submaximal exercise capacity in patients with left ventricular assist devices. Circulation. Nov 1 1996;94(9 Suppl):II222–226.
56. Mancini DM, Beniaminovitz A, Levin H, et al. Low incidence of myocardial recovery after left ventricular assist device implantation in patients with chronic heart failure. Circulation. Dec 1 1998;98(22):2383–2389.
57. Levin HR, Oz MC, Catanese KA, et al. Transient normalization of systolic and diastolic function after support with a left ventricular assist device in a patient with dilated cardiomyopathy. J Heart Lung Transplant. Aug 1996;15(8):840–842.
58. Rose EA, Gelijns AC, Moskowitz AJ, et al. Long-term mechanical left ventricular assistance for end-stage heart failure. N Engl J Med. Nov 15 2001;345(20):1435-1443.
59. Lee MS, Makkar RR. Stem-cell transplantation in myocardial infarction: a status report. Ann Intern Med. May 4 2004;140(9):729–737.
60. Klotz S, Dickstein M, Morgan J, et al. Extracellular Matrix Remodeling during Left Ventricular Assist Device Support: Relation between Collagen and Passive Pressure-Volume Relations (Abstract). JACC. 2004;March; 43(5): A225.
61. Klotz S, Foronjy R, Dickstein M, et al. Low Incidence or Myocardial Recovery in LVAD Patients due to Increased Collagen Cross-linking and Myocardial Stiffness (Abstract). Circulation. 2004;Oct 26(Suppl).

Myocardial Regeneration

2
Myocardial Regeneration: Which Cell and Why

ELMOSTAFA EL FAHIME AND JACQUES P. TREMBLAY*

1.   Background

During the development, growth of the heart is generally characterized by division of cardiac cells (cardiomyocytes) during the embryonic stages of life, followed after birth by entry into a post-mitotic state. Therefore, growth of the heart after normal development and in cases of cardiac diseases requires enlargement of individual cardiomyocytes (hypertrophy) rather than proliferation of post-mitotic cardiac myocytes.

Cardiovascular disease, including hypertensive diseases and myocardial infarction, leads to loss of cardiac tissue through death of the cells by apoptosis and necrosis. The remaining myocytes are unable to reconstitute the lost tissue, and the diseased heart deteriorates functionally with time. Current therapeutic approaches suffer from limitations and are primarily focused at limiting disease progression rather than repair and restoration of healthy tissue and function. The limited efficacy and co-morbidity of these current treatments have increased the interest to investigate other options, alternative and additional long-term therapeutic approaches.

In this perspective, cell transplantation therapy (CTT) seems to be a potential new therapeutic strategy to achieve cardiac repair.

2.   Rational

Preliminary experiments with cardiac tissue established that minced adult newt ventricular tissue could reorganize into a contractile mass when attached to the apex of an injured heart.[1] Subsequent investigations in rats indicated that minced fetal atrial tissue could form stable, contractile grafts in ectopic skeletal muscle beds.[2] A series of breakthroughs in the last few

*Elmostafa El fahime and Jacques Tremblay, Unité de Génétique humain, Centre de recherché CHUL (CR-CHUL), 2705 boulevard Laurier, Ste-Foy, G1V 4G2, Québec, Canada

years demonstrated that dispersed preparations of cardiac myocytes were stable when transplanted onto donor mouse hearts.[3] Moreover, formation of cell-to-cell contacts, complete with gap junction proteins has been reported in the fetal cardiomyocytes grafts.[4] More recent work to larger animal models have made a successful transition to clinical trial and are being considered to treat human patients.[5,6]

3.   Potential Cell Types for Heart Repair

Recent work focused on identifying suitable sources of cells for cardiac repair. Potential cells for autologous cell transplantation might be cardiomyocytes,[7] myoblasts grown from skeletal muscle,[8] smooth muscle cells from blood vessels,[9] or hematopoietic or mesenchymal stem cells either mobilized with pharmaceuticals or by biopsy from the bone marrow.[10,11] In this chapter, we have reviewed the recent literature on the remodeling of the infracted myocardium with various cell types and discussed the promises and challenges of the cell transplantation therapy for heart diseases (Figure 1).

3.1.   Cardiomyocytes

It seems logical that cardiac myocytes (cardiomyocytes) would be the best cell type to repair a myocardial infarct. However, successful cardiomyocyte engraftment depends on a complex series of parameters, including terminal differentiation of the transplanted cells and proper excitation/contraction coupling with the host myocardium. Since adult cardiomyocytes do not survive well or proliferate *in vitro*, cardiomyocytes from fetal sources have to be used in cell transplantation experiments. Initial studies generated significant excitement after they demonstrated that cardiomyocytes from fetal mice formed viable grafts after injection into normal myocardium of syngeneic hosts. Furthermore, electron microscopy of engrafted nonimmortalized fetal cardiac myocytes demonstrated that the transplanted cells could form intercalated disks and tight junctions connecting them to the host myocardium.[3] Moreover, cardiomyocytes can be proliferated easily in culture and could thus be genetically modified *in vitro*. However, fetal cardiomyocytes are highly sensitive to ischemic injury, and their therapeutic use might ultimately require additional interventions (for example, treatment with cardioprotective genes or drugs).[12] Moreover, human fetal cardiomyocytes are difficult to obtain because of the limited availability of aborted embryos and are limited with respect to their ability to be amplified in culture. Since the embryonic cardiomyocytes are necessarily allogeneic they do not survive in the host heart without adequate immunosuppression. In addition, the use of fetal cardiomyocytes may also face ethical and political difficulties in human application.[13] This problem accelerated the search of alternative cell types for the repair of the heart.

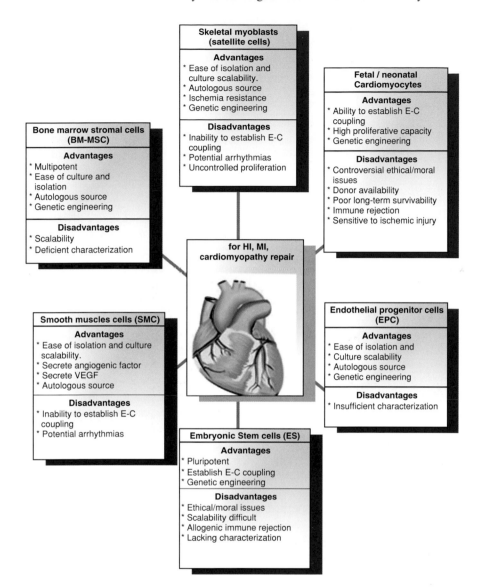

FIGURE 1. Potential cell types for cell-based therapies for the heart (E-C: electro-mechanical coupling; EPC: Endothelial progenitor cells; MI: myocardial infarction; HF: heart failure).

3.2. Myoblasts

Myoblasts or satellite cells are precursor cells attached to skeletal muscle fibers. Every myofiber is intimately associated with a number of satellite cells that lie beneath the basal lamina, closely applied to the plasmalemma. In normal muscles, satellite cells are mitotically quiescent, but become activated to divide in response to signals released following damage or in response to increased workload or following tissue dissociation (*in vitro*) in culture. After division, satellite cell progeny, termed myoblasts, undergo terminal differentiation and become incorporated into mature muscle fibers as post-mitotic myonuclei reviewed by Bischoff and Heintz.[14] Satellite cells are therefore a population of precursors that provide a reserve capacity to replace differentiated, post-mitotic cells required for the functions of adult skeletal muscles.

Researchers and clinicians took advantage of this natural ability to develop strategies aimed at forming skeletal muscle tissue *in vivo* in various normal or pathological conditions. For example, we have developed a cell therapy approach based on myoblast transplantation to treat Duchenne Muscular Dystrophy patients.[15-19]

Skeletal myoblasts exhibit many desirable qualities as donor cells for the treatment of cardiovascular diseases: (1) the ability to be amplified in large quantities and in an undifferentiated state *in vitro*, (2) the possibility of genetically engineering these cells, (3) the capacity to remain viable in ischemic tissue, (4) the potential to maintain their proliferation capacity *in vivo*, and (5) the possibility to achieve autologous transplantation. Successful engraftment of autologous skeletal myoblasts into injured myocardium has been reported in multiple animal models of cardiac injury.[20-23] These studies have demonstrated survival and engraftment of myoblasts into infracted or necrotic hearts, differentiation of the myoblasts into striated cells within the damaged myocardium and improved myocardial functional performance.

On the basis of these preliminary results and the well-established capacity to amplify primary myoblasts from humans, the potential use of skeletal myoblast grafts for treating heart disease has generated considerable interest and clinical trials have begun both in Europe and in the United States.[24,8] In these studies, the authors report the first intramyocardial transplantation of autologous skeletal myoblasts in a patient with severe ischemic cardiac failure. The encouraging results after an 8-month follow-up underline the potential of this new approach.

However, the transplantation of myoblasts in the heart has some disadvantages. The main one is that these cells do not form intercalated disks and electrical synapses with the host cardiomyocytes. Thus they cannot contract synchronously with the rest of the heart compartment. Moreover, there is conflicting evidence on whether these cells can survive for a long period in the host heart.[25] In fact, the myoblasts could produce their therapeutic benefits by secreting transiently growth factor that may prevent the atrophy of the heart wall after an infarct.[26] Thus, since the myoblasts do not form new functional cardiac tissue, they are not the best cells for an ideal tissue engineering of the heart.

3.3.   Endothelial Cell

The demonstration of the conversion of mouse and human endothelial cells (EC) into cardiomyocytes in *in vitro* co-cultures and *in vivo*[27] opened the possibility of using human endothelial cells for cardiac repair. Cell contacts between the endothelial cells and existing cardiomyocytes seem to be indispensable for such conversion. However, the plasticity of endothelial cells is reduced during development, and the fact that relatively well-differentiated endothelial cells derived from human umbilical veins did form cardiomyocytes,[27] made the umbilical cord a possible source of human endothelial cells for therapeutic purposes. Alternatively it might be possible to expand populations of circulating human endothelial progenitor cells (EPC).[28] These blood-born cells are thought to originate from a common precursor in adult bone marrow.[29] For a review, see Rafii and Lyden.[30] They express endothelial lineage markers (i.e., CD34+, Flk-1+, VE-cadherin, PECAM-1, von Willebrand factor, eNOS, and E-selectin) and can be expanded and genetically modified ex vivo to yield sufficient numbers for therapeutic applications.[31,32,28] However, these endothelial cells will have to be further characterized before they can be used for heart therapies.

3.4. Bone Marrow–Derived Mesenchymal Stem Cells (BM-MSC)

BM-MSCs have myogenic potential and are therefore promising candidates for cell-based therapies for myocardial diseases.[33-36,11] These cells can be isolated on the basis of their adhesive proprieties, they can be proliferated extensively in culture and thus be easily genetically modified.[37-40] Moreover, they exhibit a remarkable plasticity.[34] Indeed it is now well-established that these cells can differentiate into functional cardiomyocytes under specific culture conditions.[33,34,41,42] BM-MSC can be induced to differentiate into synchronously beating cardiomyocytes in vitro after treatment of primary cultures of mouse bone marrow with the cytosine analog 5-azacytidine.[42,43] They are thus an interesting source of autologous cells for cardiac repair. In the light of these reports, systemic administration of BM-MSCs to repair infarcted myocardium has been proposed as an attractive clinical strategy.[44,36] Altogether these studies indicated that bone marrow progenitors share transdifferentiation into the various cell types required for regeneration and maintenance of the myocardium.[45] These encouraging preclinical results have led to several recent small-scale feasibility and safety studies to evaluate the therapeutic potential of bone marrow cell transplantation in treatment of ischemic heart diseases and myocardial infarctions.[46-50]

Nevertheless, these results should be considered preliminary. The nature of the mobilizing, migration and homing signals for bone marrow progenitor cells and the mechanism of differentiation and incorporation into the target tissues need to be identified.

3.5. Smooth Muscle Cells

Smooth muscle cells (SMCs) have intrinsic characteristics that may be clinically important in the context of cell therapies for heart failure. Indeed, SMCs have the capacity to divide and to secrete angiogenic factors, such as nitric oxide (NO),[51] fibroblast growth factors,[52] and vascular endothelial cell growth factor (VEGF).[53] The secretion of these factors may permit to eliminate intractable angina unresponsive to coronary artery bypass and restore contractility to hibernating cardiomyocytes. Li et al. showed that fetal smooth muscle cells can be successfully transplanted into myocardial scar tissue to form smooth muscle tissue, to stimulate angiogenesis, to limit remodelling and to improve myocardial function.[9] The consequences of transplanting the smooth muscle cells in the heart have to be further investigated before a clinical trial of such transplantation is undertaken.

3.6.   Embryonic Stem Cells

It is well-established that totipotent murine embryonic stem (ES) cells can give rise to a variety of cell lineages *in vitro* and *in vivo* including cardiac myocytes. Pure cultures of cardiomyocytes with expanding capacity in culture and therefore suitable for transplantation have been obtained by simple genetic selection protocols.[54] The transplanted cells formed intra-cardiac grafts that were stable up to 7 weeks. Given the excellent potential demonstrated by mouse ES cells, much effort has been spent on the development of human ES cell lines. Kehat et al. described the generation of a reproducible cardiomyocyte differentiation system from human ES cells.[55] The generated myocytes were shown to display functional and structural properties consistent with early-stage cardiomyocytes.

However, it is very important to keep in mind the existence of striking differences between the human and murine stem cell models. Indeed, human ES cells have a very low efficiency of conversion into cardiomyocytes compared with those of mice, a slower time course of differentiation, and only a lower number of human ES cells are able to undergo differentiation and spontaneous contraction.[55]

Although, the development of the human ES cell technology holds great potential for the field of myocardial regeneration, a number of issues will need to be met before any clinical applications can be expected. First of all, the use of embryonic cell lines is still controversial in some countries. There are also many technical issues. Some of the milestones that need to be achieved include: (1) Development of strategies for directing differentiation of the human ES cells into the cardiac lineage; (2) Selection protocols should be devised to allow generation of pure population of cardiomyocytes for transplantation; (3) The differentiation process should be up-scaled to yield clinically relevant number of cells for transplantation; (4) Several technical and conceptual issues regarding *in vivo* cell transplantation should be resolved and (5) Methods for circumventing immune rejection of these allogeneic cells should be developed. In fact, approaches aimed at reduction of the mass of alloreactive T cells are being developed and these and other novel therapies with particular relevance to the anticipated immune response mounted against ES-derived cell transplants will probably be used.[56] These strategies may also include establishing 'banks' of major histocompatibility complex antigen-typed human ES cells, genetically manipulating ES cells to suppress the immune response, such as by knocking-out the major histocompatibility complexes [57] and possibly also by nuclear transfer techniques (therapeutic cloning).[58]

4. Conclusion

Treatment of damaged myocardium after myocardial infarction by cell transplantation is becoming an increasingly promising therapeutic approach. Ideally, the donor cells should be amplified efficiently in culture and would lead to regeneration of infarcted myocardial tissue, including cardiogenic differentiation with local angiogenesis. Two of the most widely used cell types for cardiac repair today are skeletal muscle-derived progenitors, or myoblasts, and bone marrow-derived progenitors. Both cell types share advantages over other cells used for cardiac repair (or at least for limiting infarcts) in that they are readily available, autologous, exhibit a high proliferative potential *in vitro* and share a low potential for tumor genesis.

However, the transplantation of autologous cells to repair the heart also has serious drawbacks. It is labor intensive since isolation and cell proliferation has to be done for each patient. This procedure also delays the treatment. The 'ideal' cell to treat the heart should be transplantable without delay to any patient without a sustained immunosupression. Such ideal cells may be obtained one day by the genetic engineering of embryonic stem cells.

Through cellular therapies, the concept of "growing" heart muscle and vascular tissue and manipulating the myocardial cellular environment may revolutionize the approach to treating heart disease.

5. References

1. Bader, D., and Oberpriller, J. O. 1978. Repair and reorganization of minced cardiac muscle in the adult newt (Notophthalmus viridescens). J Morphol 155: 349.
2. Jockusch, H., Fuchtbauer, E. M., Fuchtbauer, A., Leger, J. J., Leger, J., Maldonado, C. A., and Forssmann, W. G. 1986. Long-term expression of isomyosins and myoendocrine functions in ectopic grafts of atrial tissue. Proc Natl Acad Sci U S A 83: 7325.
3. Soonpaa, M. H., Koh, G. Y., Klug, M. G., and Field, L. J. 1994. Formation of nascent intercalated disks between grafted fetal cardiomyocytes and host myocardium. Science 264: 98.
4. Koh, G. Y., Soonpaa, M. H., Klug, M. G., Pride, H. P., Cooper, B. J., Zipes, D. P., and Field, L. J. 1995. Stable fetal cardiomyocyte grafts in the hearts of dystrophic mice and dogs. J Clin Invest 96: 2034.
5. Grounds, M. D., White, J. D., Rosenthal, N., and Bogoyevitch, M. A. 2002. The role of stem cells in skeletal and cardiac muscle repair. J Histochem Cytochem 50: 589.

6. Melo, L. G., Pachori, A. S., Kong, D., Gnecchi, M., Wang, K., Pratt, R. E., and Dzau, V. J. 2004. Gene and cell-based therapies for heart disease. Faseb J 18: 648.29.

7. Soonpaa, M. H., Daud, A. I., Koh, G. Y., Klug, M. G., Kim, K. K., Wang, H., and Field, L. J. 1995. Potential approaches for myocardial regeneration. Ann N Y Acad Sci 752: 446.

8. Menasche, P., Hagege, A. A., Scorsin, M., Pouzet, B., Desnos, M., Duboc, D., Schwartz, K., Vilquin, J. T., and Marolleau, J. P. 2001. Myoblast transplantation for heart failure. Lancet 357: 279.

9. Li, R. K., Jia, Z. Q., Weisel, R. D., Merante, F., and Mickle, D. A. 1999. Smooth muscle cell transplantation into myocardial scar tissue improves heart function. J Mol Cell Cardiol 31: 513.

10. Kocher, A. A., Schuster, M. D., Szabolcs, M. J., Takuma, S., Burkhoff, D., Wang, J., Homma, S., Edwards, N. M., and Itescu, S. 2001. Neovascularization of ischemic myocardium by human bone-marrow-derived angioblasts prevents cardiomyocyte apoptosis, reduces remodeling and improves cardiac function. Nat Med 7: 430.

11. Orlic, D., Kajstura, J., Chimenti, S., Limana, F., Jakoniuk, I., Quaini, F., Nadal-Ginard, B., Bodine, D. M., Leri, A., and Anversa, P. 2001b. Mobilized bone marrow cells repair the infarcted heart, improving function and survival. Proc Natl Acad Sci U S A 98: 10344.

12. Reinecke, H., Zhang, M., Bartosek, T., and Murry, C. E. 1999. Survival, integration, and differentiation of cardiomyocyte grafts: a study in normal and injured rat hearts. Circulation 100: 193.

13. Reinlib, L., and Field, L. 2000. Cell transplantation as future therapy for cardiovascular disease?: A workshop of the National Heart, Lung, and Blood Institute. Circulation 101: E182.

14. Bischoff, R., and Heintz, C. 1994. Enhancement of skeletal muscle regeneration. Dev Dyn 201: 41.

15. Skuk, D., Roy, B., Goulet, M., Chapdelaine, P., Bouchard, J. P., Roy, R., Dugre, F. J., Lachance, J. G., Deschenes, L., Helene, S., Sylvain, M., and Tremblay, J. P. 2004. Dystrophin expression in myofibers of Duchenne muscular dystrophy patients following intramuscular injections of normal myogenic cells. Mol Ther 9: 475.

16. Skuk, D., and Tremblay, J. P. 2003a. Cell therapies for inherited myopathies. Curr Opin Rheumatol 15: 723.

17. Skuk, D., and Tremblay, J. P. 2003b. Myoblast transplantation: the current status of a potential therapeutic tool for myopathies. J Muscle Res Cell Motil 24: 285.

18. Tremblay, D. S. a. J. P. 2001. "Engineering" Myoblast Transplantation. Graft 4: 558.

19. Tremblay, J. P., Malouin, F., Roy, R., Huard, J., Bouchard, J. P., Satoh, A., and Richards, C. L. 1993. Results of a triple blind clinical study of myoblast transplantations without immunosuppressive treatment in young boys with Duchenne muscular dystrophy. Cell Transplant 2: 99.

20. Atkins, B. Z., Lewis, C. W., Kraus, W. E., Hutcheson, K. A., Glower, D. D., and Taylor, D. A. 1999. Intracardiac transplantation of skeletal myoblasts yields two populations of striated cells in situ. Ann Thorac Surg 67: 124.

21. Dorfman, J., Duong, M., Zibaitis, A., Pelletier, M. P., Shum-Tim, D., Li, C., and Chiu, R. C. 1998. Myocardial tissue engineering with autologous myoblast implantation. J Thorac Cardiovasc Surg 116: 744.

22. Murry, C. E., Wiseman, R. W., Schwartz, S. M., and Hauschka, S. D. 1996. Skeletal myoblast transplantation for repair of myocardial necrosis. J Clin Invest 98: 2512.

23. Taylor, D. A., Atkins, B. Z., Hungspreugs, P., Jones, T. R., Reedy, M. C., Hutcheson, K. A., Glower, D. D., and Kraus, W. E. 1998. Regenerating functional myocardium: improved performance after skeletal myoblast transplantation. Nat Med 4: 929.
24. Dib, N., Diethrich, E. B., Campbell, A., Goodwin, N., Robinson, B., Gilbert, J., Hobohm, D. W., and Taylor, D. A. 2002. Endoventricular transplantation of allogenic skeletal myoblasts in a porcine model of myocardial infarction. J Endovasc Ther 9: 313.
25. Suzuki, K., Smolenski, R. T., Jayakumar, J., Murtuza, B., Brand, N. J., and Yacoub, M. H. 2000. Heat shock treatment enhances graft cell survival in skeletal myoblast transplantation to the heart. Circulation 102: III216.
26. Menasche, P. 2002. [Cell therapy: myoblast autograft]. Bull Acad Natl Med 186: 73.
27. Condorelli, G., Borello, U., De Angelis, L., Latronico, M., Sirabella, D., Coletta, M., Galli, R., Balconi, G., Follenzi, A., Frati, G., Cusella De Angelis, M. G., Gioglio, L., Amuchastegui, S., Adorini, L., Naldini, L., Vescovi, A., Dejana, E., and Cossu, G. 2001. Cardiomyocytes induce endothelial cells to trans-differentiate into cardiac muscle: implications for myocardium regeneration. Proc Natl Acad Sci U S A 98: 10733.
28. Kawamoto, A., Gwon, H. C., Iwaguro, H., Yamaguchi, J. I., Uchida, S., Masuda, H., Silver, M., Ma, H., Kearney, M., Isner, J. M., and Asahara, T. 2001. Therapeutic potential of ex vivo expanded endothelial progenitor cells for myocardial ischemia. Circulation 103: 634.
29. Asahara, T., Masuda, H., Takahashi, T., Kalka, C., Pastore, C., Silver, M., Kearne, M., Magner, M., and Isner, J. M. 1999. Bone marrow origin of endothelial progenitor cells responsible for postnatal vasculogenesis in physiological and pathological neovascularization. Circ Res 85: 221.
30. Rafii, S., and Lyden, D. 2003. Therapeutic stem and progenitor cell transplantation for organ vascularization and regeneration. Nat Med 9: 702.
31. Iwaguro, H., Yamaguchi, J., Kalka, C., Murasawa, S., Masuda, H., Hayashi, S., Silver, M., Li, T., Isner, J. M., and Asahara, T. 2002. Endothelial progenitor cell vascular endothelial growth factor gene transfer for vascular regeneration. Circulation 105: 732.
32. Kalka, C., Masuda, H., Takahashi, T., Kalka-Moll, W. M., Silver, M., Kearney, M., Li, T., Isner, J. M., and Asahara, T. 2000. Transplantation of ex vivo expanded endothelial progenitor cells for therapeutic neovascularization. Proc Natl Acad Sci U S A 97: 3422.
33. Jackson, K. A., Majka, S. M., Wang, H., Pocius, J., Hartley, C. J., Majesky, M. W., Entman, M. L., Michael, L. H., Hirschi, K. K., and Goodell, M. A. 2001. Regeneration of ischemic cardiac muscle and vascular endothelium by adult stem cells. J Clin Invest 107: 1395.
34. Jiang, Y., Jahagirdar, B. N., Reinhardt, R. L., Schwartz, R. E., Keene, C. D., Ortiz-Gonzalez, X. R., Reyes, M., Lenvik, T., Lund, T., Blackstad, M., Du, J., Aldrich, S., Lisberg, A., Low, W. C., Largaespada, D. A., and Verfaillie, C. M. 2002. Pluripotency of mesenchymal stem cells derived from adult marrow. Nature 418: 41.
35. Orlic, D., Kajstura, J., Chimenti, S., Jakoniuk, I., Anderson, S. M., Li, B., Pickel, J., McKay, R., Nadal-Ginard, B., Bodine, D. M., Leri, A., and Anversa, P. 2001a. Bone marrow cells regenerate infarcted myocardium. Nature 410: 701.
36. Toma, C., Pittenger, M. F., Cahill, K. S., Byrne, B. J., and Kessler, P. D. 2002. Human mesenchymal stem cells differentiate to a cardiomyocyte phenotype in the adult murine heart. Circulation 105: 93.

37. Blau, H. M., Brazelton, T. R., and Weimann, J. M. 2001. The evolving concept of a stem cell: entity or function? Cell 105: 829.
38. Gao, J., Dennis, J. E., Muzic, R. F., Lundberg, M., and Caplan, A. I. 2001. The dynamic *in vivo* distribution of bone marrow-derived mesenchymal stem cells after infusion. Cells Tissues Organs 169: 12.
39. Pittenger, M. F., Mackay, A. M., Beck, S. C., Jaiswal, R. K., Douglas, R., Mosca, J. D., Moorman, M. A., Simonetti, D. W., Craig, S., and Marshak, D. R. 1999. Multilineage potential of adult human mesenchymal stem cells. Science 284: 143.
40. Wakitani, S., Saito, T., and Caplan, A. I. 1995. Myogenic cells derived from rat bone marrow mesenchymal stem cells exposed to 5-azacytidine. Muscle Nerve 18: 1417.
41. Hakuno, D., Fukuda, K., Makino, S., Konishi, F., Tomita, Y., Manabe, T., Suzuki, Y., Umezawa, A., and Ogawa, S. 2002. Bone marrow-derived regenerated cardiomyocytes (CMG Cells) express functional adrenergic and muscarinic receptors. Circulation 105: 380.
42. Makino, S., Fukuda, K., Miyoshi, S., Konishi, F., Kodama, H., Pan, J., Sano, M., Takahashi, T., Hori, S., Abe, H., Hata, J., Umezawa, A., and Ogawa, S. 1999. Cardiomyocytes can be generated from marrow stromal cells *in vitro*. J Clin Invest 103: 697.
43. Tomita, S., Li, R. K., Weisel, R. D., Mickle, D. A., Kim, E. J., Sakai, T., and Jia, Z. Q. 1999. Autologous transplantation of bone marrow cells improves damaged heart function. Circulation 100: II247.
44. Orlic, D., Hill, J. M., and Arai, A. E. 2002. Stem cells for myocardial regeneration. Circ Res 91: 1092.
45. Kamihata, H., Matsubara, H., Nishiue, T., Fujiyama, S., Tsutsumi, Y., Ozono, R., Masaki, H., Mori, Y., Iba, O., Tateishi, E., Kosaki, A., Shintani, S., Murohara, T., Imaizumi, T., and Iwasaka, T. 2001. Implantation of bone marrow mononuclear cells into ischemic myocardium enhances collateral perfusion and regional function via side supply of angioblasts, angiogenic ligands, and cytokines. Circulation 104: 1046.
46. Assmus, B., Schachinger, V., Teupe, C., Britten, M., Lehmann, R., Dobert, N., Grunwald, F., Aicher, A., Urbich, C., Martin, H., Hoelzer, D., Dimmeler, S., and Zeiher, A. M. 2002. Transplantation of Progenitor Cells and Regeneration Enhancement in Acute Myocardial Infarction (TOPCARE-AMI). Circulation 106: 3009.
47. Perin, E. C., Dohmann, H. F., Borojevic, R., Silva, S. A., Sousa, A. L., Mesquita, C. T., Rossi, M. I., Carvalho, A. C., Dutra, H. S., Dohmann, H. J., Silva, G. V., Belem, L., Vivacqua, R., Rangel, F. O., Esporcatte, R., Geng, Y. J., Vaughn, W. K., Assad, J. A., Mesquita, E. T., and Willerson, J. T. 2003. Transendocardial, autologous bone marrow cell transplantation for severe, chronic ischemic heart failure. Circulation 107: 2294.
48. Stamm, C., Westphal, B., Kleine, H. D., Petzsch, M., Kittner, C., Klinge, H., Schumichen, C., Nienaber, C. A., Freund, M., and Steinhoff, G. 2003. Autologous bone-marrow stem-cell transplantation for myocardial regeneration. Lancet 361: 45.
49. Strauer, B. E., Brehm, M., Zeus, T., Kostering, M., Hernandez, A., Sorg, R. V., Kogler, G., and Wernet, P. 2002. Repair of infarcted myocardium by autologous intracoronary mononuclear bone marrow cell transplantation in humans. Circulation 106: 1913.
50. Tse, H. F., Kwong, Y. L., Chan, J. K., Lo, G., Ho, C. L., and Lau, C. P. 2003. Angiogenesis in ischaemic myocardium by intramyocardial autologous bone marrow mononuclear cell implantation. Lancet 361: 47.

51. Koide, M., Y. Kawahara, et al. (1993). "Cyclic AMP-elevating agents Induce an inducible type of nitric oxide synthase in cultured vascular smooth muscle cells. Synergism with the induction elicited by inflammatory cytokines." J Biol Chem 268(33): 24959-66.

52. Ali, N. and D. K. Agrawal (1994). "Guanine nucleotide binding regulatory proteins: their characteristics and identification." J Pharmacol Toxicol Methods 32(4): 187-96.

53. Stavri, G. T., I. C. Zachary, et al. (1995). "Basic fibroblast growth factor upregulates the expression of vascular endothelial growth factor in vascular smooth muscle cells. Synergistic interaction with hypoxia." Circulation 92(1): 11-4.

54. Klug, M. G., Soonpaa, M. H., Koh, G. Y., and Field, L. J. 1996. Genetically selected cardiomyocytes from differentiating embronic stem cells form stable intracardiac grafts. J Clin Invest 98: 216.

55. Kehat, I., Kenyagin-Karsenti, D., Snir, M., Segev, H., Amit, M., Gepstein, A., Livne, E., Binah, O., Itskovitz-Eldor, J., and Gepstein, L. 2001. Human embryonic stem cells can differentiate into myocytes with structural and functional properties of cardiomyocytes. J Clin Invest 108: 407.

56. Bradley, J. A., Bolton, E. M., and Pedersen, R. A. 2002. Stem cell medicine encounters the immune system. Nat Rev Immunol 2: 859.

57. Grusby, M. J., Auchincloss, H., Jr., Lee, R., Johnson, R. S., Spencer, J. P., Zijlstra, M., Jaenisch, R., Papaioannou, V. E., and Glimcher, L. H. 1993. Mice lacking major histocompatibility complex class I and class II molecules. Proc Natl Acad Sci U S A 90: 3913.

58. Lanza, R. P., Chung, H. Y., Yoo, J. J., Wettstein, P. J., Blackwell, C., Borson, N., Hofmeister, E., Schuch, G., Soker, S., Moraes, C. T., West, M. D., and Atala, A. 2002. Generation of histocompatible tissues using nuclear transplantation. Nat Biotechnol 20: 689.

Cardiac Stem Cells

3
Cardiac Stem Cells for Myocardial Regeneration

BERNARDO NADAL-GINARD AND SIMÓN MÉNDEZ-FERRER*

1. Introduction

Until the turn of this century, the accepted paradigm in cardiac biology and medicine considered the adult myocardium a post-mitotic organ without intrinsic regenerative capacity with a relatively constant but diminishing number of myocytes from shortly after birth to adulthood and senescence.[1-3] This belief has been based on the twin notions that (a) in the adult heart all myocytes, the cells that generate the contractile force responsible for the cardiac output, are terminally differentiated and, therefore, cannot be recalled into the cell cycle, and (b) that the myocardium, in contrast to other tissues such as bone marrow, liver, skin and even brain, lacks a stem cell population capable of generating new myocytes. These two concepts have affected cardiovascular research and clinical cardiology in significant ways. If no new myocytes can be formed in adult life, it follows that all therapeutic interventions designed to preserve or improve cardiac function need to be oriented toward the preservation of the remaining myocytes. According to this point of view, myocyte death should normally be a very rare event if cardiac mass and an acceptable level of function have to be preserved throughout the lifespan of the individual. Moreover, by necessity, in a given heart all myocytes had to be as old as the individual. Thus, although often overlooked, according to the prevalent view, each and every myocyte of a 90 year-old person had to be at least 90 years old.

Despite several early observations documenting the existence of some cycling ventricular and atrial myocytes,[4,5] the prevalent static view of the myocardium implied that both myocyte death and myocyte regeneration had little role in cardiac homeostasis. Although in recent years stem cells have been identified in and isolated from many adult tissues, including the blood, skin, liver, brain, skeletal muscle, and intestinal tract among others,[3,6] the search for a cardiac stem cell (CSC) had been considered futile because of the widely accepted lack of regeneration potential of this organ (Figure 1).

---

* Cardiovascular Research Institute. Department of Medicine. Vosburgh Pavilion. New York Medical College, Valhalla, NY 10595. USA.

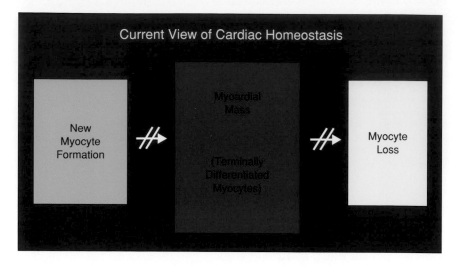

FIGURE 1. Most currently accepted view of cardiac cellular homeostasis. The myocardium is viewed as a closed box composed of terminally differentiated myocytes where there is little, if any, new input of newly formed myocytes and negligible output due to myocyte death.

2.   Myocyte Death and Regeneration

Myocyte death and regeneration are proposed as central events determining adult cardiac cellular homeostasis. Evidence challenging the accepted wisdom has been accumulating, albeit slowly. First, it is obvious that if the heart lacks self-renewal properties, over time, even moderate rates of myocyte death would lead to the disappearance of the myocardial mass. Not surprisingly, therefore, the existence of myocyte death in the normal myocardium has been quite controversial.[7-9] Nevertheless, there is now a consensus that myocyte death occurs in the normal and pathological heart of both human and experimental animals. Even the most conservative values indicate that, in the absence of new myocyte formation, the normal heart would lose most of its mass in a few decades and the senile and failing heart would disappear in a matter of several months or, at most, a few years.[10-12] There is no doubt that myocyte death occurs throughout the lifespan of the organism, independently from cardiac disease. Therefore, the demonstration of cycling ventricular myocytes in the normal and pathological adult mammalian heart of several species, including humans, was particularly intriguing.[10,11]

In the normal heart, the rate of cell death increases with age. From birth to middle age this cell loss is compensated by the rate of new myocyte formation that until puberty exceeds the myocyte death. From middle age on, however, the increased myocyte death is not balanced by an equivalent increase in myocyte formation. This excess in cell death over new myocyte formation results in a net reduction in myocyte number. This smaller number of myocytes hypertrophies to preserve the size of the myocardial mass and results in an old heart of normal or slightly decreased size but with enlarged parenchymal cells. Thus, myocyte death, hypertrophy and new myocyte formation characterize normal cardiac homeostasis and its evolution through time might explain why coronary artery disease and its complications are major risk factors in the elderly and why myocardial infarction is associated with increased morbidity and mortality in this population.[10-12]

Although the data summarized above provided an alternative view of adult cardiac homeostasis, it was not readily accepted because it lacked a proper biological context[13] and also failed to reconcile two apparently contradictory bodies of evidence: on one hand, the well-documented irreversible withdrawal of cardiac myocytes from the cell cycle soon after birth, producing a heart constituted mainly by terminally differentiated myocytes[1,2] and, on the other hand, the presence of cycling myocytes undergoing mitosis and cytokinesis in the adult heart. Interestingly, the number of these cycling myocytes and, therefore, the rate of new myocyte formation, increases dramatically in old age[14] and in response to acute[15] and chronic overload,[16] suggesting that their generation responds to physiological demands. Together, these observations raised questions about the nature of these cycling myocytes, their origin, as well as their physiological relevance.

It was soon noted that the cycling myocytes in the adult myocardium, as detected by expression of cell cycle related proteins and/or BrdU incorporation, were cells significantly smaller than the average myocyte[10,11] and that many expressed functional telomerase activity,[17] an enzyme that so far has only been detected in cells that are either in or capable of entering the cell cycle. There was also an inverse correlation between DNA replication and expression of cell cycle inhibitors, such as p16, expressed in terminally differentiated myocytes. This phenotype raised the possibility that the cycling myocytes represented a subpopulation of newly born, immature cells, which had not yet irreversibly withdrawn from the cell cycle. This point of view was reinforced by the finding that in the acute phase of human myocardial infarction, the border zone and the myocardium remote from the damage exhibited very high levels of myocyte replication with newly formed myocytes of small size.[15] However, it was the cases of sex mismatched cardiac transplants in humans, in which a female heart is transplanted into a male host,[18] that shed light on the origin of these cycling myocytes and paved the way for the identification of CSCs.

3. Bone Marrow Cells Form Myocardial Cells and Integrate Within the Myocardium

Despite the increasing evidence that the adult myocardium was not a post-mitotic and terminally differentiated tissue but that, on the contrary, was able to produce new myocytes, it was also clear that this potential regenerative capacity was not sufficient to change the course of the adverse myocardial remodeling and the development of cardiac failure following the loss of a significant number of ventricular myocytes, such as a result of a myocardial infarction (MI). Thus, at the turn of the century the question arose on how to complement the endogenous myocardial regenerative capacity to replace a significant fraction of the myocytes lost after an MI.

At the time there had been several reports indicating that hematopoietic stem cells (HSCs), in addition to giving rise to blood cells, could also differentiate into several other cell types, particularly in response to tissue damage.[19-23] Although the interpretation of many of these early results has recently been questioned,[25,26,41] at the time created great excitement. Therefore, we tested whether genetically tagged (from transgenic eGFP mice) lineage-negative (Lin[neg]) bone marrow cells (BMCs) expressing c-kit, the membrane receptor for stem cell factor, isolated from syngeneic males could adopt the myocardial phenotype when injected into the border of recent acute MIs produced in females by ligation of the anterior descending coronary artery.[24] Surprisingly, the injected BMCs regenerated most of the necrosed myocardium with biochemically and anatomically differentiated myocytes, arterioles and capillaries. The number of regenerated cells was more than three orders of magnitude higher than the number of injected cells, demonstrating that they were not only able to differentiate into myocytes, endothelial and smooth muscle cells but were also able to amplify until a number slightly higher than the cells lost had been regenerated. These new cells restored contractility to the infarcted area and improved the ventricular performance of the affected hearts.

Although these results demonstrated that c-kit[pos] cells from the bone marrow can become engrafted and contribute to physiologically meaningful myocardial regeneration, they left unanswered the questions about the precise identity of the regenerating cells and whether or not they were multipotential, since the production of different cell types could equally be the result of the presence of different cell types in the injected cell mixture. Although it was never stated that the regenerating cells were HSCs, the results have been recently challenged by groups claiming their inability to obtain similar results.[25,26] That these discrepancies are likely due to different methodologies is reinforced by a more recent demonstration that c-kit[pos] bone marrow-derived cells are highly efficient in the regeneration of the post-infarcted myocardium.[27] All these experiments suggest that the regenerating cells have a strong tropism for the damaged tissue since they colonize only the ischemic myocardium and are not found in the neighboring healthy tissue.

The finding that bone marrow-derived cells are able to regenerate the post-ischemic myocardium when directly injected into the damaged tissue, together with their tropism for the ischemic tissue, raised the question of whether it would be possible to home these cells directly into the damaged myocardium by increasing their concentration in the peripheral circulation by stimulating the bone marrow. To test this possibility, post-infarcted mice were injected with stem cell factor (SCF) and granulocyte-colony-stimulating factor (G-CSF) using a protocol known to increase the number of circulating stem cells from ~29 in the non-treated controls to ~7,200 in the cytokine treated mice.[28] This cytokine-stimulation protocol resulted in a significant degree of tissue regeneration 27 days later. The cytokine-induced myocardial regeneration decreased mortality by 68%, infarct size by ~40%, cavitary dilation by ~26% and diastolic wall stress by ~70%. Ejection fraction progressively increased and hemodynamics improved as a consequence of the formation of ~15×10^6 new myocytes with arterioles and capillaries connected to the coronary circulation. These results strongly suggest that the ischemic myocardium can be colonized by circulating cells whose number can be increased by the proper cytokine stimulation of the bone marrow. Unfortunately, because the animals used for these experiments did not have their bone marrow genetically tagged, it was not possible to unambiguously state that the regenerating cells originated from the bone marrow. Although this probability is low, the regenerating cells could have originated from other tissues, the vascular endothelium or even the myocardium itself.

Bone marrow-derived stem/progenitor cells are normally found in the circulation.[29] Stimulation with cytokines only enhances dramatically this natural phenomenon.[30] Therefore, if these circulating stem/progenitor cells upon bone marrow stimulation can colonize the ischemic myocardium and produce a significant functional and anatomical regeneration, it stands to reason that, during the normal lifespan of an organism, there should be a low level myocardial colonization from these circulating cells when there is myocardial damage. This hypothesis can be tested in humans because of the availability of two clinically relevant cases of human chimerism: cases of sex mismatched cardiac and bone marrow transplants. The relevance of these "clinical experimental models" was first demonstrated in a series of cardiac transplants where a female heart was transplanted into a male recipient.[18] The colonization and differentiation of host cells homed to the transplanted female heart can be identified by the presence of a Y chromosome in the host-derived cells. It was shown that as early as a few days after the transplant the female hearts contained a significant number of male (Y chromosome-positive) myocytes, as well as endothelial and smooth muscle cells organized into arterioles and capillaries. Although there has been some discrepancy between research groups about the extent of this colonization,[18,31-34] most likely due to methodological differences,[35] there is full agreement on the validity of the observation. In those cases, it can be argued that the stimulus for the colonization of circulating cells are the dispersed areas of myocardial damage in the donor heart secondary to the ischemic and physical trauma of the transplant procedure. In addition, these observations have been strengthened by the data obtained from sex-mismatched bone marrow transplants where a similar phenomenon of myocardial colonization of the myocardium from the donor bone marrow was also observed. Similarly to the cardiac transplant cases, the donor BMCs produced myocytes, endothelial and smooth muscle cells organized into arterioles and capillaries.[36-40]

These observations in the human strongly support the notion that the myocardium can be colonized by bone marrow-derived cells that, most likely, reach the myocardium through the circulation. Once in the myocardium these cells are able to differentiate into the three main myocardial cell types: myocytes, endothelial and smooth muscle cells. Interestingly, in the case of the sex-mismatched cardiac transplants, cells with the immunological and morphological characteristics of stem cells where identified.[18] These cells, however, were of both donor and recipient origin, and some of them could be seen in the process of commitment to the myogenic phenotype because of their expression of myocyte transcription factors and initial accumulation of sarcomeric proteins. Similar cells were found in the age-matched control heart, indicating that these cells were normally present in the myocardium. These results indicated that stem/precursor cells of the main myocardial cell types could colonize the myocardium through the circulation, but whatever their origin, they also seemed to be present in the adult myocardium. The identification of these undifferentiated and/or early differentiating cells not only suggested the presence of stem cells in the myocardium but could also provide a satisfactory explanation for the existence of a small population of cycling myocytes which could be looked upon as the amplifying cells in the process of myocyte maturation before their irreversible withdrawal from the cell cycle.

4.   Identification of Cardiac Primitive Cells

As indicated above, previous work had shown that BMCs injected directly into ischemic myocardium[24] or mobilized into the peripheral circulation by systemic administration of cytokines[28] were able to home to acutely infarcted myocardium, undergo significant expansion, differentiate into the three main cardiac cell types – myocytes, smooth and endothelial vascular cells– and organize into an anatomical and functional new myocardium. These results, which have created significant controversy,[25,26,41] strongly suggested that circulating cells colonize the myocardium and contribute to myocyte renewal. This hypothesis was confirmed by the cases of sex-mismatched transplants in humans where there is no argument that these male cells in the female hearts originated from host cells that colonized the heart after the transplant and subsequently differentiated. The existence of these cells is an irrefutable proof of new myocyte formation in the adult heart and presupposes the existence of mobile stem-like cells able to differentiate into the three main cardiac cell types: myocytes, smooth muscle and endothelial vascular cells. We hypothesized that these migrating myocyte-generating cells were likely to have many of the characteristics of stem or precursor cells that should make them identifiable in the transplanted heart myocardium.

Cells of donor and recipient origin that express stem cell-related surface antigens – c-kit, Sca-1 and MDR1 – but negative for markers of the blood cell lineages (Lin[neg]) were identified in each of the transplanted donor hearts.

Most importantly, identical cells were found in the control hearts. Additionally, cardiac progenitor and precursor cells of male and female origin were detected by co-expression of stem cell antigens and transcription factors of the cardiocyte lineage or markers characteristic of endothelial and smooth muscle cells.[18] Taken together, these observations identified stem-like cells which have the potential to regenerate the main components of the myocardium: contractile cardiocytes and coronary vasculature. The data, however, did not offer information on whether all cell types originated from one multipotential precursor or from several different precursors, each with a narrower differentiation potential.

5.   Primitive Cells in Adult Heart are True Cardiac Stem Cells

To determine whether the putative CSCs detected in the human heart transplants and normal control hearts were true stem cells with cardiogenic potential, we isolated them from the hearts of experimental animals and tested their differentiation potential *in vitro* and *in vivo*. Undifferentiated cardiac cells expressing the stem cell market c-kit (the receptor for SCF) and negative for all the blood lineage markers (Lin[neg]) were isolated from the ventricles of adult rats and cloned. These cells have continued to proliferate more than 48 months after their original isolation without reaching growth arrest or senescence and >90% of cells maintain a diploid chromosomal complement. When cultured in bacteriological plates, these cells do not attach and form clones in suspension analogous to the pseudoembryoid bodies, neurospheres, formed by the neural stem cells.[42,43] By analogy, we have termed these clones "cardiospheres". Each cardiosphere represent the progeny of a single cell. When allowed to differentiate, each cardiosphere produced three different cell types, each expressing biochemical markers characteristic either of myocytes, smooth muscle or endothelial cells. However, the morphological and functional differentiation of these cells was incomplete. At no time did we detect spontaneous contractions of the cells expressing myocytes markers. Conversely, skeletal muscle, blood cell lineages, and neural markers were not detected. Similar results were obtained when attached clones were allowed to form.

Despite the aborted differentiated phenotype, the continuous growth of these cells over extended periods of time and their very high frequency of differentiation in the three main myocardial cell types, are a strong indication of their self-renewal potential. The fact that the progeny of a single clone gives origin to cells with biochemical markers of the myocyte, smooth muscle and endothelial cell lineages demonstrates that these cells are multipotent. Taken together, these results indicate that the Lin[neg] c-kit[pos] cells isolated from the adult myocardium have the *in vitro* properties expected from CSCs: they are self-renewing, clonogenic, and multipotent.[44] Similar results have been obtained with the cardiac Sca-1 and MDR1 positive cells. Cells isolated from mice, rats, dogs an human have very similar phenotypes. Other authors have also identified similar cells.[45,46]

6.   Cardiac Stem Cells Regenerate a Functional Myocardium

The abortive differentiation of the CSCs when grown *in vitro* suggested that the culture medium was deficient in factors required for complete differentiation. To determine the ability of the CSCs to fully differentiate and reconstitute the myocardium when injected into syngeneic rats acutely after myocardial infarction, 1×10^5 cells derived from a single clone and marked either with BrdU or by expression of the transgene coding for the enhanced green fluorescent protein (eGFP) were injected into the myocardium. Cells were introduced in two sites of the border of a five hour-old infarct in two groups of animals. Infarcted animals injected with equal volumes of PBS and sham-operated animals injected with the same number of cells were used as controls.

A band of BrdU-labeled or eGFP-positive regenerating myocardium was identified in ~50% of the cell-treated infarcted hearts and was absent from all the controls. The regenerated myocardium had the infarct size reduced by ~25% and was constituted by labeled small myocytes, capillaries, and arterioles that matured over time. The new myocytes expressed cardiac sarcomeric proteins, N-cadherin and connexin 43 (main components of the zone adherens and gap junctions that allow mechanical and electrical coupling, respectively). The injected cells underwent an impressive degree of amplification. At 10 days after injection, the regenerating band contained $~14 \times 10^6$ myocytes with an average cell volume of $1,500~\mu m^3$, while at 20 days the band had $~13 \times 10^6$ larger myocytes with an average volume of $3,400~\mu m^3$, as compared to the average volume of $20,000\text{-}25,000~\mu m^3$ for adult rat myocytes. In addition, arteriolar density in the regenerating myocardium had reached mature values ($55\text{-}60/mm^2$) in these animals, while capillary density ($1,130/mm^2$) was more comparable to the neonatal than to the adult heart ($4,000/mm^2$), even at the later time point. All these characteristics reinforced the notion that at 20 days, the regenerated myocardium, constituted by new blood carrying vessels and myocytes, resembled the neonatal heart.[44]

The regenerating myocardial cells positively affected cardiac performance and contraction reappeared in the infarcted ventricular wall. Cell implantation reduced infarct size and cavitary dilation; wall thickness, ejection fraction, + and − dP/dt significantly improved at 20 days. End-diastolic pressure and diastolic stress was 52% lower in treated rats. Thus, at 20 days the treated animals had a decreased diastolic load and improved overall pump function.[44]

The improved functional performance of the post-infarcted hearts suggested that the newly generated myocytes were functional and contributed to the overall contractility of the treated hearts. This point of view was further reinforced by the appearance of synchronous motility of the treated ventricular wall, as detected by echocardiography and the contractility parameters of isolated cells. Despite the dramatic size difference between new and surviving myocytes (new myocytes were ~1/10 the size of the spared ones), the contractility parameters of the new cells exhibited similar time to peak shortening, but with higher values of peak and velocity of shortening than spared myocytes.

Therefore, from a structural and functional point of view, *in vivo* the CSCs generate *bona fide* myocardial tissue composed of cardiac myocytes and vasculature[44] (Figure 2).

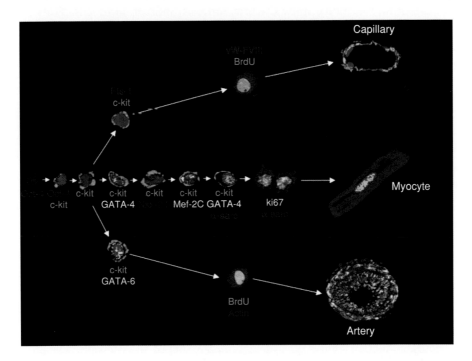

FIGURE 2. Cardiac stem cells are multipotent and regenerate a functional myocardium. In the adult heart, the activation of a multipotent CSC expressing the POU transcription factor Oct-4 (unpublished data), an essential regulator of embryonic stem cells pluripotency, induces successive rounds of symmetrical and asymmetrical divisions that generate a pool of multipotent, c-kit positive cells that progressively differentiate into the main cell types of the heart, as revealed by the expression of transcription factors indicating commitment and differentiation into the myogenic (GATA-4, Nkx-2.5, MEF-2C), endothelial (Ets-1) and smooth muscle (GATA-6) lineages, as well as by the expression of cytoplasmic proteins characteristic of cardiomyocytes (α-sarcomeric actin, α-sarc), endothelial (von Willebrand factor VIII, vW-FVIII) and smooth muscle (actin) cells. The differentiated cells, including small cardiomyocytes, continue proliferating, as shown by the incorporation of bromodeoxyuridine (BrdU) into the DNA or by the expression of the nuclear protein ki67, a marker of cells that are either or have recently been in the cell cycle, being able to form capillaries, cardiomyocytes and arteries organized into a functional regenerated myocardium.

The injected CSCs also exhibited a tropism for the ischemic tissue because all the regenerating cells were located in the necrotic area and not in the spared myocardium, despite the fact that the cells had been injected in the border zone between ischemic and healthy myocardium. The stimulating role of ischemia is further highlighted by the rapid disappearance of the transplanted cells when injected into the healthy myocardium of the mock-infarcted animals.

As was the case of the myocardial regeneration produced by the bone marrow derived cells, there was no evidence of any significant cell fusion between the donor and host cells using the same criteria outlined in ref. 10. Whether or not the CSCs fulfill all the criteria that some believe are required before the label of "stemness" can be applied to a given cell type[6,47] is beside the point. Independently of what is the appropriate name for these cells, the evidence is convincing that the progeny of a single cell is able to produce the three main cardiac cell types and organize them into a functional myocardium.[44]

The presence of cells with CSC properties in the adult myocardium conclusively dispels the notion that the heart is a terminally differentiated organ without self-renewal potential and points toward this endogenous renewal potential as a tool for the treatment of heart diseases with a significant loss of myocytes. Because these CSCs regenerate both myocytes and small vessels, they might provide the new myocardium with self-renewing capabilities and might be attractive candidates for clinical myocardial regeneration.

7.   Distribution of Cardiac Stem Cells

The demonstration of a cohort of CSCs in the myocardium raised the question of their location and distribution in the myocardium. CSCs are distributed unevenly throughout the heart. Although the majority is in the body of the left ventricle, their concentration per unit volume is significantly higher in the atria and apex than at the base and mid-region of the ventricle. The atria and the apex are the regions of the heart that are exposed to lower levels of wall stress. On the average there is one CSC per ~10,000 myocytes in a healthy myocardium or one CSC per every ~30,000 to 40,000 myocardial cells (does not include the cells with markers for progenitors and precursors, see below). This myocardial concentration of CSCs approximates that of HSCs in the bone marrow[48] and is very similar in different species, including the humans.

Hepatocyte growth factor (HGF) and insulin-like growth factor (IGF-1) are produced by ischemic myocardium[49] and also synthesized by the CSCs, which also possess receptors for these cytokines.[50] *In vitro* and *in vivo* studies have documented that HGF is a chemoattractant for the CSCs.[50] IGF-1 promotes cell survival, proliferation and differentiation. In addition, the activation of c-Met and IGF-1R receptors on these primitive cells results in the induction of a characteristic set of integrins that might be responsible for the mobilization and growth of CSCs. The induction of the $\alpha_V\beta_3$ and $\alpha_6\beta_4$ in the early stages of myocardial damage might facilitate the interaction with fibrinogen/fibrin and plasma fibronectin as well as mobilization toward the areas of damage. The late activation of $\alpha_4\beta_1$, $\alpha_2\beta_1$, and $\alpha_6\beta_4$ integrin receptors favors interaction with collagen and fibronectin during the organization of the scar. Thus, it was of interest to test whether local intra-myocardial administration of HGF and IGF-1 shortly after coronary artery ligation would result in the accumulation and activation of these cells in the infarcted area. As discussed in more detail elsewhere,[50] the results of local cytokine administration are indistinguishable from those obtained after the transplantation of the *in vitro* expanded CSCs. These results, together with the isolation and *in vitro* expansion of the CSCs, have obvious potential for clinical applicability.

8.   Cardiac Stem Cells and Heart Aging

If cardiac cell homeostasis is dependent on myocyte and vascular cell regeneration from the CSCs, it can be predicted that loss of CSCs function, either as a consequence of death or because they have become non-productive, should result in progressive myocyte loss and impaired ventricular function. This is exactly what happens in experimental animals and humans.[14,51,52]

Proliferation of mammalian cells, including human, is dependent on having functional telomeres. Telomere shortening in the absence of telomerase activity is one of the major causes of loss of proliferative capacity in mammalian cells.[53-55] Telomere attrition occurs with age and is proposed to be causal for replicative cell aging. To test the effect of this type of aging in the heart, we analyzed the phenotype of telomerase knock out mice, Terc-/-. Progressive loss of telomere sequences in these animals eventually leads to loss of organismal viability after 3-6 generations.[52] Telomerase shortening at the second and fifth generation of Terc-/- mice was coupled with a profound attenuation in new myocyte formation, increased apoptosis and hypertrophy of the remaining myocytes. These cellular changes were concomitant with ventricular dilatation, wall thinning and ventricular dysfunction resulting in de-compensated eccentric hypertrophy and heart failure.[52] These results were confirmed in two additional animal models.

9.   Cardiac Stem Cell's Role in Heart Homeostasis

Despite the increasing body of data documenting the formation of new cardiac myocytes in the normal and diseased adult mammalian heart, the idea that normal and pathological cardiac homeostasis represents a balance between myocyte death and renewal has been met with significant resistance by the cardiovascular community. At least in part this resistance has been due to the fact that until now there has been a lack of biological understanding about the origin and fate of the cycling myocytes detected in the normal and pathological heart. The existence in the myocardium of stem cells capable of committing to the myocyte lineage provides an explanation and a biologically satisfactory context for the existence of cycling myocytes in the adult myocardium. The finding that some of these primitive cells *in situ* have already activated the myogenic program, their ability to generate a progeny of millions of myocytes from a single cell, together with the small size of the cycling myocytes in the normal, pathological, and regenerating heart indicate that these cycling myocytes are the progeny of the CSCs that have not yet reached a mature and terminally differentiated state. Unpublished data indicate that, once committed to the myocyte lineage, the progeny of a stem cell can undergo only three or four rounds of cell replication before withdrawing permanently from the cell cycle. Taken together, all these data highlight a mechanism for the continuous renewal of the myocardium –both myocytes and coronary vessels– throughout the lifespan of the individual. The CSCs are the source of new myocytes and vascular cells that throughout adult life regenerate those lost by normal wear and tear. These CSCs go on overdrive in pathological conditions characterized by significant myocyte loss. Additionally, they provide a basis for the increase in myocardial contractile cells (hyperplasia) that complements the hypertrophic response when physiological and/or pathological demands impose an increased workload on the heart[7,16] (Figure 3). Thus, the adult heart, which, like the brain, is composed of mainly terminally differentiated parenchymal cells that do not re-enter the cell cycle, is not a terminally differentiated organ because it also contains stem cells that support its regeneration.

10.   Prospects for Myocardial Regeneration in Humans

Over the past two decades there have been significant advances in the management of acute and chronic myocardial infarction. Despite this progress, there remains a very large population of post-infarct survivors who will develop cardiac failure, leading to early death. Cardiac transplant remains the only therapeutic option available to many of these patients. Because of the ingrained concept of the myocardium as a terminally differentiated organ in the cardiovascular community, it has been assumed that any attempt to replace the lost myocytes using cellular therapy would require the introduction of exogenous cells with myogenic potential into the myocardium. Recently, there has been a flurry of clinical trials of human myocardial therapy using bone marrow-derived cells and skeletal myoblasts.[3,56-63] The preliminary results of the clinical trials have unambiguously demonstrated two things: cellular transplants into the myocardium are well-tolerated at least for the first year and have not adverse effect on ventricular performance. Whether this procedure has a clinically significant beneficial effect remains to be demonstrated, despite

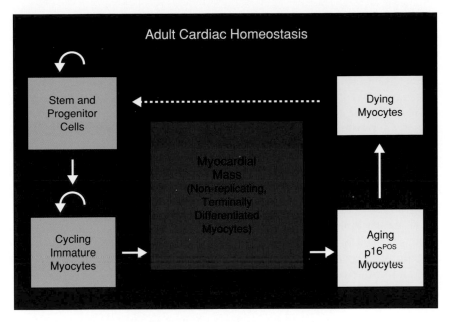

FIGURE 3. Proposed new view of adult cardiac cellular homeostasis. The presence of stem cells in the adult myocardium has revealed the vigorous self-renewal of this tissue. Although the contractile mass is mainly constituted of non-replicating terminally differentiated myocytes, they are constantly replaced. New myocytes are continuously formed by the stem/progenitor cells. These immature myocytes can cycle 2-4 times and they become terminally differentiated. At the same there is a continuous loss of old and hypertrophied myocytes. When the myocyte loss is intense, there is a stimulation of the stem/progenitor cells to increase the production of myocytes. In many pathologies this increase is not sufficient to compensate for the myocyte loss.

early indications that the cell transplanted patients appear to do slightly better than a similar cohort. The reasons for this cautious evaluation are three fold: (1) With one exception,[60] all the clinical trials presently in the public domain have been open label, with a small number of patients who, at the time of the transplant, have also received a revascularization procedure. This setting makes it difficult to fairly evaluate the contribution of the cell transplants. (2) The similarity in results among all the clinical trials is striking, given the disparity of cell preparations used, number of transplanted cells and methods of transplantation. (3) If account is taken of the prevalence of stem/progenitor cells in the transplanted cell populations (as well as the number of skeletal myoblast used) it is clear that the number of cells transplanted is very small and extremely unlikely to directly contribute to the ventricular performance post-transplant. The human left ventricle has a mass of ≥ 400 g while a mouse left ventricle is ≤ 200 mg. To regenerate the mass lost in a 30% infarct in the two species would require the production of 120 g and 60 mg of myocardium, respectively. Despite the more than three orders of magnitude difference in the task required of the transplanted cells, number of stem/progenitor cells used in the human experiments are similar or even lower than those used in the murine experiments.[24,27,44] These murine experiments, however, have been used as the basis for the human trials. These facts argue against a direct contribution of the transplanted cells to the ventricular performance and they favor a transient paracrine effect for the reported improvement in ventricular function, if proven to be real. For all these reasons, the evaluation of the clinical significance of cardiac stem/progenitor cell transplantation will have to wait for the results of double-blind clinical trials, probably using larger numbers of cells.

These early attempts at myocardial regeneration are very valuable as proof of concept and to uncover the hurdles facing myocardial regenerative therapies. However, given the complexity of the procedures and their cost, both in time and resources, it seems unlikely that this approach could become available to the millions of patients that have or will develop terminal heart failure. For myocardial regeneration to become a standard of care treatment will require the development of a simpler an "of the shelf" method to induce myocardial regeneration. The demonstration that the heart harbors stem cells capable of regenerating large amounts of functional myocardium[44] and the possibility to stimulate those cells by means of commercially available cytokines offers an intriguing opportunity for developing a simpler and cheaper procedure that can become available to a large number of patients at a reasonable cost. The next few years will demonstrate whether these objectives are realistic.

The existence of endogenous cardiac stem/progenitor cells, whatever their origin, also explains the earlier observation of a robust regenerative capacity in response to work overload[16] and in the acute post-infarct,[15] but raises the question of why this regenerative response stops before the completion of the repair. The identification of the CSCs[44-46] offers an opportunity to address this clinically important question and opens the tantalizing possibility that in the near future we might manipulate the human CSCs *in situ* to home to the areas of damaged myocardium, proliferate, and differentiate and, therefore, promote a functional cardiac repair without the need of introducing exogenous cells, as shown feasible in the rodents.[50] Elucidation of the regulation of new myocyte formation will provide not only a better understanding of normal and pathological cardiac homeostasis but will open new avenues for therapeutic intervention. The extraordinary clinical need for some form of myocardial functional repair makes the understanding of the biological properties of these cells and harnessing their regenerative capacity an exciting possibility that might help to maintain and restore cardiac function and, perhaps, reduce the need for cardiac transplantation.

11.   Acknowledgments

The authors thank G.M. Ellison and D. Torella for their help with figures.

12.   References

1. Pasumarthi, K.B. and Field, L.J. Cardiomyocyte cell cycle regulation. Circ. Res. 2002; 90: 1004–1054.
2. Chien, K.R. and Olson, E.N. Converging pathways and principles in heart development and disease. Cell. 2002; 110: 153–162.
3. Rosenthal, N. Prometheus's vulture and the stem cell promise. N. Engl. J. Med. 2003; 346: 5–15.
4. Linzbach, A.J. Heart failure from the point of view of quantitative anatomy. Am. J. Cardiol. 1960; 5: 370–382.
5. Rumyantsev, P.P. DNA synthesis and nuclear division in embryonical and postnatal histogenesis of myocardium. Arch. Anat. 1964; 47: 59–65.
6. Anderson, D.J. Gage, F.H. and Weissman, I.L. Can stem cells cross lineage boundaries? Nat. Med. 2001; 7: 393–395.
7. Schaper, J. Elsasser, A. and Kostin, S. The role of cell death in heart failure. Circ. Res. 1999; 85: 867–869.
8. Anversa, P. Myocyte death in the pathological heart. Circ. Res. 2000; 86: 121–124.
9. Kang, P.M. and Izumo, S. Apoptosis and heart failure: a critical review of the literature. Circ. Res. 2000; 86: 1107–1113.
10. Nadal-Ginard, B., Kajstura, J., Leri, A. and Anversa, P. Myocyte death, growth, growth and regeneration in cardiac hypertrophy and failure. Circ. Res. 2003; 92: 139–150.
11. Anversa, P. and Nadal-Ginard, B. Myocyte renewal and ventricular remodeling. Nature, 2002; 415: 240–243.
12. Nadal-Ginard, B., Kajstura, J., Anversa, P. and Leri, A. A matter of life and death: cardiac myocyte apoptosis and regeneration. J. Clin. Invest. 2003; 111: 1457–1459.
13. Anversa P. and Kajstura, J. Ventricular myocytes are not terminally differentiated in the adult mammalian heart. Circ. Res. 1998; 83: 1–14.
14. Chimenti, C., Kajstura, J., Torella, D., Urbanek, K., Heleniak, H., Colussi, C., Di Meglio, F., Nadal-Ginard, B., Frustaci, A., Leri, A., Maseri, A. and Anversa, P. Senescence and death of primitive cells and myocytes lead to premature cardiac aging and heart failure. Circ. Res. 2003; 93: 604–613.
15. Beltrami, A. P. Urbanek, K., Kajstura, J., Yan, S. M., Finato, N., Bussani, R., Nadal-Ginard, B., Silvestri, F., Leri, A., Beltrami, C. A. and Anversa, P. Evidence that human cardiocytes divide after myocardial infarction. N. Engl. J. Med. 2001; 344: 1750–1757.
16. Urbanek, K., Quaini, F., Tasca, G., Torella, D., Castaldo, C., Nadal-Ginard, B., Leri, A., Kajstura, J., Quaini, E. and Anversa, P. Intense myocyte formation from cardiac stem cells in human cardiac hypertrophy. Proc. Natl. Acad. Sci. U.S.A. 2003; 100: 10440–10445.
17. Leri, A., Barlucchi, L., Limana, F., Deptala, A., Darzynkiewicz, Z., Hintze, T. H., Kajstura, J., Nadal-Ginard, B. and P. Anversa. Telomerase expression and activ-

ity are coupled with myocyte proliferation and preservation of telomeric length in the failing heart. Proc. Natl. Acad. Sci. USA. 2001; 98: 8626–8631.

18. Quaini, F., Urbanek, K., Beltrami, A. P., Finato, N., Beltrami, C. A., Nadal-Ginard, B., Kajstura, J., Leri, A. and Anversa, P. Chimerism of the transplanted heart. N. Engl. J. Med. 2002. 346: 5–15.

19. Ferrari G., Cusella-De Angelis G., Coletta M., Paolucci E., Stornaiuolo A., Cossu G. and Mavilio F. Muscle regeneration by bone marrow-derived myogenic progenitors. Science. 1998; 279: 1528–1530.

20. Lagasse E., Connors H., Al-Dhalimy M., Reitsma M., Dohse M., Osborne L., Wang X., Finegold M., Weissman I.L. and Grompe M. Hematopoietic stem cells can differentiate into hepatocytes *in vivo*. Nat. Med. 2000; 6: 1229–1234.

21. Brazelton T.R., Rossi F.M., Keshet G.I. and Blau H.M. From marrow to brain: expression of neuronal phenotypes in adult mice. Science. 2000; 290: 1775–1779.

22. Mezey, E., Chandross, K.J., Harta, G., Maki, R.A. and McKercher, S.R. Turning blood into brain: cells bearing neuronal antigens generated *in vivo* from bone marrow. Science. 2000; 290: 1779–1782.

23. Krause D.S., Theise N.D., Collector M.I., Henegariu O., Hwang S., Gardner R., Neutzel S. and Sharkis S.J. Multi-organ, multi-lineage engraftment by a single bone marrow-derived stem cell. Cell. 2001; 105: 369–377.

24. Orlic, D., Kajstura, J., Chimenti, S., Jakonuik, I., Li, B. Pickel, J., McKay, R., Nadal-Ginard, B., Bodine, D., Leri, A. and Anversa, P. Bone marrow cells regenerate infarcted myocardium. Nature. 2001; 410: 701–705.

25. Balsam, L.B., Wagers, A.J., Christensen, J.L., Kofidis, T., Weissman, I.L. and Robbins, R.C. Hematopoietic stem cells adopt mature hematopoietic fates in ischemic myocardium. Nature. 2004; 428: 668–673.

26. Murry, C.E., Soonpaa, M.H., Reinecke, H., Nakajima, H.O., Rubart, M., Pasumarthi, K.B., Virag, J.I., Bartelmez, S.S., Poppa, V., Bradford, G., Dowell, J.D., Williams, D.A. and Field, L.J. Hematopoietic stem cells do not transdifferentiate into cardiac myocytes in myocardial infarcts. Nature. 2004; 428: 664–668.

27. Kajstura, J., Rota, M., Whang, B., Cascapera, S., Hosoda, T., Bearzi, C., Nurzynska, D., Kasahara, H., Zias, E., Bonafe, M., Nadal-Ginard, B., Torella, D., Nascimbene, A., Quaini, F., Urbanek, K., Leri, A. and Anversa, P. Bone marrow cells differentiate in cardiac cell lineages after infarction independently of cell fusion. Circ. Res. Published online November 29, 2004.

28. Orlic, D., Kajstura, J., Chimenti, S., Limana, F., Jakoniuk, I., Quaini, F., Nadal-Ginard, B., Bodine, D., Leri, A. and Anversa, P. Mobilized bone marrow cells repair the infarcted heart, improving function and survival. Proc. Natl. Acad. Sci. USA. 2001; 98: 10344–10349.

29. Urbich C. and Dimmeler S. Endothelial progenitor cells: characterization and role in vascular biology. Circ Res. 2004; 95: 343–53.

30. Bodine, D. M., Seidel, N. E., Gale, M. S., Nienhuis, A. W. and Orlic, D. Efficient retrovirus transduction of mouse pluripotent hematopoietic stem cells mobilized into the peripheral blood by treatment with granulocyte colony-stimulating factor and stem cell factor. Blood. 1994; 84: 1482–1491.

31. Laflamme M.A., Meyerson D., Saffitz J.E. and Murry, C.E. Evidence for cardiomyocyte repopulation by extracardiac progenitors in transplanted human hearts. Circ. Res. 2002; 90: 634–640.

32. Müller P., Pfeiffer P., Koglin J., Schafers, H.J., Seeland, U., Janzen, I., Urbschat, S. and Bohm, M. Cardiomyocytes of noncardiac origin in myocardial biopsies of human transplanted hearts. Circulation. 2002; 105: 31–35.

33. Glaser R., Lu M.M., Narula N. and Epstein, J.A. Smooth muscle cells, but not myocytes, of host origin in transplanted human hearts. Circulation. 2002; 106: 17–19.
34. Bayes-Genis A., Salido M., Sole Ristol F., Puig M., Brossa V., Camprecios M., Corominas J.M., Marinoso M.L., Baro T., Vela M.C., Serrano S., Padro J.M., Bayes de Luna A. and Cinca J. Host cell-derived cardiomyocytes in sex-mismatch cardiac allografts. Cardiovasc. Res. 2002; 56: 404–410.
35. Anversa, P. and Nadal-Ginard, B. Cardiac chimerism: methods matter. Circulation. 2002; 106: e129–e131.
36. Deb A., Wang S., Skelding K.A., Miller D., Simper D. and Caplice N.M. Bone marrow-derived cardiomyocytes are present in adult human heart: A study of gender-mismatched bone marrow transplantation patients. Circulation. 2003; 107: 1247–1249.
37. Thiele J., Varus E., Wickenhauser C., Kvasnicka H.M., Lorenzen J., Gramley F., Metz K.A., Rivero F. and Beelen D.W. Mixed chimerism of cardiomyocytes and vessels after allogeneic bone marrow and stem-cell transplantation in comparison with cardiac allografts. Transplantation. 2004; 77: 1902–1905.
38. Soukiasian H.J., Czer I.S., Avital I., Aoki T., Kim Y.H., Umehara Y., Pass J., Tabrizi R., Magliato K., Fontana G.P., Cheng W., Demetriou A.A. and Trento A. A novel sub-population of bone marrow-derived myocardial stem cells: potential autologous cell therapy in myocardial infarction. J. Heart Lung Transplant. 2004; 23: 873–880.
39. Bayes-Genis A., Muniz-Diaz E., Catasus L., Arilla M., Rodriguez C., Sierra J., Madoz P.J. and Cinca J. Cardiac chimerism in recipients of peripheral-blood and bone marrow stem cells. Eur. J. Heart Fail. 2004; 6: 399–402.
40. Thiele J., Varus E., Wickenhauser C., Kvasnicka H.M., Metz K.A. and Beelen D.W. Regeneration of heart muscle tissue: quantification of chimeric cardiomyocytes and endothelial cells following transplantation. Histol. Histopathol. 2004; 19: 201–209.
41. Chien, K.R. Stem cells: lost in translation. Nature. 2004; 428: 607–608.
42. Reynolds, B.A. and Weiss, S. Generation of neurons and astrocytes from isolated cells of the adult mammalian central nervous system. Science. 1992; 255: 1707–1710.
43. Gritti, A., Parati, E.A., Cova, L., Frolichsthal, P., Galli, R., Wanke, E., Faravelli, L., Morassutti, D.J., Roisen, F., Nickel, D.D. and Vescovi, A.L. Multipotential stem cells from adult mouse brain proliferate and self-renew in response to basic fibroblast growth factor. J. Neurosci. 1996; 16: 1091–1100.
44. Beltrami, A. P., Barlucchi, L., Torella, D., Baker, M., Limana, F., Climenti, S., Kasahara, H., Rota, M., Musso, E., Urbanek, K., Leri, A., Kajstura, J., Nadal-Ginard, B. and Anversa, P. Adult cardiac stem cells are multipotent and support myocardial regeneration. Cell. 2003; 114:763–776.
45. Oh H., Bradfute S.B., Gallardo T.D., Nakamura T., Gaussin V., Mishina Y., Pocius J., Michael L.H., Behringer R.R., Garry D.J., Entman M.L. and Schneider M.D. Cardiac progenitor cells from adult myocardium: homing, differentiation, and fusion after infarction. Proc. Natl. Acad. Sci. U.S.A. 2003; 100: 12313–12318.
46. Matsuura K., Nagai T., Nishigaki N., Oyama, T., Nishi, J., Wada, H., Sano, M., Toko, H., Akazawada, H., Sato, T., Nakaya, H., Kasanuki, H. and Komuro, I. Adult cardiac Sca-1-positive cells differentiate into beating cardiomyocytes. J. Biol. Chem. 2004; 279: 11384–11391.
47. Wagers, A.J. and Weissman, I.L. Plasticity of adult stem cells. Cell. 2004; 116: 639–648.
48. Spangrude, G.J., Perry, S.S. and Slayton, W.B. Early stages of hematopoietic differentiation. Ann. N.Y. Acad. Sci. 2003; 996: 186–194.

49. Ono, K., Matsumori, A., Shioi, T., Furukawa, Y. and Sasayama S. Enhanced expression of HGF/c-Met by myocardial ischemia and reperfusion in a rat model. Circulation. 1997; 95: 2552–2558.
50. Torella, D., Urbanek, K., Rota, M., Nurzynska, D., Climenti, S., Barlucchi, L., Baker, M., Cascapera, S., Bearzi, C., Musso, E., Rastaldo, R., Limana, F., Nadal-Ginard, B., Leri, A., Kajstura, J. and Anversa, P. Local activation of cardiac stem cells repairs the infarcted heart and improves survival. Submitted. 2004.
51. Torella, D., Rota, M., Nurzynska, D., Musso, E., Monsen, A., Shiraishi, I., Zias, E., Walsh, K., Rosenzweig, A., Sussman, M.A. Urbanek, K., Nadal-Ginard, B., Kajstura, J., Anversa, P. and Leri, A. Cardiac stem cell and myocyte aging, heart failure, and insulin-like growth factor-1 overexpression. Circ. Res. 2004; 94: 514–524.
52. Leri, A., Franco, S., Zacheo, A., Barlucchi, L., Climenti, S., Limana, F., Nadal-Ginard, B., Kajstura, J., Anversa, P. and Blasco, M.A. Ablation of telomerase and telomere loss leads to cardiac dilatation and heart failure associated with p53 upregulation. EMBO J. 2003; 22: 131–139.
53. Collins, K. and Mitchell, J.R. Telomerase in the human organism. Oncogene. 2002; 21: 564–579.
54. Harley, C.B., Futcher, A.B. and Greider, C.W. Telomeres shorten during aging of human fibroblasts. Nature. 1990; 345: 458–460.
55. Lee, H.W., Blasco, M.A., Gottlieb, G.J., Horner, J.W., Greider, C.W. and DePinho, R.A. Essential role of mouse telomerase in highly proliferative organs. Science. 1998; 392: 569–574.
56. Kang H.J., Kim H.S., Zhang S.Y., Park K.W., Cho H.J., Koo B.K., Kim Y.J., Soo Lee D., Sohn D.W., Han K.S., Oh B.H., Lee M.M. and Park Y.B. Effects of intra-coronary infusion of peripheral blood stem-cells mobilised with granulocyte-colony stimulating factor on left ventricular systolic function and restenosis after coronary stenting in myocardial infarction: the MAGIC cell randomised clinical trial. Lancet. 2004; 363: 751–756.
57. Strauer B.E., Brehm M., Zeus T., Kostering M., Hernandez A., Sorg R.V., Kogler G. and Wernet P. Repair of infarcted myocardium by autologous intracoronary mononuclear bone marrow cell transplantation in humans. Circulation. 2002; 106: 1913–1918.
58. Schachinger V., Assmus B., Britten M.B., Honold J., Lehmann R., Teupe C., Abolmaali N.D., Vogl T.J., Hofmann W.K., Martin H., Dimmeler S. and Zeiher A.M. Transplantation of progenitor cells and regeneration enhancement in acute myocardial infarction: final one-year results of the TOPCARE-AMI Trial. J. Am. Coll. Cardiol. 2004; 44: 1690–1699.
59. Perin E.C., Dohmann H.F., Borojevic R., Silva S.A., Sousa A.L., Mesquita C.T., Rossi M.I., Carvalho A.C., Dutra H.S., Dohmann H.J., Silva G.V., Belem L., Vivacqua R., Rangel F.O., Esporcatte R., Geng Y.J., Vaughn W.K., Assad J.A., Mesquita E.T. and Willerson J.T. Transendocardial, autologous bone marrow cell transplantation for severe, chronic ischemic heart failure. Circulation. 2003; 107: 2294–2302.
60. Stamm, C., Westphal, B., Kleine, H.-D., Petzsch, M., Kittner, C., Klinge, H., Schümichen, C., Nienaber, C.A., Freund, M. and Steinhoff, G. Autologous bone-marrow stem-cell transplantation for myocardial regeneration. Lancet. 2003; 361: 45–46.

61. Menasche P., Hagege A.A., Scorsin M., Pouzet B., Desnos M., Duboc D., Schwartz K., Vilquin J.T. and Marolleau J.P. Myoblast transplantation for heart failure. Lancet. 2001; 357: 279–280.
62. Smits P.C., van Geuns R.J., Poldermans D., Bountioukos M., Onderwater E.E., Lee C.H., Maat A.P. and Serruys P.W. Catheter-based intramyocardial injection of autologous skeletal myoblasts as a primary treatment of ischemic heart failure: clinical experience with six-month follow-up. J. Am. Coll. Cardiol. 2003; 42: 2063–2069.
63. Pagani F.D., DerSimonian H., Zawadzka A., Wetzel K., Edge A.S., Jacoby D.B., Dinsmore J.H., Wright S., Aretz T.H., Eisen H.J. and Aaronson K.D. Autologous skeletal myoblasts transplanted to ischemia-damaged myocardium in humans. Histological analysis of cell survival and differentiation. J. Am. Coll. Cardiol. 2003; 41: 879–888.

Skeletal Myoblast

4
A Historic Recapitulation of Myoblast Transplantation

DANIEL SKUK AND JACQUES P. TREMBLAY*

1. Introduction

The term "myoblast transplantation" defines the implantation into the body of precursor cells able to differentiate into striated muscle, i.e., myoblasts. It integrates into the new medical field of cell transplantation, which includes other important disciplines such as bone marrow, islet, neuron or hepatocyte transplantation. Bone marrow transplantation, that is a standard therapeutic tool since the decade of the 70s, is in fact the best example of a cell-transplantation strategy used successfully in the clinics. Although all cell-transplantation strategies generically imply the implantation into the body of cells isolated from their original tissues, there are substantial differences between them. As an example, donor cells could be either differentiated cells that are not proliferated in culture (islet transplantation) or precursor cells that are proliferated in culture (myoblast transplantation); they can delivered systemically by intravascular injection (bone-marrow transplantation), infused in the specific blood supply of an organ (the portal vein in the case of hepatocytes) or must need stereotaxic local delivery to a precise minute region in the brain (dopaminergic neurons in the treatment of Parkinson disease), and so forth.

Myoblast transplantation was born as an attempt to develop a treatment for the diseases of the skeletal muscle, mainly those myopathies of genetic recessive etiology, and the point of departure of this research can be situated in 1978. Among these diseases, Duchenne muscular dystrophy (DMD), both by its relative frequency (1 affected in 3500 male newborns) and severity (progression to severe generalized paresis and paralysis in the adolescence and death around the age of 20 to 30), was the main target of this potentially therapeutic tool. The idea of using myoblast transplantation to reengineer contractile tissues in the scars of infarcted hearts was tributary of the original skeletal muscle application, and appeared at the end of the 80's.[1]

*Daniel Skuk and Jacques P. Tremblay, Unité de recherche en Génétique humaine, Centre de Recherche du Centre Hospitalier de l'Université Laval, Québec, Canada G1V 4G2.

Collaterally to these two main targets of myoblast transplantation, other anecdotic uses were proposed. Genetically modified myoblasts are considered promising vehicles for the systemic delivery of hormones or factors, such as factor IX,[2] erytropoietin,[3] growth hormone,[4] proinsulin[5] and the granulocyte colony stimulating factor-1.[6] Implantation of transgenic myoblasts for the local delivery of therapeutic factors was proposed for the treatment of joint pathologies[7] and neurodegenerative diseases.[8] Local injection of myoblasts expressing Fas ligand was proposed to destroy solid tumors.[9]

2.   A Brief History of Myoblast Culture

As mentioned above, donor cells for cell transplantation could be either the differentiated cells that normally constitute the parenchyma of an organ, or precursor cells with the ability to differentiate into those cells. By their characteristics, the differentiated cells of skeletal muscles cannot be used for transplantation: myofibers are very long and highly specialized syncytia that cannot be implanted as isolated elements in a recipient. Thus, the only possibility of using a donor cell for the treatment of myopathies is finding a precursor cell able to differentiate into myofibers. These precursors (myoblasts) exist during the embryological development but are also present in the adult skeletal muscles in the form of quiescent stem cells called "satellite cells". This is the reason why skeletal muscles, contrary to myocardium, can regenerate following necrosis. However, since the quantity of satellite cells that can be obtained freshly from a skeletal muscle is very low, these cells need to be expanded prior to transplantation, and in this case, the proliferating myogenic cells are also called "myoblasts". The discipline of myoblast transplantation is thus tributary of the techniques of *in vitro* culture, and an historical recapitulation of myoblast transplantation must begin with the origin of these techniques.

2.1.   First Observations of Myoblasts in Culture

The technique of myoblast culture can be traced to the origins of the art of tissue culture in the beginnings of the XX century, when Ross G. Harrison published in 1907 a method to maintain tissues from frog embryos *in vitro* up to 4 weeks "when reasonable aseptic precautions are taken".[10] Specially interesting for the history of muscle-cell culture is his pioneer observation of myoblasts *in vitro*, as inferred from his observation that "masses of cells taken from the myotomes differentiate into muscle fibers showing fibrillae with typical striations".[10] Thereafter, among the first studies describing myoblasts in culture, we found those of Margaret Reed Lewis in 1915.[11] She used explants taken from the legs of 4 to 10 day chick embryos maintained in a Locke's solution supplemented with 0.5% dextrose and 10% bouillon, where, according to her own words, "the growth of cells is rapid and luxuriant".[11] She described that "numerous isolated fibers and many primitive myoblasts are scattered throughout the new growth" and she noted that there was no mitosis in the myofibers while she observed mitosis in the myoblasts. This was probably the first statement that *in vitro* myofibers are post-mitotic, and that the only myogenic cells able to proliferate were the mononucleated myoblasts. However, she mentioned a report of Champy in 1913 (*Archivos de Zoologia Experimental*, liii, 42) as the first describing that "the striated muscle fiber of the rabbit, when explanted into plasma, differentiates into an indifferent mass of cells".[11]

2.2.   The Beginnings of the Modern Technique for Myoblast Culture

While those first myoblast cultures were made by the technique of explants, putting small fragments of muscle in culture, the development of the techniques of tissue dissociation by enzymatic treatment allowed the *in vitro* cultivation of muscle cells in monolayers.[12-15] In the 60's, skeletal muscle culture is a well-established technique. David Yaffe was one of the main experts at that time, since he used extensively myoblast cultures to study many aspects of the cell biology of these cells, such as their differentiation.[16-20] To increase the percentage of myoblasts in skeletal-muscle cultures, that he defined as "a heterogeneous population of mononucleated cells",[16] he took advantage of the different attachment times of the different cells: since fibroblasts attached to the substrate faster than myoblasts, he used sequential preplattings of 40 to 60 minutes to enrich his primary cultures in myoblasts.[16,20] This simple technique of increasing the percentage of myoblasts in primary cultures of skeletal muscle by preplatting is still in use, and we use it in our current clinical trial.[21]

2.3.   Discovering the Origin of Cultured Myoblasts

It must be noted that the origin of the mononucleated myogenic cells obtained from skeletal muscle cultures was not clear until the 60's. It was Alexander Mauro who described for the first time, during electronic microscopic studies on frog skeletal muscles, a cell that he denominated "satellite cell".[22] According to this author, previous to his discovery, most cytologists believed that the mononuclear cells that participate in muscle regeneration were surviving nuclei of the damaged myofibers, that "gathered up" sarcoplasmic cytoplasm to became single cells. Mauro immediately proposed that the satellite cells could be "remnants from the embryonic development of the multinucleate muscle cell", and that they could be "merely dormant myoblasts" that "are ready to recapitulate the embryonic development of skeletal muscle fiber when the main multinucleate cell is damaged". The concept that the satellite cell is the committed stem cell of the myofibers was becoming the established paradigm since that original observation, however recent studies have suggested that some myoblasts obtained from skeletal muscle could have other origins, such as vascular-associated cells.[23,24] In spite of that, satellite cells remains the main source of cell precursors for myofiber regeneration.[25]

3.   Pioneer Myoblast Transplantation Experiments

Terence Partridge, Miranda Grounds and John C. Sloper set the basis of myoblast transplantation in 1978 when they expressed that "in subjects suffering from inherited recessive myopathies, muscle function might be restored if normal myoblasts could be made to fuse with defective muscle fibers during muscle growth or regeneration".[26] This is probably the first mention of a potential therapeutic use of myoblasts following strategies of cell transplantation, although their study consisted of transplantation of minced muscles. It is interesting to note that, to prevent the rejection of the graft in this early experiments, the authors developed immune tolerance by injecting lymphoid cells.[26]

3.1.   *The Two First Studies on Myoblast Transplantation*

The first studies on intramuscular transplantation of cultured myoblasts were published in 1979, when this technique was used as an experimental tool to analyze some aspects of the myogenic differentiation. Paul Jones used it in rats to develop "an experimental system which would include the advantages of both *in vivo* and *in vitro* systems", and he suggested the term *culturegraft* "to describe the implantation of cultured cells back into an animal".[27] He was also the first to describe the acute rejection response that follows myoblast transplantation in allogeneic conditions: he detected important lymphocyte accumulations in muscles that received allotransplantation of myoblasts at days 5 and 14 post-graft, followed by the disappearance of donor nuclei at 3 weeks post-graft. On the contrary, autotransplantation led to the presence of donor nuclei up to 28 weeks post-graft, without lymphocyte infiltration. Simultaneously, Bruce H. Lipton and Edward Schultz published also interesting observations following the injections of myoblasts in muscles and non-muscular sites of rats and quails.[28] They observed yet that donor myoblasts either form new small myofibers or are incorporated in the large recipient myofibers after their intramuscular injection, and they described donor-cell migration into the host muscle. Injected in a subcutaneous site, they observed that donor myoblasts were able to form new myofibers in a disorganized fashion, but that fibrosis developed among them. One year later, cloned chick myoblasts were also transplanted in quail embryos to study their fusion in vivo.[29]

3.2.   The Pioneer Work of Partridge's Group

Following their original idea of developing a therapeutic tool for hereditary myopathies, Partridge's team did a pioneer series of studies on myoblast transplantation in mice in the beginning of the '80s (Partridge and many of his collaborators at that time are still active in the field). Their studies confirmed that the intramuscular injection of myoblast from neonatal mice can introduce donor genes into the host muscles, forming that they called "mosaic" or "hybrid" myofibers (i.e., myofibers expressing proteins coded by donor and recipient nuclei).[30,31] Through this classical series of experiments, they confirmed the fusion of donor myoblasts with host myofibers by using strains of mice that expressed different isoenzymes of glucose-6-phosphate isomerase. The long-term aim of these researchers was clearly stated: "Our hope is that these normal myonuclei, by supplying the muscle fiber with normal gene products, will alleviate the myopathy".[30]

In 1987, a great step was done in the field of neuromuscular diseases when the group of Louis M. Kunkel reported the discovery of the protein that is absent or altered in DMD patients, which they called "dystrophin".[32] Following this discovery, it was also Partridge's team that reported that the intramuscular injection of normal myoblasts in dystrophin-deficient mice (called *mdx*) was able to induce the expression of this protein in some host myofibers.[33] This property of myoblast transplantation to induce the expression of normal proteins in dystrophic myofibers was demonstrated later in mouse models of other muscular dystrophies, following the molecular characterization of each individual disease. This was the case of merosin expression following normal myoblast transplantation in the *dy/dy* mouse, a model of the congenital muscle dystrophy produced by the absence of merosin,[34,35] and dysferlin in the case of the SJL mouse, a model of a limb-girdle muscular dystrophy produced by the absence of dysferlin.[36]

4.   Early Clinical Trials on Myopathic Patients

Once the first animal experiments reported some potentially useful results, several groups rapidly undertook clinical trials of myoblast transplantation in myopathic patients, whose results were published between 1991 and 1998. Most of these early clinical trials were performed in DMD patients,[37-46] although brief essays in patients suffering of Becker muscular dystrophy[46] and McArdle's disease[43] were also reported. The overall results of theses clinical trials were quite disappointing. Some potentially positive but generally not-significant results in the molecular level (detection of the dystrophin gene, transcript or protein by PCR, Western blot and immunodetection) did not correspond with a significant clinical benefit of the patients.

This rapid transition from mouse experiments to the clinics was justified by the absence of other effective treatments for a progressive disease that is severely disabling and lethal. However, researchers bypassed the differences between mice and humans, and misinterpreted and/or overestimated the few experimental data. In fact, these early clinical trials were based on the hope that some myoblasts injected at isolated points in the skeletal muscle of a patient would proliferate and migrate throughout the muscle, fusing with most of the myofibers. The research developed later in animal models demonstrated that this hope was not realistic. Technical, important parameters such as the inter-injection distance, the number of cells per injection or the protocols of immunosuppression were improvised. This failure of not well-planned clinical trials due to absence of enough animal experiments, justified those researchers that claimed at the beginning of human experiments that the clinical trials needed to be stopped because they required more experimental support.[47]

5.   Continuation of Animal Experiments

The absence of positive results in the first clinical trials discouraged most groups to pursue research to understand how myoblast transplantation works and how it could be improved for clinical applications.

5.1.   *Several Research Axes to Improve Myoblast Transplantation*

However, some groups attempted to demonstrate that myoblast transplantation in mice can restore the mass and force of muscles submitted to severe irreversible damage.[48-52] Others addressed the important question of whether exogenous myoblasts injected into muscles provide a permanent source of mononuclear muscle precursor cells able to be recruited later in myofiber regeneration, because in this case the effect of myoblast transplantation would not be limited to the early fusion of the donor cells but would also insure a permanent source of normal muscle-precursor cells able to participate in muscle hypertrophy and regeneration. This was confirmed in mice,[53,54] where it was recently shown that some donor myoblasts can form new satellite cells.[55]

Some groups tried different methods to improve the success of myoblast transplantation, i.e., to obtain the largest hybrid myofibers in a muscle as possible following the injection of the donor myoblasts. A frequent approach was to produce increased muscle damage concomitant to the myoblast injections, in order to increase the number of regenerating fibers able to incorporate the injected myoblasts. This was obtained in mice by injection of myotoxins, such as snake venoms[56-58] or local anesthetics.[5,9,60] The inhibition of host satellite cells to favor the uptake of the exogenous myoblasts was done in mice by using high doses of ionizing radiation.[48,49,56-58,61] Cryodamage was used to produce muscle necrosis while also killing satellite cells.[50,51,62]

The possibility to deliver myogenic cells to the skeletal muscles by the blood stream was studied since the beginning of the '90s in mice. Partridge's team tried unsuccessfully to deliver primary-cultured myoblasts by intravenous and intraperitoneal injection.[63] Others tried the intra-arterial route in mice, but in this case the donor cells fused with a significant number of host myofibers only after a mechanical muscle injury not different from that produced by the intramuscular injections.[64,65]

5.2.   A New Problem: the Hyperacute Donor-Cell Death

A new problem on the field was raised in 1994, when two groups reported simultaneously that most of the donor myoblasts die very rapidly after the intramuscular transplantation.[66,67] It was frequently claimed thereafter that a massive donor-cell death limits the success of myoblast transplantation,[68,69] but it became clear that this phenomenon is not sufficient to prevent the success of myoblast transplantation in mice, both because not all cells die and the proliferation of the surviving cells compensates the cell death.[70] Presently, the early survival of donor myoblasts is not well-understood and some aspects remain controversial. Some studies have suggested indirectly that the cellular components of the acute inflammatory reaction could be involved in an early donor-cell killing,[71-74] but this idea was recently challenged by some evidence suggesting the contrary.[75] The importance of the treatments of the donor-cell survival between their collection from the culture flasks and the moment of transplantation was signaled.[76] On the other end, Partridge's group suggested that high mortality of the transplanted myoblasts could be explained by the hypothetical existence of a specific subpopulation among the donor myoblasts, which would be the only one with the ability to survive and proliferate following transplantation.[70]

5.3.   Understanding the Immunology of Myoblast Transplantation

A lot of attention was given to the immunological aspects of myoblast transplantation, i.e., to the phenomenon of acute rejection and the use of immunosuppression. Acute rejection is the mechanism by which donor-alloantigen-reactive cytolytic T-lymphocytes of the recipient destroy an allograft by a response implicating recognition of the MHC (Major Histocompatibility Complex) class I on the donor cells. Some researchers first thought that there is no acute rejection after myoblast transplantation, since MHC class I is not present on normal mature myofibers.[77-79] However, MHCs are expressed during muscle regeneration and in the muscles of DMD patients.[78-80] Moreover, since myoblasts and myotubes always express MHC class I,[81-83] they can be attacked by cytotoxic T-lymphocytes. Indeed, since the beginning of the 90's there was a cumulus of observations suggesting that myoblasts may act as professional antigen-presenting cells,[84] since under specific conditions they also expressed MHC class II[81,82,85-89] and co-stimulatory molecules.[90] However, this immunological property of myoblasts remains controversial.

As previously said, the first description of lymphocyte infiltration following myoblast allotransplantation in mice dates from 1979.[27] Indeed, Partridge's group already considered in the beginning of the 80's that "the main obstacle to the therapeutic use of grafts of muscle precursor cells would be allograft rejection",[30] and they used central tolerance development[31] or immunosuppression[91] to avoid acute rejection during their early experiments in mice. Most of the attention to this phenomenon, however, dates from the middle of the 90's, when researches tried to explain in animal models the failure of the early clinical trials. The identification of Mac-1+, CD8+ and CD4+ cells among the leukocyte infiltrates observed following myoblast allotransplantation in immunocompetent mice was simultaneously reported by two groups.[62,92,93] Expression of IL-2 receptors, Th-1 cytokine and granzyme B confirmed that these lymphocytes were activated.[94,95] Acute rejection was also described following myoblast transplantation in dogs[96] and monkeys.[97-99]

5.4. Progress in the Control of Acute Rejection

A series of studies was also attempted to develop ideal protocols to control acute rejection of myoblast transplantation. In fact, it was observed that the degree of control of the immune response after myoblast allotransplantation in mice varied between different immunosuppressive drugs.[100] Cyclophosphamide gave negative results, and it was suggested that this antiproliferative drug kills the donor myoblasts because they proliferate after transplantation.[101] Cyclosporine A was the first immunosuppressant to be used for myoblast transplantation in mice[91] and was effective in later experiments,[50,93,102,103] but untoward properties for myoblast transplantation were reported *in vitro*.[104,105] Mycophenolate mofetil alone was not useful for myoblast transplantation.[106] Sirolimus was effective in mice,[58] but the best results in this model were reported with tacrolimus.[57] Tacrolimus was also very efficient for myoblast transplantation in monkeys,[97-99,107,108] where its benefits were observed for up to 1 year.[108] More recent avenues are exploring the possibility to avoid immunosuppression for myoblast transplantation, either by developing donor-specific tolerance,[109,110] or by autotransplantation of myoblast genetically corrected *in vitro*.[111-114]

6.   Recent Pre-clinical and Clinical Progress

Based on the premise that therapeutic approaches must be tested under conditions, that can be extrapolated to humans, our group was the only one that, since the middle of the 90's, focused studies of myoblast transplantation in non-human primates. We considered this model especially important, since mouse experiments provide a lot of information that either do not apply to humans or use parameters difficult to apply in myoblast transplantation to humans. In transplantation research it is known that humans and monkeys share immunological characteristics[115-118] that differ from mice. Moreover, skeletal muscle regeneration is better in rodents than in primates, probably due to the evolutionary retention of some characteristics of early mammals, which evolved from reptile ancestors with a high regenerative capacity.[119] Moreover, the size and structure of the skeletal muscles in the monkey is by far more appropriate than those of mice to design strategies of myogenic-cell delivery.[99,108] Finally, some specific aspects in the biology of myoblast transplantation seem to be different between humans and mice, such as the importance of the compatibility of functional phenotype between the donor myoblasts and the host muscles.[120,121]

6.1. Pre-Clinical Progress

Our series of myoblast transplantation studies in non-human primates allowed us to advance towards our current clinical trials by many steps. In 1995 and 1996, we published the first reports demonstrating the usefulness of tacrolimus as an immunosuppressor for myoblast allotransplantation in primates.[97,107] Three years later, we published the best success ever obtained in primate skeletal muscles in terms of high percentages of myofibers expressing an exogenous protein introduced by any method, and in this case we used very close injections of myoblasts in a limited volume of muscle, with or without concomitant injection of myotoxins.[98] The third step was the demonstration that we were able to obtain significant percentages of hybrid myofibers throughout whole large limb muscles in primates, by a method that consists of performing close parallel equidistant injections of myoblasts, percutaneously, throughout the muscle.[108] We confirmed at the same time that the method did not produce hazardous local or systemic consequences. Parallel, we showed that an appropriate immunosuppression with tacrolimus allowed a graft survival for up to one year (the longer period studied).[108] Finally, in a recent study, we began to quantitatively define the parameters that are important to obtain a reproducible success following myoblast transplantation by this technique.[99]

6.2. A New Clinical Trial

A corollary of this series of primate experiments is an ongoing clinical trial of normal-myoblast allotransplantation in DMD patients testing the two main parameters previously determined in monkeys, i.e., a tacrolimus-based immunosuppression and a method of cell injection by multiple close parallel injections.[21] Our allogeneic myoblast transplantations in DMD patients were initially done in a small volume of muscle that was sampled 1 month later. The parameters of these transplantations allowed, for the first time, to consistently observe the expression of donor dystrophin in the myofibers of the patients.[21] Up to the moment of writing this chapter, this was the only report of a method insuring normal-dystrophin expression in significant percentages of myofibers in DMD patients.

7.   Switching From Skeletal Muscle to The Heart

The idea of using cultured myoblasts in the treatment of the heart infarcts was proposed in 1989 by Kao et al.[1,122] They hypothesized at that time that myoblasts injected into a recently damaged region of the myocardium would differentiate into myocardial cells once exposed to this new environment. In 1992, Marelli et al. published the results of a first experiment of myoblast autotransplantation in dogs.[123] They produced a cryoinjury in the heart muscle, followed by the injection at the same place of cultured myoblasts proliferated from a skeletal muscle biopsy of the same animal. Six and 8 weeks later, they observed the formation of striated muscle in the center of the scar tissue formed by the cryodamage, which they attributed to the grafted cells. In this first observation, the authors reported the presence of intercalated discs. In fact, this was the first observation of a "transdifferentiation" of the injected myoblasts into a cardiac phenotype,[124] reported later by other investigators.[125] This potential conversion of the donor myoblasts into cardiomyocytes, however, was not observed by other researchers.[126] Taylor et al. were the first to publish, in 1998, evidence of myocardial performance improvements following myoblast transplantation in acutely injured hearts.[127] The authors observed that the striated muscle cells produced by the grafts in the scars were isolated from the myocardial tissue by the fibrotic tissue (thus, direct electrical interaction with the myocardium was not possible). Moreover, the muscle cells resulting from the graft "did not look as healthy as cells in the normal zone", concluding that the graft did not offer a contractile benefit, and the improvements in the cardiac function were explained by an increasing compliance in the scar.[127] In fact, the mechanisms by which myoblast transplantation improves the performance of the infarcted heart are still not elucidated, although some hypothesis were suggested.[128] The corollary of the first series of experiments was the initiation of a first phase I clinical trial by the team of Philippe Menasché in 2000,[129] which initiated a series of clinical essays in other centers.[130,131]

8.   At The Beginning of The XXI Century

Presently, the original research of myoblast transplantation as a treatment for genetic myopathies seems being overtaken by the cumulus of publications in the field of ischemic cardiomyopathies. The reason can be found in the higher incidence of cardiovascular diseases, with both the public health and economical concerns that derive from this fact. Presently, both applications are being tested in humans and the success, although promising, are still quite modest and need to be further improved. In the ischemic heart, myoblast transplantation is far from reaching the reengineering of the myocardial structure, and the functional improvements in animals and patients are more related to an improvement in the physical characteristics of the scar than from reconstitution of functional tissue. Myoblast transplantation in myopathies have demonstrated recently to be able to restore dystrophin expression in DMD patients,[21] but an efficient cell delivery to most of skeletal muscles remains a challenge, and it is not clear (as in the infarcted heart) whether this technique could restore a functional structure in muscles that have already degenerated to fibrosis and fat substitution. However, although the ultimate goal of a therapy is to restore normality in a patient suffering from a disease, any significant benefit obtained by a therapeutic tool should be useful as long as the ultimate goal has not been reached. As in other medical treatments, this would also depend on a balance between the risks and benefits of the procedure.

To reach the ultimate goal of myoblast transplantation as an optimal therapeutic tool, some aspects of the problem need to be further investigated. According to our personal experience in myoblast transplantation in skeletal muscles, we recommend to give priority to the following items:

(1) The development of efficient methods of donor-cell delivery applicable to the clinics.
(2) The development of procedures able to increase the efficiency of each single cell injection.
(3) The understanding of the early donor-cell death following transplantation.
(4) An analysis of whether myoblast transplantation can reengineer a functional structure in skeletal muscles that degenerated by fibrosis and fat substitution (or in the scar of an infarcted heart).
(5) Further analysis of whether other sources of myogenic cells (such as any kind of less differentiated multi- or pluripotent stem cells) could produce a better improvement of the heart function
(6) In the case of allotransplantation, the development of protocols to control or to avoid acute rejection with the lowest adverse effects.

9. References

1. Kao RL, Rizzo C and. Magovern GI, Satellite cell for myocardial regeneration., Physiologist 32, 220 (1989).
2. Wang JM, Zheng H, Blaivas M and Kurachi R, Persistent systemic production of human factor IX in mice by skeletal myoblast-mediated gene transfer: feasibility of repeat application to obtain therapeutic levels, Blood 90(3), 1075–1082 (1997).

3. Hamamori Y, Samal B, Tian J and Kedes L, Persistent erythropoiesis by myoblast transfer of erythropoietin cDNA, Hum. Gene Ther. 5(11), 1349–1356 (1994).

4. Dhawan J, Pan LC, Pavlath GK, Travis MA, Lanctot AM and Blau HM, Systemic delivery of human growth hormone by injection of genetically engineered myoblasts, Science 254(5037), 1509–1512 (1991).

5. Simonson GD, Groskreutz DJ, Gorman CM and MacDonald MJ, Synthesis and processing of genetically modified human proinsulin by rat myoblast primary cultures, Hum. Gene Ther. 7(1), 71–78 (1996).

6. Moisset PA, Bonham L, Skuk D, Koeberl D, Brussee V, Goulet M, Roy B, Asselin I, Miller AD and Tremblay JP, Systemic production of human granulocyte colony-stimulating factor in nonhuman primates by transplantation of genetically modified myoblasts, Hum. Gene Ther. 11(9), 1277–1288. (2000).

7. Day CS, Kasemkijwattana C, Menetrey J, Floyd Jr SS, Booth D, Moreland MS, Fu FH and Huard J, Myoblast-mediated gene transfer to the joint, J. Orthop. Res. 15(6), 894–903 (1997).

8. Deglon N, Heyd B, Tan SA, Joseph JM, Zurn AD and Aebischer P, Central nervous system delivery of recombinant ciliary neurotrophic factor by polymer encapsulated differentiated C2C12 myoblasts, Hum. Gene Ther. 7(17), 2135–2146 (1996).

9. Hofmann A and Blau HM, Death of solid tumor cells induced by Fas ligand expressing primary myoblasts, Somat. Cell Mol. Genet. 23(4), 249–257 (1997).

10. Harrison RG, Observations on the living developing nerve fiber, Proc. Soc. Exp. Biol. Med. 4, 140–143 (1907).

11. Lewis MR, Rhythmical contraction of the skeletal muscle tissue observed in tissue cultures, Am. J. Physiol. 38, 153–161 (1915).

12. Herrmann H, Konigsberg UR and Robinson G, Observations on culture in vitro of normal and dystrophic muscle tissue, Proc. Soc. Exp. Biol. Med. 105, 217–221 (1960).

13. Konigsberg IR, The differentiation of cross-striated myofibrils in short term cell culture, Exp. Cell Res. 21, 414–420 (1960).

14. Konigsberg IR, Some aspects of myogenesis in vitro, Circulation 24, 447–457 (1961).

15. Konigsberg IR, Cellular differentiation in colonies derived from single cells platings of freshly isolated chick embryo muscle cells, Proc Natl Acad Sci U S A 47, 1868–1872 (1961).

16. Yaffe D, Retention of differentiation potentialities during prolonged cultivation of myogenic cells, Proc Natl Acad Sci U S A 61(2), 477–483 (1968).

17. Yaffe D and Feldman M, The Formation of Hybrid Multinucleated Muscle Fibers from Myoblasts of Different Genetic Origin, Dev Biol 11, 300–317 (1965).

18. Yaffe D, Developmental changes preceding cell fusion during muscle differentiation in vitro, Exp Cell Res 66(1), 33–48 (1971).

19. Yaffe D and Fuchs S, Autoradiographic study of the incorporation of uridine-3H during myogenesis in tissue culture, Dev Biol 15(1), 33–50 (1967).

20. Richler C and Yaffe D, The in vitro cultivation and differentiation capacities of myogenic cell lines, Dev Biol 23(1), 1–22 (1970).

21. Skuk D, Roy B, Goulet M, Chapdelaine P, Bouchard JP, Roy R,. Dugré FJ, Lachance JG, Deschênes L, Senay H, Sylvain M and Tremblay JP, Dystrophin expression in myofibers of Duchenne muscular dystrophy patients following

intramuscular injections of normal myogenic cells., Molecular Therapy 9, 475–482 (2004).

22. Mauro A, Satellite cell of skeletal muscle fibers, J Biophys Biochem Cytol 9493–495 (1961).

23. Tamaki T, Akatsuka A, Ando K, Nakamura Y, Matsuzawa H, Hotta T, Roy R and Edgerton VR, Identification of myogenic-endothelial progenitor cells in the interstitial spaces of skeletal muscle, J. Cell Biol. 157(4), 571–577 (2002).

24. Asakura A, Seale P, Girgis-Gabardo A and Rudnicki MA, Myogenic specification of side population cells in skeletal muscle, J. Cell Biol. 159(1), 123–134 (2002).

25. Zammit PS, Heslop L, Hudon V, Rosenblatt JD, Tajbakhsh S, Buckingham ME, Beauchamp JR and Partridge TA, Kinetics of myoblast proliferation show that resident satellite cells are competent to fully regenerate skeletal muscle fibers, Exp. Cell Res. 281(1), 39–49 (2002).

26. Partridge TA, Grounds M and Sloper JC, Evidence of fusion between host and donor myoblasts in skeletal muscle grafts, Nature 273(5660), 306–308 (1978).

27. Jones PH, Implantation of cultured regenerate muscle cells into adult rat muscle, Exp. Neurol. 66(3), 602–610. (1979).

28. Lipton BH and Schultz E, Developmental fate of skeletal muscle satellite cells, Science 205(4412), 1292–1294 (1979).

29. Womble MD and Bonner PH, Developmental fate of a distinct class of chick myoblasts after transplantation of cloned cells into quail embryos, J. Embryol. Exp. Morphol. 58, 119–130 (1980).

30. Watt DJ, Morgan JE and Partridge TA, Use of mononuclear precursor cells to insert allogeneic genes into growing mouse muscles, Muscle Nerve 7(9), 741–750 (1984).

31. Watt DJ, Lambert K,. Morgan JE, Partridge TA and Sloper JC, Incorporation of donor muscle precursor cells into an area of muscle regeneration in the host mouse, J. Neurol. Sci. 57(2–3), 319–331 (1982).

32. Hoffman EP, Brown Jr RH, and Kunkel LM, Dystrophin: the protein product of the Duchenne muscular dystrophy locus, Cell 51(6), 919–928 (1987).

33. Partridge TA, Morgan Je, Coulton GR, Hoffman EP and Kunkel LM, Conversion of mdx myofibres from dystrophin-negative to -positive by injection of normal myoblasts, Nature 337(6203), 176–179 (1989).

34. Vilquin JT, Kinoshita I, Roy B, Goulet M, Engvall E, Tome F, Fardeau M and Tremblay JP Partial laminin alpha2 chain restoration in alpha2 chain-deficient dy/dy mouse by primary muscle cell culture transplantation, J. Cell Biol. 133(1), 185–197 (1996).

35. Vilquin JT, Guerette B, Puymirat J, Yaffe D, Tome FM, Fardeau M, Fiszman M, Schwartz K and Tremblay JP, Myoblast transplantations lead to the expression of the laminin alpha 2 chain in normal and dystrophic (dy/dy) mouse muscles, Gene Ther. 6(5), 792–800 (1999).

36. Leriche-Gueri K, Anderson LV, Wrogemann K, Roy B, Goulet M and Tremblay JP, Dysferlin expression after normal myoblast transplantation in SCID and in SJL mice, Neuromuscul. Disord. 12(2), 167–173. (2002).

37. Gussoni E, Pavlath GK, Lanctot AM, Sharma KR, Miller RG, Steinman L and Blau HM, Normal dystrophin transcripts detected in Duchenne muscular dystrophy patients after myoblast transplantation, Nature 356(6368), 435–438 (1992).

38. Huard J, Bouchard JP, Roy R, Malouin F, Dansereau G, Labrecque C, Albert N, Richards CL, Lemieux B and Tremblay JP, Human myoblast transplantation: preliminary results of 4 cases, Muscle Nerve 15(5), 550–560 (1992).

39. Huard J, Bouchard JP, Roy R, Labrecque C, Dansereau G, Lemieux B and Tremblay JP, Myoblast transplantation produced dystrophin-positive muscle fibres in a 16-year-old patient with Duchenne muscular dystrophy, Clin. Sci. (Colch.) 81(2), 287–288 (1991).
40. Tremblay JP, Bouchard JP, Malouin F, Theau D, Cottrell F, Collin H, Rouche A, Gilgenkrantz S, Abbadi N, Tremblay M and et al., Myoblast transplantation between monozygotic twin girl carriers of Duchenne muscular dystrophy, Neuromuscul. Disord. 3(5–6), 583–592 (1993).
41. Tremblay JP, Malouin F, Roy R, Huard J, Bouchard JP, Satoh A and Richards CL, Results of a triple blind clinical study of myoblast transplantations without immunosuppressive treatment in young boys with Duchenne muscular dystrophy, Cell Transplant. 2(2), 99–112 (1993).
42. Karpati G, Ajdukovic D, Arnold D, Gledhill RB, Guttman R, Holland P, Koch PA, Shoubridge E, Spence D, Vanasse M, Watters GV, Abrahamowicz M, Duff C and Worton RG, Myoblast transfer in Duchenne muscular dystrophy, Ann. Neurol. 34, 8–17 (1993).
43. Karpati G, Johnston W, Ajdukovic G, Arnold D, Vanasse M, Guttmann R, Crerar M, Carpenter S and Shoubridge E, Myoblast transfer (MT) in McArdle's disease (McD), Neurology 42 (Suppl 3), 387 (1992).
44. Mendell JR, Kissel JT, Amato AA, King W, Signore L, Prior TW, Sahenk Z, Benson S, McAndrew PE, Rice R, Nagaraja H, Stephens R, Lantry L, Morris GE and Burghes AHM, Myoblast transfer in the treatment of Duchenne's muscular dystrophy, N. Engl. J. Med. 333, 832–838 (1995).
45. Miller RG, Sharma KR, Pavlath GK, Gussoni E, Mynhier M, Lanctot AM, Greco CM, Steinman L and Blau HM, Myoblast implantation in Duchenne muscular dystrophy: the San Francisco study, Muscle Nerve 20(4), 469–478 (1997).
46. Neumeyer AM, Cros D, McKenna-Yasek D, Zawadzka A, Hoffman EP, Pegoraro E, Hunter RG, Munsat TL and Brown Jr RH, Pilot study of myoblast transfer in the treatment of Becker muscular dystrophy, Neurology 51(2), 589–592 (1998).
47. Thompson L, Researchers call for time out on cell-transplant research, Science 257(5071), 738 (1992).
48. Alameddine HS, Louboutin JP, Dehaupas M, Sebille A and Fardeau M, Functional recovery induced by satellite cell grafts in irreversibly injured muscles, Cell Transplant. 3(1), 3–14 (1994).
49. Wernig A, Zweyer M and Irintchev A, Function of skeletal muscle tissue formed after myoblast transplantation into irradiated mouse muscles, J. Physiol. (Lond.) 522(Pt 2), 333–345 (2000).
50. Wernig A, Irintchev A and Lange G, Functional effects of myoblast implantation into histoincompatible mice with or without immunosuppression, J. Physiol. (Lond.) 484(Pt 2), 493–504 (1995).
51. Irintchev A, Langer M, Zweyer M, Theisen R and Wernig A, Functional improvement of damaged adult mouse muscle by implantation of primary myoblasts, J. Physiol. (Lond.) 500(Pt 3), 775–785 (1997).
52. Arcila ME, Ameredes BT, DeRosimo JF, Washabaugh CH, Yang J, Johnson PC and Ontell M, Mass and functional capacity of regenerating muscle is enhanced by myoblast transfer, J. Neurobiol. 33(2), 185–198 (1997).
53. Yao SN and Kurachi K, Implanted myoblasts not only fuse with myofibers but also survive as muscle precursor cells, J. Cell Sci. 105(Pt 4), 957–963 (1993).

54. Gross JG and Morgan JE, Muscle precursor cells injected into irradiated mdx mouse muscle persist after serial injury, Muscle Nerve 22(2), 174–185 (1999).

55. Heslop L, Beauchamp JR, Tajbakhsh S, Buckingham ME, Partridge TA and Zammit PS, Transplanted primary neonatal myoblasts can give rise to functional satellite cells as identified using the Myf5(nlacZl+) mouse, Gene Ther. 8(10), 778–783 (2001).

56. Huard J, Verreault S, Roy R, Tremblay M and Tremblay JP, High efficiency of muscle regeneration after human myoblast clone transplantation in SCID mice, J. Clin. Invest. 93(2), 586–599 (1994).

57. Kinoshita I, Vilquin JT, Guerette B, Asselin I, Roy R and Tremblay JP, Very efficient myoblast allotransplantation in mice under FK506 immunosuppression, Muscle Nerve 17(12), 1407–1415 (1994).

58. Vilquin JT, Asselin I, Guerette B, Kinoshita I, Roy R and Tremblay JP, Successful myoblast allotransplantation in mdx mice using rapamycin, Transplantation 59(3), 422–426 (1995).

59. Cantini M, Massimino ML, Catani C, Rizzuto R, Brini M and Carraro U, Gene transfer into satellite cell from regenerating muscle: bupivacaine allows beta-Gal transfection and expression in vitro and in vivo, In Vitro Cell Dev. Biol. Anim. 30A(2), 131–133 (1994).

60. Pin CL and Merrifield PA, Developmental potential of rat L6 myoblasts in vivo following injection into regenerating muscles, Dev. Biol. 188(1), 147–166 (1997).

61. Morgan JE, Hoffman EP and. Partridge TA, Normal myogenic cells from newborn mice restore normal histology to degenerating muscles of the mdx mouse, J Cell Biol 111(6 Pt 1), 2437–2449 (1990).

62. Wernig A and Irintchev A, "Bystander" damage of host muscle caused by implantation of MHC-compatible myogenic cells, J. Neurol. Sci. 130(2), 190–196 (1995).

63. Partridge TA, Invited review: myoblast transfer: a possible therapy for inherited myopathies?, Muscle Nerve 14(3), 197–212 (1991).

64. Neumeyer AM, DiGregorio DM and Brown Jr RH, Arterial delivery of myoblasts to skeletal muscle, Neurology 42(12), 2258–2262 (1992).

65. Torrente Y, Tremblay JP, Pisati F, Belicchi M, Rossi B, Sironi M, Fortunato F, El Fahime M, Grazia D'Angelo MG, Caron NJ, Constantin G, Paulin D, Scarlato G and Bresolin N, Intraarterial Injection of Muscle-derived CD34+Sca-1+ Stem Cells Restores Dystrophin in mdx Mice, J. Cell. Biol. 152(2), 335–348 (2001).

66. Beauchamp JR, Morgan JE, Pagel CN and Partridge TA, Quantitative studies of efficacy of myoblast transplantation, Muscle Nerve 4(Suppl.), S261 (1994).

67. Huard J, Acsadi G, Jani A, Massie B and Karpati G, Gene transfer into skeletal muscles by isogenic myoblasts, Hum. Gene Ther. 5(8), 949–958 (1994).

68. Smythe GM, Hodgetts SI and Grounds MD, Immunobiology and the future of myoblast transfer therapy, Mol. Ther. 1(4), 304–313 (2000).

69. Tremblay JP and Guérette B, Myoblast transplantation: a brief review of the problems and of some solutions, Basic Appl. Myol. 7 (1997).

70. Beauchamp JR, Morgan JE, Pagel CN and Partridge TA, Dynamics of myoblast transplantation reveal a discrete minority of precursors with stem cell-like properties as the myogenic source, J. Cell. Biol. 144(6), 1113–1122 (1999).

71. Guerette B, Asselin I, Skuk D, Entman M and Tremblay JP, Control of inflammatory damage by anti-LFA-1: increase success of myoblast transplantation, Cell Transplant. 6(2), 101–107 (1997).

72. Guerette B, Skuk D, Celestin F, Huard C, Tardif F, Asselin I, Roy B, Goulet M, Roy R, Entman M and Tremblay JP, Prevention by anti-LFA-1 of acute myoblast death following transplantation, J. Immunol. 159(5), 2522–2531 (1997).

73. Merly F, Huard C, Asselin I, Robbins PD and Tremblay JP, Anti-inflammatory effect of transforming growth factor-beta1 in myoblast transplantation, Transplantation 65(6), 793–799 (1998).

74. Qu Z, Balkir L, van Deutekom JC, Robbins PD, Pruchnic R and Huard J, Development of approaches to improve cell survival in myoblast transfer therapy, J. Cell Biol. 142(5), 1257–1267 (1998).

75. Sammels LM, Bosio E, Fragall CT, Grounds MD, van Rooijen N and Beilharz MW, Innate inflammatory cells are not responsible for early death of donor myoblasts after myoblast transfer therapy, Transplantation 77(12), 1790–1797 (2004).

76. Rando TA, Pavlath GK and Blau HM, The fate of myoblasts following transplantation into mature muscle, Exp. Cell Res. 220(2), 383–389 (1995).

77. Ponder BA, Wilkinson MM, Wood M and Westwood JH, Immunohistochemical demonstration of H2 antigens in mouse tissue sections, J. Histochem. Cytochem. 31(7), 911–919 (1983).

78. Appleyard ST, Dunn MJ, Dubowitz V and Rose ML, Increased expression of HLA ABC class I antigens by muscle fibres in Duchenne muscular dystrophy, inflammatory myopathy, and other neuromuscular disorders, Lancet 1(8425), 361–363 (1985).

79. Karpat G, Pouliot Y and Carpenter S, Expression of immunoreactive major histocompatibility complex products in human skeletal muscles, Ann. Neurol. 23(1), 64–72 (1988).

80. Emslie-Smith AM, Arahata K and Engel AG, Major histocompatibility complex class I antigen expression, immunolocalization of interferon subtypes, and T cell-mediated cytotoxicity in myopathies, Hum. Pathol. 20(3), 224–231 (1989).

81. Mantegazza R, Hughes SM, Mitchell D, Travis M, Blau HM and Steinman L, Modulation of MHC class II antigen expression in human myoblasts after treatment with IFN-gamma, Neurology 41(7), 1128–1132 (1991).

82. Cifuentes-Diaz C, Delaporte C, Dautreaux B, Charron D and Fardeau M, Class II MHC antigens in normal human skeletal muscle, Muscle Nerve 15(3), 295–302 (1992).

83. Michaelis D, Goebels N and Hohlfeld R, Constitutive and cytokine-induced expression of human leukocyte antigens and cell adhesion molecules by human myotubes, Am. J. Pathol. 143(4), 1142–1149 (1993).

84. Goebels N, Michaelis D, Wekerle H and Hohlfeld R, Human myoblasts as antigen-presenting cells, J. Immunol. 149(2), 661–667. (1992).

85. Hohlfeld R and Engel AG, Induction of HLA-DR expression on human myoblasts with interferon-gamma, Am. J. Pathol. 136(3), 503–508. (1990).

86. Roy R, Dansereau G, Tremblay JP, Belles-Isles M, Huard J, Labrecque C and Bouchard JP, Expression of major histocompatibility complex antigens on human myoblasts, Transplant. Proc. 23(1 Pt 1), 799–801. (1991).

87. Bao S, dos Remedios CG and King NJ, Ontogeny of major histocompatibility complex antigen expression on cultured human embryonic skeletal myoblasts, Transplantation 58(5), 585–591. (1994).

88. Curnow SJ, Willcox N and Vincent A, Induction of primary immune responses by allogeneic human myoblasts: dissection of the cell types required for proliferation, IFNgamma secretion and cytotoxicity, J. Neuroimmunol. 86(1), 53–62 (1998).

89. Hardiman O, Faustman D, Li X, Sklar RM and Brown Jr RH, Expression of major histocompatibility complex antigens in cultures of clonally derived human myoblasts, Neurology 43(3 Pt 1), 604–608 (1993).

90. Behrens L, Kerschensteiner M, Misgeld T, Goebels N, Wekerle H and Hohlfeld R, Human muscle cells express a functional costimulatory molecule distinct from B7.1 (CD80) and B7.2 (CD86) in vitro and in inflammatory lesions, J. Immunol. 161(11), 5943–5951 (1998).

91. Watt DJ, Morgan JE and Partridge TA, Long term survival of allografted muscle precursor cells following a limited period of treatment with cyclosporin A, Clin Exp Immunol 55(2), 419–426 (1984).

92. Guerette B, Asselin I, Vilquin JT, Roy R and Tremblay JP, Lymphocyte infiltration following allo- and xenomyoblast transplantation in mdx mice, Muscle Nerve 18(1), 39–51 (1995).

93. Irintchev A, Zweyer M and Wernig A, Cellular and molecular reactions in mouse muscles after myoblast implantation, J. Neurocytol. 24(4), 319–331 (1995).

94. Guerette B, Roy R, Tremblay M, Asselin I, Kinoshita I, Puymirat J and Tremblay JP, Increased granzyme B mRNA after alloincompatible myoblast transplantation, Transplantation 60(9), 1011–1016 (1995).

95. Guerette B, Tremblay G, Vilquin JT, Asselin I, Gingras M, Roy R and Tremblay JP, Increased interferon-gamma mRNA expression following alloincompatible myoblast transplantation is inhibited by FK506, Muscle Nerve 19(7), 829–835 (1996).

96. Ito H, Vilquin JT, Skuk D, Roy B, Goulet M, Lille S, Dugre FJ, Asselin I, Roy R, Fardeau M and Tremblay JP, Myoblast transplantation in non-dystrophic dog, Neuromuscul. Disord. 8(2), 95–110 (1998).

97. Kinoshita I, Roy R, Dugre FJ, Gravel C, Roy B, Goulet M, Asselin I and Trembla JP, Myoblast transplantation in monkeys: control of immune response by FK506, J. Neuropathol. Exp. Neurol. 55(6), 687–697 (1996).

98. Skuk D, Roy B, Goulet M and Trembla JP, Successful myoblast transplantation in primates depends on appropriate cell delivery and induction of regeneration in the host muscle, Exp. Neurol. 155(1), 22–30 (1999).

99. Skuk D, Goulet M, Roy B and Trembla JP, Efficacy of myoblast transplantation in nonhuman primates following simple intramuscular cell injections: toward defining strategies applicable to humans, Exp. Neurol. 175(1), 112–126. (2002).

100. Vilquin JT, Asselin I, Guerette B, Kinoshita I, Lille S, Roy R and Tremblay JP, Myoblast allotransplantation in mice: degree of success varies depending on the efficacy of various immunosuppressive treatments, Transplant. Proc. 26(6), 3372–3373 (1994).

101. Vilqui JT, Kinoshita I, Roy R and Tremblay JP, Cyclophosphamide immunosuppression does not permit successful myoblast allotransplantation in mouse, Neuromuscul. Disord. 5(6), 511–517 (1995).

102. Pavlath GK, Rando TA and Blau HM, Transient immunosuppressive treatment leads to long-term retention of allogeneic myoblasts in hybrid myofibers, J. Cell Biol. 127(6 Pt 2), 1923–1932 (1994).

103. Asselin I, Tremblay M, Vilquin JT, Guerette B, Roy R and Tremblay, JP, Quantification of normal dystrophin mRNA following myoblast transplantation in mdx mice, Muscle Nerve 18(9), 980–986 (1995).

104. Hardiman O, Sklar RM and Brown Jr RH, Direct effects of cyclosporin A and cyclophosphamide on differentiation of normal human myoblasts in culture, Neurology 43(7), 1432–1434 (1993).

105. Hong F, Lee J, Song JW, Lee SJ, Ahn H, Cho JJ, Ha J and Kim SS, Cyclosporin A blocks muscle differentiation by inducing oxidative stress and inhibiting the peptidyl-prolyl-cis-trans isomerase activity of cyclophilin A: cyclophilin A protects myoblasts from cyclosporin A-induced cytotoxicity, Faseb J. 16(12), 1633–1635 (2002).

106. Camirand G, Caron NJ, Asselin I and Tremblay JP, Combined immunosuppression of mycophenolate mofetil and FK506 for myoblast transplantation in mdx mice, Transplantation 72(1), 38–44. (2001).

107. Kinoshita I, Vilquin JT, Gravel C, Roy R and Tremblay JP, Myoblast allotransplantation in primates, Muscle Nerve 18(10), 1217–1218 (1995).

108. Skuk D, Goulet M, Roy B and Tremblay JP, Myoblast transplantation in whole muscle of nonhuman primates, J. Neuropathol. Exp. Neurol. 59(3), 197–206 (2000).

109. Camirand G, Caron NJ, Turgeon NA, Rossini AA and Tremblay JP, Treatment with anti-CD154 antibody and donor-specific transfusion prevents acute rejection of myoblast transplantation, Transplantation 73(3), 453–461. (2002).

110. Camirand G, Rousseau J, Ducharme ME, Rothstein DM and Tremblay JP, Novel Duchenne Muscular Dystrophy Treatment Through Myoblast Transplantation Tolerance with Anti-CD45RB, Anti-CD154 and Mixed Chimerism, Am. J. Transplant. 4(8), 1255–1265 (2004).

111. Floyd Jr SS, Clemens PR, Ontell MR, Kochanek S, Day CS, Yang J, Hauschka SD, Balkir L, Morgan J, Moreland MS, Feero GW, Epperly M and Huard J, Ex vivo gene transfer using adenovirus-mediated full-length dystrophin delivery to dystrophic muscles, Gene Ther. 5(1), 19–30 (1998).

112. Moisset PA, Gagnon Y, Karpati G and Tremblay JP, Expression of human dystrophin following the transplantation of genetically modified mdx myoblasts, Gene Ther. 5(10), 1340–1346 (1998).

113. Bujold M, Caron N, Camiran G, Mukherjee S, Allen PD, Tremblay JP and Wang Y, Autotransplantation in mdx mice of mdx myoblasts genetically corrected by an HSV-1 amplicon vector, Cell Transplant. 11(8), 759–767 (2002).

114. Moisset PA, Skuk D, Asselin I, Goulet M, Roy B, Karpati G and Tremblay JP, Successful transplantation of genetically corrected DMD myoblasts following ex vivo transduction with the dystrophin minigene, Biochem. Biophys. Res. Commun. 247(1), 94–99 (1998).

115. Slierendregt BL, van Noort JT, Bakas RM, Otting N, Jonker M and Bontrop RE, Evolutionary stability of transspecies major histocompatibility complex class II DRB lineages in humans and rhesus monkeys, Hum. Immunol. 35(1), 29–39. (1992).

116. Geluk A, Elferink DG, Slierendreg BL, van Meijgaarden KE,. de Vries RR, Ottenhoff TH and Bontrop RE, Evolutionary conservation of major histocompatibility complex-DR/peptide/T cell interactions in primates, J. Exp. Med. 177(4), 979–987 (1993).

117. Jaeger EE, Bontrop RE and Lanchbury JS, Structure, diversity, and evolution of the T-cell receptor VB gene repertoire in primates, Immunogenetics 40(3), 184–191 (1994).

118. Levinson G, Hughes AL and Letvin NL, Sequence and diversity of rhesus monkey T-cell receptor beta chain genes, Immunogenetics 35(2), 75–88 (1992).

119. Borisov AB, Regeneration of skeletal and cardiac muscle in mammals: do non-primate models resemble human pathology?, Wound Repair Regen. 7(1), 26–35 (1999).

120. Qu Z and Huard J, Matching host muscle and donor myoblasts for myosin heavy chain improves myoblast transfer therapy, Gene Ther. 7(5), 428–437 (2000).
121. Bonavaud S, Agbulut O, Nizard R, D'Honneur G, Mouly V and Butler-Browne G, A discrepancy resolved: human satellite cells are not preprogrammed to fast and slow lineages, Neuromuscul. Disord. 11(8), 747–752 (2001).
122. Kao RL, Regeneration of injured myocardium from implanted satellite cells., Circulation 84(Suppl. II), 386 (1991).
123. Marelli D, Desrosiers C, el-Alfy M, Kao RL and Chiu RC, Cell transplantation for myocardial repair: an experimental approach, Cell Transplant. 1(6), 383–390 (1992).
124. Kessler PD and Byrne BJ, Myoblast cell grafting into heart muscle: cellular biology and potential applications, Annu. Rev. Physiol. 61, 219–242 (1999).
125. Yoon PD, Kao RL and Magovern GJ, Myocardial regeneration. Transplanting satellite cells into damaged myocardium, Tex. Heart Inst. J. 22(2), 119–125 (1995).
126. Murry CE, Wiseman RW, Schwartz SM and Hauschka SD, Skeletal myoblast transplantation for repair of myocardial necrosis, J. Clin. Invest. 98(11), 2512–2523 (1996).
127. Taylor DA, Atkins BZ, Hungspreugs P, Jones TR, Reedy MC, Hutcheson KA, Glower DD and Kraus WE, Regenerating functional myocardium: improved performance after skeletal myoblast transplantation, Nat. Med. 4(8), 929–933 (1998).
128. Menasche P, Skeletal muscle satellite cell transplantation, Cardiovasc. Res. 58(2), 351–357 (2003).
129. Menasche P, Hageg AA, Scorsin M, Pouzet B, Desnos M, Duboc D, Schwartz K, Vilquin JT and Marolleau JP, Myoblast transplantation for heart failure, Lancet 357(9252), 279–280 (2001).
130. Siminiak T, Fiszer D, Jerzykowska O, Grygielska B, Kalmucki P and Kurpisz M, Percutaneous autologous myoblast transplantation in the treatment of post-infarction myocardial contractility impairment–report on two cases, Kardiol. Pol. 59(12), 492–501 (2003).
131. Herreros J, Prosper F, Perez A, Gavira JJ, Garcia-Velloso MJ, Barba J, Sanchez PL, Canizo C, Rabago G,. Marti-Climent JM, Hernandez M, Lopez-Holgado N, Gonzalez-Santos JM, Martin-Luengo C and Alegria E, Autologous intramyocardial injection of cultured skeletal muscle-derived stem cells in patients with non-acute myocardial infarction, Eur. Heart J. 24(22), 2012–2020 (2003).

5
Myoblast Cell Transplantation: Preclinical Studies

HARALD C. OTT AND DORIS A. TAYLOR*

1. Introduction

The theory behind cell therapy, the concept of organ repair by substitution of its functional components, is centuries old. Phillippus Aureolus Paracelsus (1493-1541), a German-Swiss physician and alchemist wrote in his *Der grossen Wundartzney* ("Great Surgery Book") in 1536 that "the heart heals the heart, lung heals the lung, spleen heals the spleen; like cures like." However, the way from basic research to clinical application was several centuries long and held insurmountable hurdles until less than 50 years ago. In 1958 the cornerstone for successful cell therapy was finally laid by Jean Dausset by describing the first of many human leukocyte antigens (HLA). Ten years later the first successful bone marrow transplant took place at the University of Minnesota. The recipient was a child with severe combined immunodeficiency disease and the donor was a sibling.

Over 20 years later, the concept of cell transplantation expanded into the field of cardiovascular medicine. The need for new therapeutic options developed with a newly evolving patient collective. Thanks to broader access to better medical therapies, a growing population of patients began surviving the acute event of myocardial infarction. However, an increasing number of these patients also suffered from decreased organ function as a consequence of ischemic damage. Thus it became obvious that, in most cases, the adult heart had insufficient potential for effective endogenous repair. Instead, the damaged myocardium eventually progressed through a cascade of events including inflammation, cardiocyte apoptosis, fibrous scar formation, alteration in the workload of the surviving myocardium, and, if the infarct was large enough, ultimately decompensation and deterioration to heart failure (HF). The tantalizing goal of treating the underlying pathology causing this

---

*Medtronic Bakken Professor, Director, Center for Cardiovascular Repair, Departments of Physiology and Medicine, University of Minnesota, 312 Church St. SE, Minneapolis MN 55455

detrimental cascade, the loss of cardiomyocytes, was the initial impulse for the development of cell therapy concepts. Potential regeneration of viable tissue opened new vistas, at least in theory, for the treatment of ischemic heart diseases and chronic heart failure.

2.   Skeletal Myoblasts–A Pioneer in Cell Therapy

The idea of using skeletal muscle to support the injured heart evolved before the introduction of cell therapy into this field. As early as 1987, the latissimus dorsi muscle, after being preconditioned by chronic pacing, was surgically wrapped around the failing heart to provide contractile support to the left ventricle, a procedure described as dynamic cardiomyoplasty.[1] Within a few years, cardiomyoplasty was introduced on a cellular level when the C2C12 skeletal myoblast cell line was first successfully transplanted into healthy mouse hearts.[2]

These myoblasts were derived from muscle "satellite cells," first described in 1961 as cells that regenerate damaged skeletal muscle.[3] These skeletal myoblasts (SKM) expand and form neofibres after muscle injury. Thus, it is not surprising that they were the first candidates for cardiac repair. In 1994, the first successful experimental transplantation of skeletal myoblasts into injured dog hearts was reported.[4] The promising finding that transplanted skeletal myoblasts survived and formed striated grafts within the hostile damaged cardiac tissue was followed by a number of experimental studies investigating the regenerative potential of these cells. Yet, it was not until the report that the successful engraftment of SKM into injured myocardium improved left ventricular contractile performance and attenuated left ventricular remodeling[5] that the field exploded (see table 1 for overview). How these successfully engrafted skeletal myoblasts improved function was unclear. It appeared that the muscle cells could improve contractility of the previously scarred heart without transdifferentiating into cardiomyocytes. Instead, skeletal myoblasts appeared to adapt to the surrounding myocardium by forming slow twitch myofibers that appeared electrically isolated from host cardiomyocytes (Figure 1).[6] At the same time however, these cells appeared to recruit non-transplanted cells to the infarct.[7] These results, showing an improvement in cardiac function without full integration of transplanted cells into host myocardium, and with recruitment of endogenous cells, raised questions about potential mechanisms that underlie the functional benefit. Numerous mechanisms have been suggested, ranging from passive changes in wall stress and cardiac geometry to active contraction of the injected cells, but the exact mechanism(s) underlying the beneficial effect are still debated. It is likely that the benefits involve both a direct effect of the transplanted muscle cells on performance and an indirect "paracrine" effect that likely includes an endogenous cell recruitment component.

TABLE 1. Early experimental studies on cardiac skeletal myoblast transplantation, 1993-2001

Study	Species	Model	Cell type	Outcome
Koh et al. J Clin Invest. 1993;92:1548-54[2]	Mouse	Uninjured heart	C2C12 myoblasts	Differentiated multinucleated myofibers, no arrhythmias, no coupling to host.
Zibaitis et al. Transplant Proc. 1994;26:3294[4]	Dog	Cryoinjury	Autologous skeletal myoblasts	Intercalated discs, skeletal muscle, mosaic cardioskeletal fibers.
Chiu et al. Ann Thorac Surg. 1995;60:12-8[8]	Dog	Cryoinjury	Autologous skeletal myoblasts	Histology: striated muscle grafts (differentiation into cardiac cells? central nuclei).
Murry et al. J Clin Invest. 1996;98:2512-23[6]	Rat	Cryoinjury	Neonatal skeletal myoblasts	No coupling to graft but conversion to β-MHC mature myofibers after 2-7w (slow twitch fibers, cardiac cell-like).
Robinson et al. Cell Transplant 1996; 5: 77[9]	Mouse	Uninjured heart	C2C12 myoblasts	Fast twitch to slow twitch/ cardiac protein (phospholamban) after 4 months, gap junctions (Connexin43) to host cardiocytes.
Taylor et al. Proc Assoc Am Physicians. 1997;109:245-53[10]	Rabbit	Uninjured heart	Autologous skeletal myoblasts	Integration into cardiac environment, lymphocyte infiltration with injection.
Dorfman et al. J Thorac Cardiovasc Surg. 1998;116:744-51[11]	Rat	Uninjured heart	Adult skeletal myoblasts	Four of 24 rats are successfully transplanted.
Taylor et al. Nat Med. 1998;4:929-33[5]	Rabbit	Cryoinjury	Autologous skeletal myoblasts	In 7/12 functional improvement, combined features of skeletal (myogenin pos.) and cardiac cells (mononucleated, gap junctions).
Atkins et al. Ann Thorac Surg. 1999;67:124[13]	Rabbit	Cryoinjury	Autologous skeletal myoblasts	Thirteen of 18 engraftment pos. Two cell types: central multinucleated cells, peripheral immature cardiocytes. Myotubes are surrounded by scar.
Atkins et al. J Surg Res. 1999;85:234-42[12]	Rabbit	Cryoinjury	Autologous skeletal myoblasts	Nine of 15 engraftment pos. Diastolic improvement in all 9 hearts.
Atkins et al. 1999;18:1173-80[7]	Rabbit	Cryoinjury	Autologous skeletal myoblasts	No coupling to cardiac cells. Systolic improvement in 3 hearts with greater engraftment. Diastolic in all.
Reinecke et al. J CellBiol 2000; 149:731-40[14]	Rat	Cryoinjury	Neonatal skeletal myoblasts	Myoblasts express N-cadherin/Cx43, functionally active junction between cardiac & myocytes.

(*Continues*)

TABLE 1. *Continued*

Study	Species	Model	Cell type	Outcome
Hutcheson et al. *Cell Transplant.* 2000;9:359-68[15]	Rabbit	Cryoinjury	Autologous skeletal myoblasts, dermal fibroblasts	SKM improved systolic performance; fibroblasts improved only diastolic function.
Scorsin et al. J Thorac Cardiovasc Surg. 2000; 119:1169-75[16]	Rat	LAD ligation	Neonatal skeletal myoblasts, fetal cardiomy-ocytes	Multinucleated myotubes embr. MHC pos, no Connexin43. EF increases SKM > cardiomyocyte transplantation.
Pouzet et al. Circulation. 2000; 102:III210-5[17]	Rat	LAD ligation	Autologous skeletal myoblasts	Engraftment, but no Connexin43. Functional improvement.
Suzuki et al. Circulation. 2000; 102:III216-21[18]	Rat	Uninjured trans-planted hearts	Skeletal myoblasts	Multinucleated myotubes and myoblasts.
Suzuki et al. Circulation. 2000; 102:III359-64[19]	Rat	Uninjured trans-planted hearts	Skeletal myoblasts	Cx43 between myotubes and cardiac cells. No arrhythmogenicity.
Pouzet et al. Circulation. 2001;104:I223-8[20]	Rat	LAD ligation	Autologous skeletal myoblasts	Engraftment, but no Connexin43. Combination of ACE-Inhibitor SKM
Pouzet et al. Ann Thorac Surg. 2001;71:844-50[21]	Rat	LAD ligation	Autologous skeletal myoblasts	Engraftment; Bubivacain increases cell harvest by 20x.
Rajnoch et al. J Thorac Cardiovasc Surg. 2001; 121:871-8.[22]	Sheep	Cardiotoxin	Autologous skeletal myoblasts	Fast MHC myotubes in 3 of 6 sheep. Increase in local and global EF.
Suzuki et al. J Thorac Cardiovasc Surg. 2001;122:759-66[23]	Rat	Uninjured trans-planted hearts	Skeletal myoblasts Cx43 c DNA trans-fection	Cell culture, dye transfer, GJIC and myogenic differentiation increased, proliferation decreased.
Suzuki et al. Circulation. 2001;104:I213-7[24]	Rat	Doxo rubicin CMP in trans-planted hearts	Skeletal myoblasts	Multinucleated myotubes throughout the heart. Improved function.
Suzuki et al. Circulation. 2001;104:I207-12[25]	Rat	LAD ligation	Skeletal myoblasts, VEGF transfected	Reduction of infarct size and increased angiogenesis. Improved function
Jain et al. Circulation 2001;103:1920-7[26]	Rat	LAD ligation	Skeletal myoblasts	Skeletal MHC myotubes in 13 of 14. Exercise capacity increased

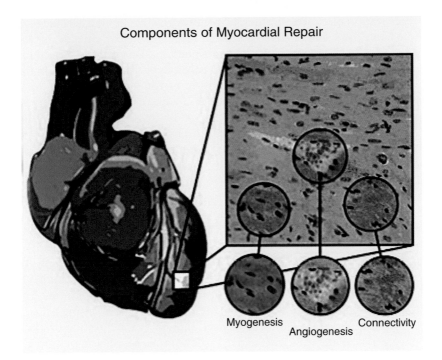

FIGURE 1. Cellular components of myocardial repair

Despite the remaining questions, approximately 15 years of preclinical data have shown that autologous skeletal myoblast transplantation can augment both diastolic and systolic myocardial performance in a number of animal species after both acute and chronic injury. These preclinical data opened the field of cardiovascular disease to this new therapeutic approach, showing that the centuries old idea of organ repair may soon become clinical reality.

3.   Skeletal Myoblasts – Current Role in Cardiac Cell Therapy

Preclinical studies laid a strong foundation for the potential role of autologous skeletal myoblasts in the treatment of patients suffering from ischemic heart disease. In addition, the use of autologous cells offered several practical benefits. By using self-derived (autologous) skeletal myoblasts it is possible to overcome the major limitations associated with allogeneic cell-based treatments: a shortage of donor tissue, the need for immunosuppression and the ethical dilemma associated with the use of allogeneic or even embryonic stem cells. By using primary cells rather than immortalized or totipotent stem cells, the likelihood of tumor formation[27] after cell transplantation is decreased. By using muscle-forming, myogenic (versus non-myogenic) cells, the regeneration of contractile muscle in a previously infarcted cardiac region is more likely. By using relatively ischemia-resistant skeletal myoblasts rather than cardiocytes, a higher level of engraftment and survival can be obtained in infarcted regions – where transplanted cardiocytes perish.[28] Based on these results and the suggestions that regeneration of functional muscle in infarct is possible after myoblast transplantation, clinical studies have begun both in Europe and in the United States.

Although the preclinical and initial clinical data appear encouraging, myoblast transplantation is not without potential limitations. The first limitation is that the use of autologous cells necessitates sufficient time between injury and injection to allow cell expansion *in vitro*. In normal healthy donors and many heart failure patients, this is a two to three week period which does not seem problematic if treatment is not emergent. In the case of acute MI where early treatment may be supposed to be beneficial, either alternative cells can be chosen, or if myoblasts are truly superior, allogeneic cells may ultimately offer a solution. Of note, the 2-3 week period after acute myocardial injury is one of heightened inflammation, which in preclinical studies has been associated with increased loss of cells after transplantation. Thus, delayed autologous delivery could be beneficial even in this setting.

A second potential limitation to any cell therapy is the question of electrical integration of the cells with native myocardium. Myoblasts are the most well studied cell type, yet it is not clear if, and how, myoblasts electrically integrate into surrounding myocardium. Nor is it completely clear what impact integration may have on either function or rhythmicity. Menasche and colleagues report no electrical integration of myoblasts preclinically; yet, early clinical data suggest that myoblast transplantation may be associated with a transient period of electrical instability within the first weeks after cell transplantation. However, the treated patient population (MADIT population) is known to be highly susceptible to arrhythmia, and it remains to be seen whether the recorded events reflect a cell-associated event (e.g. cell integration, differentiation or even death) or some other phenomenon related to the patient population or the injection itself. Our group has shown preliminarily that direct injection of cells into the center of an infarct decreases electrical instability when compared with injection into the peri-infarct zone or both regions; yet in the early clinical studies the peri-infarct and infarct zones were both major therapeutic targets, which could have influenced outcome. In more recent results, the prevalence of arrhythmia in treated patients is significantly lower than in initial studies,[29] which may reflect the administration of low dose anti-arrhythmic agents during the susceptible period[30] or the use of human serum for skeletal myoblast culture[29] in the later studies.

Even though myoblast transplantation is the most well-defined technique for myocardial regeneration, other important questions remain – questions that will need to be answered for any cellular cardiomyoplasty technique. Again, these questions primarily revolve around long term safety and efficacy. For example, if cellular cardiomyoplasty is to be viewed as a long-term solution to myocardial injury, cells must be able to mediate a positive functional effect for years in heart; yet the long-term fate of skeletal myoblasts, or any transplanted cell, is untested.

4.   Skeletal Myoblasts – Still the Best Choice?

The field of cellular cardiomyoplasty, as with many other promising approaches, has moved from bench to bedside extremely rapidly, and with it many questions have arisen. Probably the most prevalent question is the choice of cell type, which currently seems to have very little basis in science and seems to depend more on investigator access or preference. Yet, considering that patients suffering from heart disease are a heterogeneous population, the choice of cell type may ultimately matter greatly and may differ depending upon the injury to be treated. In conditions where chronic ischemia prevails, or where reperfusion is the primary objective, the angiogenic potential of non-myogenic bone marrow derived cells may be of high priority. Under these conditions, bone marrow mononuclear cells,[31] endothelial or vascular progenitor cells from bone marrow or blood,[32] marrow angioblasts[33] or blood-derived multi-potent adult progenitor cells[36] may be useful. However, in patients where restoration of contractile function is the clinical goal, such as those with end-stage ischemic heart failure or those at early times post infarction when blood flow has been restored but cardiocytes have died, then delivering cells with contractile potential seems a more reasonable approach. Under these conditions, myoblasts appear the logical first choice, although cardiac stem cells or other mesenchymal progenitors driven down a muscle lineage may also be of use. However, ultimate proof of any cell superiority will require side by side comparisons of cells in similar disease states.

Recently, several preclinical studies have been performed to compare the beneficial effects of different cell types for cellular cardiomyoplasty (see Table 2).

According to these, skeletal myoblast transplantation is more effective than transplantation of adult cardiomyocytes and dermal or cardiac fibroblasts.[15,37] This presumably reflects the greater survival of myoblasts than of cardiocytes as discussed earlier; and reflects an active impact of myoblasts on cardiac systolic function as compared to a passive effect of fibroblasts on compliance. Surprisingly, there is no functional difference between animals treated with skeletal myoblasts and animals treated with bone marrow stromal cells[35] but in this case, a portion of the stromal cells were shown to differentiate into muscle-like cells within the infarct so the similarities may not be too unexpected. More surprising is the similar outcome in animals treated with myoblasts or with AC133+ stem cells.[36] Of particular interest is the finding that a combined transplantation of bone marrow mononuclear cells with skeletal myoblasts increased the efficacy of each, suggesting a potential synergistic effect between the two cell types.[38]

As the mechanisms underlying the positive effects of myoblast transplantation are still not fully understood, there is some debate as to whether

TABLE 2. Experimental studies comparing different cell types in cellular cardiomyoplasty

Study	Species	Model	Cell type	Outcome
Hutcheson et al. Cell Transpl 2000; 9;359-368[15]	Rabbit	Cryoinjury	Skeletal myoblasts vs. fibroblasts	SKM superior to Fb. SKM improve systolic and diastolic function. Fb only improves diastolic.
Thompson et al. Circulation. 2003 Sep 9;108 Suppl 1:II264-71[35]	Rabbit	Cryoinjury	Skeletal myoblasts vs. mononuclear bone marrow stem cells	No difference between SKM and mononuclear bone marrow stem cells regarding LV function.
Agbulut et al. J Am Coll Cardiol. 2004 Jul 21;44(2):458-63[36]	Rat	LAD ligation	Human skeletal myoblasts vs. human AC133+	Myotubes in SKM treated group. No difference regarding LV function.
Horackova et al. Am J Physiol Heart Circ Physiol. 2004 Oct;287(4): H1599-608. Epub 2004 May 27[37]	Guinea pig	LAD ligation	Skeletal myoblasts vs. Cardiac fibroblasts vs. cardiomy-ocytes	Myotube formation in SKM treated animals. SKM superior to CM and CFs regarding remodeling. Functional improvement in SKM treated animals. No comparison regarding LV function.
Ott et al. Eur J Cardiothorac Surg. 2004 Apr;25(4):627-34[38]	Rat	LAD ligation	Autologos skeletal myoblasts vs. mononu-clear bone marrow stem cells	SKM superior to isolated BM-MNC regarding LV function. Combination of these cell types shows synergy.

myoblasts improve contraction or just prevent further deterioration of the injured heart. Although either may be desirable in the clinical setting, a better understanding of this process will help to define optimal time points for treatment – in both acute or chronic myocardial injury. These debates are being resolved with more research, and the future for myoblast transplantation appears promising. Furthermore, the understandings gained about myoblast transplantation will provide a basis for developing second and third generation cells for cardiac repair.

5.   Skeletal Myoblasts – Future Perspectives

Developing the best cell(s) for cardiac repair is a moving target and one that may vary with the injury. Chronically infarcted myocardium lacks functional vessels as well as functional contractile elements. Therefore, to repair it (i.e., yield the greatest functional effect with minimal electrical abnormalities), there is a need for angiogenesis, myogenesis and electrical reintegration of the delivered cells (Figure 1). The ideal cell then for post-infarction cardiac repair would be an ischemia resistant electrically compatible cell capable of directing new vessel growth and new muscle integration. This could occur either via a direct effect of the cell(s) or by an indirect mechanism whereby the injected cells promote myogenesis and angiogenesis via stimulation or recruitment of endogenous cells in those processes. In non ischemic injury, where dilated cardiomyopathy is present, cells that alter wall stress and unload the surrounding heart might suffice. Contraction may not be required.

Identifying an ideal cell is not straightforward, because again it may depend on the injury. However, when examining the effects of current cell candidates for myocardial repair, a relationship between extent of differentiation, degree of successful engraftment and final effect on left ventricular function becomes apparent (Figure 2). The dilemma is obvious, injected cells are exposed to a hostile, ischemic environment. The more flexible (i.e undifferentiated) and ischemia-resistant a cell is, the higher its engraftment rate will be. However, the more differentiated a cell is toward a cardiac phenotype, the lower its ischemia resistance and engraftment will be. The perfect cell then either will be ischemia resistant initially and become fully functional after it engrafts or alternatively, some combination of cells or genes plus cells will be used to modify the local environment to promote engraftment of fully functional cells. Attempts to design candidate cells that both are ischemia resistant and able to electrically integrate have been performed by overexpressing connexin-43 in skeletal

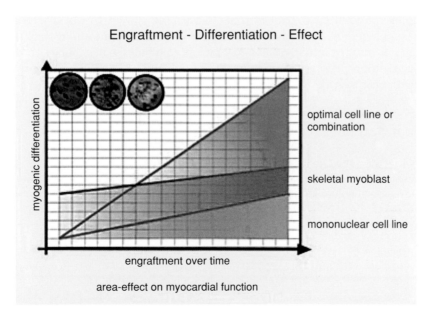

FIGURE 2. Engraftment effect and differentiation of candidate cell lines

myoblasts. Even though the it remains controversial whether these ionic channels are able to allow full communication on a single cell level, this is a first step towards engineering the optimal cell.[23] In order to increase the angiogenic potential of skeletal myoblasts, multiple attempts have been made to induce the expression of the pro-angiogenic molecule vascular endothelial growth factor in skeletal myoblasts.[5,25] In the next generation studies, investigators are transplanting combinations of angiogenic bone marrow and myogenic muscle-derived cells to promote both greater engraftment and increased functional capacity.[38] These early studies all suggest that the better we understand the required mechanisms for cardiac repair, the easier it will be to define and potentially design the optimal cell or cell combinations needed.

6. Summary

Skeletal myoblast transplantation opened the field of cellular cardiomyoplasty and remains its best studied procedure. Preclinical studies have moved to randomized clinical trials; lessons have been learned and questions remain. Cell transplantation offers the promise of a new era in the treatment of cardiovascular disease, but only if this new modality is carefully evaluated. Combining genomics, tissue engineering and advanced imaging methods to understand the mechanisms by which cell engraftment improves function, to promote graft longevity, and to improve electromechanical graft integration are the next preclinical frontiers. Basing clinical trials on good pre-clinical data, carefully defining the best cell type for a given clinical situation and performing randomized controlled trials that can be compared world-wide are the tasks before us as a field. Accepting the challenge, and pushing back this frontier is our opportunity. Changing patient outcomes will be our prize. Yet, doing it improperly could relegate this promising field to failure before its potential is realized.

7. References

1. Chachques JC, Grandjean PA, Tommasi JJ, Perier P, Chauvaud S, Bourgeois I, Carpentier A. Dynamic cardiomyoplasty: a new approach to assist chronic myocardial failure. Life Support Syst. 1987 Oct-Dec;5(4):323–7.
2. Koh GY, Klug MG, Soonpaa MH, Field LJ. Differentiation and long-term survival of C2C12 myoblast grafts in heart. J Clin Invest. 1993 Sep;92(3):1548–54.
3. Mauro A. Satellite cell of skeletal muscle fibers. J Biophys Biochem Cytol. 1961 Feb;9:493–5.
4. Zibaitis A, Greentree D, Ma F, Marelli D, Duong M, Chiu RC. Myocardial regeneration with satellite cell implantation. Transplant Proc. 1994 Dec;26(6):3294.
5. Taylor DA, Atkins BZ, Hungspreugs P, Jones TR, Reedy MC, Hutcheson KA, Glower DD, Kraus WE. Regenerating functional myocardium: Improved performance after skeletal myoblast transplantation. Nat Med 4 1998,8:929–933.

6. Murry CE, Wiseman RW, Schwartz SM, Hauschka SD. Skeletal myoblast transplantation for repair of myocardial necrosis. J Clin Invest 1996;98:2512–2523.
7. Atkins BZ, Hueman MT, Meuchel JM, Cottman MJ, Hutcheson KA, Taylor DA. Myogenic cell transplantation improves in vivo regional performance in infarcted rabbit myocardium. J Heart Lung Transplant. 1999 Dec;18(12):1173–80.
8. Chiu RC, Zibaitis A, Kao RL. Cellular cardiomyoplasty: myocardial regeneration with satellite cell implantation. Ann Thorac Surg. 1995 Jul;60(1):12–8.
9. Robinson SW, Cho PW, Levitsky HI, Olson JL, Hruban RH, Acker MA, Kessler PD. Arterial delivery of genetically labelled skeletal myoblasts to the murine heart: long-term survival and phenotypic modification of implanted myoblasts. Cell Transplant. 1996 Jan-Feb;5(1):77–91.
10. Taylor DA, Silvestry SC, Bishop SP, Annex BH, Lilly RE, Glower DD, Kraus WE. Delivery of primary autologous skeletal myoblasts into rabbit heart by coronary infusion: a potential approach to myocardial repair. Proc Assoc Am Physicians. 1997 May;109(3):245–53.
11. Dorfman J, Duong M, Zibaitis A, Pelletier MP, Shum-Tim D, Li C, Chiu RC. Myocardial tissue engineering with autologous myoblast implantation. J Thorac Cardiovasc Surg. 1998 Nov;116(5).744–51.
12. Atkins BZ, Hueman MT, Meuchel J, Hutcheson KA, Glower DD, Taylor DA. Cellular cardiomyoplasty improves diastolic properties of injured heart. J Surg Res. 1999 Aug;85(2):234–42.
13. Atkins BZ, Lewis CW, Kraus WE, Hutcheson KA, Glower DD, Taylor DA. Intracardiac transplantation of skeletal myoblasts yields two populations of striated cells in situ. Ann Thorac Surg. 1999 Jan;67(1):124–9.
14. Reinecke H, Murry CE. Transmural replacement of myocardium after skeletal myoblast grafting into the heart. Too much of a good thing? Cardiovasc Pathol. 2000 Nov-Dec;9(6):337–44.
15. Hutcheson KA Atkins BZ, Hueman MT, Hopkins MB, Glover DD, Taylor DA. Comparison of benefits on myocardial performance of cellular cardiomyoplasty with skeletal myoblasts and fibroblasts. Cell Transpl 2000;9;359–368.
16. Scorsin M, Hagege A, Vilquin JT, Fiszman M, Marotte F, Samuel JL, Rappaport L, Schwartz K, Menasche P. Comparison of the effects of fetal cardiomyocyte and skeletal myoblast transplantation on postinfarction left ventricular function. J Thorac Cardiovasc Surg. 2000 Jun;119(6):1169–75.
17. Pouzet B, Vilquin JT, Hagege AA, Scorsin M, Messas E, Fiszman M, Schwartz K, Menasche P. Intramyocardial transplantation of autologous myoblasts: can tissue processing be optimized? Circulation. 2000 Nov 7;102(19 Suppl 3):III210–5.
18. Suzuki K, Smolenski RT, Jayakumar J, Murtuza B, Brand NJ, Yacoub MH. Heat shock treatment enhances graft cell survival in skeletal myoblast transplantation to the heart. Circulation. 2000 Nov 7;102(19 Suppl 3):III216–21.
19. Suzuki K, Brand NJ, Smolenski RT, Jayakumar J, Murtuza B, Yacoub MH. Development of a novel method for cell transplantation through the coronary artery. Circulation. 2000 Nov 7;102(19 Suppl 3):III359–64.
20. Pouzet B, Ghostine S, Vilquin JT, Garcin I, Scorsin M, Hagege AA, Duboc D, Schwartz K, Menasche P. Is skeletal myoblast transplantation clinically relevant in the era of angiotensin-converting enzyme inhibitors? Circulation. 2001 Sep 18;104(12 Suppl 1):I223–8.
21. Pouzet B, Vilquin JT, Hagege AA, Scorsin M, Messas E, Fiszman M, Schwartz K, Menasche P. Factors affecting functional outcome after autologous skeletal

myoblast transplantation. Ann Thorac Surg. 2001 Mar;71(3):844–50; discussion 850–1.

22. Rajnoch C, Chachques JC, Berrebi A, Bruneval P, Benoit MO, Carpentier A. Cellular therapy reverses myocardial dysfunction. J Thorac Cardiovasc Surg. 2001 May;121(5):871–8.

23. Suzuki K, Brand NJ, Allen S, Khan MA, Farrell AO, Murtuza B, Oakley RE, Yacoub MH. Overexpression of connexin 43 in skeletal myoblasts: Relevance to cell transplantation to the heart. J Thorac Cardiovasc Surg. 2001 Oct;122(4):759–66.

24. Suzuki K, Murtuza B, Suzuki N, Smolenski RT, Yacoub MH. Intracoronary infusion of skeletal myoblasts improves cardiac function in doxorubicin-induced heart failure. Circulation. 2001 Sep 18;104(12 Suppl 1):I213–7.

25. Suzuki K, Murtuza B, Smolenski RT, Sammut IA, Suzuki N, Kaneda Y, Yacoub MH. Cell transplantation for the treatment of acute myocardial infarction using vascular endothelial growth factor-expressing skeletal myoblasts. Circulation. 2001 Sep 18;104(12 Suppl 1):I207–12.

26. Jain M, DerSimonian H, Brenner DA, Ngoy S, Teller P, Edge AS, Zawadzka A, Wetzel K, Sawyer DB, Colucci WS, Apstein CS, Liao R. Cell therapy attenuates deleterious ventricular remodeling and improves cardiac performance after myocardial infarction. Circulation. 2001 Apr 10;103(14):1920–7.

27. Tremblay JP, Roy B, Goulet M. Human myoblast transplantation: a simple model for tumorigenicity. Neuromuscul Disord 1991.1:341–343.

28. Field L. Future therapy for cardiovascular disease. NHLBI Workshop Cell Transplantation: Future Therapy for Cardiovascular Disease 1998. Columbia, MD.

29. Chachques JC, Herreros J, Trainini J, Juffe A, Rendal E, Prosper F, Genovese J. Autologous human serum for cell culture avoids the implantation of cardioverter-defibrillators in cellular cardiomyoplasty. Int J Cardiol. 2004 Jun;95 Suppl 1:S29–33.

30. Siminiak T, Kalawski R, Fiszer D, Jerzykowska O, Rzezniczak J, Rozwadowska N, Kurpisz M. Autologous skeletal myoblast transplantation for the treatment of postinfarction myocardial injury: phase I clinical study with 12 months of follow-up. Am Heart J. 2004 Sep;148(3):531–7.

31. Stamm C, Westphal B, Kleine HD, Petzsch M, Kittner C, Klinge H, Schumichen C, Nienaber CA, Freund M, Steinhoff G. Autologous bone-marrow stem-cell transplantation for myocardial regeneration. Lancet. 2003 Jan 4;361(9351):45–6.

32. Assmus B, Schachinger V, Teupe C, Britten M, Lehmann R, Dobert N, Grunwald F, Aicher A, Urbich C, Martin H, Hoelzer D, Dimmeler S, Zeiher AM. Transplantation of Progenitor Cells and Regeneration Enhancement in Acute Myocardial Infarction (TOPCARE-AMI). Circulation. 2002 Dec 10;106(24):3009–17.

33. Itescu S, Kocher AA, Schuster MD. Myocardial neovascularization by adult bone marrow-derived angioblasts: strategies for improvement of cardiomyocyte function. Heart Fail Rev. 2003 Jul;8(3):253–8.

34. Jiang Y, Jahagirdar BN, Reinhardt RL, Schwartz RE, Keene CD, Ortiz-Gonzalez XR, Reyes M, Lenvik T, Lund T, Blackstad M, Du J, Aldrich S, Lisberg A, Low WC, Largaespada DA, Verfaillie CM. Pluripotency of mesenchymal stem cells derived from adult marrow. Nature. 2002 Jul 4;418(6893):41–9.

35. Thompson RB, Emani SM, Davis BH, van den Bos EJ, Morimoto Y, Craig D, Glower D, Taylor DA. Comparison of intracardiac cell transplantation: autologous skeletal myoblasts versus bone marrow cells. Circulation. 2003 Sep 9;108 Suppl 1:II264–71.

36. Agbulut O, Vandervelde S, Al Attar N, Larghero J, Ghostine S, Leobon B, Robidel E, Borsani P, Le Lorc'h M, Bissery A, Chomienne C, Bruneval P, Marolleau JP, Vilquin JT, Hagege A, Samuel JL, Menasche P. Comparison of human skeletal myoblasts and bone marrow-derived CD133+ progenitors for the repair of infarcted myocardium. J Am Coll Cardiol. 2004 Jul 21;44(2):458–63.
37. Horackova M, Arora R, Chen R, Armour JA, Cattini PA, Livingston R, Byczko Z. Cell transplantation for treatment of acute myocardial infarction: unique capacity for repair by skeletal muscle satellite cells Am J Physiol Heart Circ Physiol. 2004 Oct;287(4):H1599–608. Epub 2004 May 27.
38. Ott HC, Bonaros N, Marksteiner R, Wolf D, Margreiter E, Schachner T, Laufer G, Hering S. Combined transplantation of skeletal myoblasts and bone marrow stem cells for myocardial repair in rats. Eur J Cardiothorac Surg. 2004 Apr;25(4):627–34.

6
Skeletal Myoblasts: The European Experience

PHILIPPE MENASCHÉ[*]

1. Introduction

It is in the "Old Europe" that cellular transplantation for heart disease has
entered the clinical arena when, on June 15, 2000, we performed the first
intramyocardial transplantation of autologous skeletal myoblasts in a 75-
year old patient suffering from severe ischemic left ventricular dysfunction.[1]
Two weeks before, he had undergone a muscular biopsy at the thigh. Expansion of this tissue specimen in a dedicated medium and according to customized GMP-compliant procedures yielded a total of 800×10^6 cells, of
which 65% were CD-56-positive myoblasts. These cells were then implanted
in multiple sites in the core and at the borders of a postinfarction posterior
nonviable scar while 2 bypass grafts were placed on the left anterior descending and diagonal coronary arteries under conventional cardiopulmonary
bypass. The postoperative course was uneventful. The patient's condition
subsequently improved and repeat echocardiograms documented the clear
restoration of some systolic thickening in the once akinetic area. This patient
died 18 months after the operation from a stroke and autopsy provided evidence for the reality of cell engraftment under the form of scar-embedded
clusters of myotubes, featuring typical cross-striations and aligned parallel to
the host cardiomyocytes.[2] This case initiated a phase I trial primarily designed
to assess the feasibility and safety of the procedure and ultimately included
10 patients.[3] Since then, 4 additional studies of myoblast transplantation
have been reported in Europe, of which two entailed surgical implantations.[4,5]
The two others used catheters for cell delivery and only one has been published at the time of this writing.[6] The purpose of this chapter is to critically
summarize the main lessons gained from these early trials, to highlight
the issues that remain to be addressed and to place myoblasts in the more

[*]Department of Cardiovascular Surgery & INSERM U 633, Hôpital Européen
Georges Pompidou, 20, rue Leblanc, 75015 Paris, France, phone: +33 1 56 09 3622,
Fax: +33 1 56 09 2219, email: philippe.menesche@hop.egp.ap-hop-paris.fr

general perspective of cell transplantation for repair of chronically infarcted myocardium.

2.   Lessons Gained from Clinical Trials

From the onset, it should be stressed that, at the time of this writing, the number of European patients for whom data are available through published reports is still limited to 47: 10, 10 and 12 in the French, Polish and Spanish surgical trials, respectively; 5 and 10 in the Dutch and Polish catheter-based trials, respectively. This clearly calls for caution in the interpretation of the results until they can be validated by a larger database.

The 10 patients comprising our phase I trial[3] were included on the basis of the following criteria: severe left ventricular dysfunction reflected by an ejection fraction ≤35%); the presence of a postinfarction akinetic and nonviable scar, as assessed by dobutamine echocardiography and 18-fluorodeoxyglucose positron emission tomography (PET); and an indication of coronary bypass in remote areas. An average of 871×10^6 cells (86% of myoblasts) were obtained from a biopsy taken at the thigh after a mean period of 16 days and implanted uneventfully across the scar at the time of bypass with the use of a customized right-angled 27 gauge needle allowing tangential injections. Except for one patient whose early death was unrelated to the cell transplantation, all patients had an uncomplicated postoperative course. At an average follow-up of 10.9 months, the mean New York Heart Association functional class improved from 2.7 ± 0.2 preoperatively to 1.6 ± 0.1 postoperatively ($p < 0.0001$), and the ejection fraction increased from $24 \pm 1\%$ to $32 \pm 1\%$ ($p < 0.02$). A blinded echocardiographic analysis showed that 63% of the cell-implanted scars (14 of 22) demonstrated improved systolic thickening. As previously stated, one non-cardiac death occurred 17.5 months after transplantation and the pathological examination of the heart demonstrated the presence of myotubes,[2] which has also been observed in that portion of the US trial where myoblasts were implanted at the time of left ventricular device insertion in patients bridged for heart transplantation.[7] At the time of this writing, all the other patients are still alive (maximal follow-up: 3 years and 8 months) and should be soon reassessed extensively.

Whereas the inclusion criteria of the 12-patient Spanish study were similar to ours,[4] the protocol differed by two major aspects: the biopsy was grown in autologous, not fetal calf, serum, which yielded an average number of 221×10^6 cells; and the cell-transplanted segments were *also* bypassed. Left ventricular ejection fraction improved from $35.5 \pm 2.3\%$ before surgery to $53.5 \pm 4.98\%$ at 3 months ($p = 0.002$). Likewise, regional contractility was found by echocardiography to markedly improve in the skeletal myoblast-grafted segments, as reflected by a wall motion score index which decreased from 2.64 ± 0.13 at baseline to 1.64 ± 0.16 at 3 months ($p = 0.0001$). Quantitative 18-fluorodeoxyglucose PET also showed a significant ($p = 0.012$) increase in cardiac viability in the infarct zone 3 months after surgery while 13N-ammonia PET studies failed to show differences in perfusion between the two groups.

So far, the third surgical trial reported by Siminiak et al.[5] has only been reported in an abstract form. Basically, it entailed in-scar transplantation of autologous skeletal myoblasts in 10 patients with ischemic heart failure and associated revascularization in the non cell-implanted areas. In keeping with the two previous studies, both global and regional function were reported to have improved postoperatively.

In the setting of catheter-based trials, only that of Smits et al.[6] has been published. It included 5 patients with symptomatic heart failure after an anterior wall infarction. At the end of the culture process, autologous skeletal myoblasts (196 ± 105 million cells) were transendocardially injected into the infarcted area under electromagnetic guidance. All procedures went on uneventfully. Compared with baseline, the left ventricular ejection fraction increased from $36 \pm 11\%$ to $41 \pm 9\%$ at 3 months ($p = 0.009$) and $45 \pm 8\%$ at 6 months ($p = 0.23$). Regional wall analysis by magnetic resonance imaging showed significantly increased wall thickening at the target areas (at 3 months: 0.9 ± 2.3 mm vs. 1.8 ± 2.4 mm, $p = 0.008$) and less wall thickening in remote areas.

A second catheter-based study was recently reported in the clinical late-breaking sessions of the 2004 American College of Cardiology by Siminak and coworkers. Ten patients received autologous myoblasts by the transvenous technique, which basically entails percutaneous catheterization of the coronary venous system and transvenous puncture by an extendable nitinol needle. This provides a direct access to the targeted myocardial area where staged injections of cells are then performed through a microcatheter advanced along the needle under endovascular ultrasound guidance. The procedure was reported to be technically successful in all but one patient and did not cause any adverse event. Of note, none of these catheter-based studies did address some specific and clinically relevant issues such as cell viability and long-term functionality following passage through the catheter and exposure to the lubricants that coat the lumen of the devices.

Altogether, analysis of these data leads to two major conclusions. First, the procedure is technically feasible in that it is possible to grow hundreds of millions of cells from a small biopsy using clinical-grade media and reagents and under Good Manufacturing Practice-compliant procedures. In our experience, the use of cell factories and of a dedicated myogenic-specific medium have been two critical factors for consistently providing an effective scale-up and a high myoblast yield, respectively. Furthermore, the reimplantation of the final cell therapy product in multiple sites across the scar area has turned out to be quite safe and devoid from specific procedural complications like bleeding from the needle punctures. Second, in spite of the overall positive tone of the various reports, it still remains uncertain whether myoblast transplantation can restore viability in scarred areas to the point that it favorably impacts on global left ventricular function and patient outcomes. Our caution about the published data, including ours, is motivated by the multiple confounding factors that tend to cloud them. They include the small size of the various patient cohorts; the lack of parallel, placebo-controlled groups; differences in cell culture processes, which may influence myoblast viability and differentiation; the variable type of examinations used for assessing viability (stress echocardiography, nuclear angiograms, magnetic resonance imaging, PET); the kinetic patterns of the grafted area, which have encompassed hypo-, a- and dyskinesia; the revascularization or lack of revascularization of the grafted scar; and the usual lack of blindness in the assessment of results.

The above considerations clearly converge to justify the implementation of prospective, randomized, placebo-controlled, blinded trials to allow an accurate assessment of efficacy. The Myoblast Autologous Grafting in Ischemic Cardiomyopathy (MAGIC) study that we have now started is designed to meet these criteria. This 3-arm trial, which should include 300 patients basically matching the inclusion criteria of our phase I, involves a dose-ranging protocol (control medium, 400×10^6 cells, 800×10^6 cells), two production sites with fully standardized procedures and 1 core lab for the assessment of the primary end point (changes in the contractility of the scarred cell- or placebo-injected segments, as assessed by echocardiography). The additional assessment of left ventricular ejection fraction and major cardiac adverse events should help in determining the extent, if any, to which improved regional wall kinetics impact on global function and clinical outcomes.

3.   Remaining Key Issues

3.1.   Arrhythmias

From the onset, ventricular arrhythmias have been identified as a potential drawback of myoblast transplantation. This issue was initially raised by the observation of sustained (non-lethal) ventricular tachycardias in 4 of our phase I patients. Similar events were reported by Siminiak et al.[5] In contrast, no cardiac arrhythmias were detected during early follow-up in the Spanish study.[4] The authors attributed this lack of complications to the use of autologous serum, but this hypothesis has not yet been validated. Finally, although the catheter study of Smits et al.[6] was claimed to be free from adverse events, it should be mentioned that the 5 patients reported in this paper are actually part of a larger hospital- and industry-sponsored trial in which 13 patients received myoblasts by the endoventricular or the transvenous coronary sinus routes. In this cohort, 2 sudden deaths presumably attributable to arrhythmias occurred and led to stopping the trial, which has been resumed after protocol changes involving the systematic implantation of a defibrillator in all cell transplant recipients.

Theoretically, there are several mechanisms which could account for these cell-related arrhythmias, including the inflammatory reaction to needle punctures, intrinsic automaticity of cells and even sympathetic nerve sprouting.[8] However, our electrophysiological studies have also highlighted the major differences in membrane electrical properties between engrafted myoblasts and host cardiomyocytes, which, for example, feature action potential durations almost ten times longer than those of skeletal muscle cells.[9] Furthermore, a recent study[10] has described fusion events between donor and recipient cells at the host-graft interface and although the electrical behavior of these chimeric cells remains to be characterized, it is sound to hypothesize that they might exhibit repolarization patterns dyssynchronous from those of the surrounding native cardiac cells. Altogether, this cellular heterogeneity could set the stage for re-entry circuits and subsequent arrhythmias, a hypothesis indirectly supported by the efficacy of amiodarone, which, among other effects, makes intracardiac conduction more homogeneous. However, the relationship between myoblast grafting and ventricular tachycardias may not be as straightforward because of the intrinsically arrhythmogenic nature of the scarred substrate the cells are implanted in and which accounts for the high incidence of sudden deaths in heart failure patients. This has been an additional arguments for implanting a defibrillator in all the MAGIC patients as the device should not only represent a safety net and provide, based on the MADIT II trial, a survival benefit,[11] but is also expected to generate, through reading of its records, meaningful information of the incidence, timing and type of arrhythmias in both control and transplanted patients.

3.2.   Cell Death

A major limitation of cell transplantation remains death of the grafted cells, whichever they are, during the early post-implantation period. In the case of myoblasts, the percentage of dead cells can be as high as 90% and is only partly compensated for by multiplication of those that have survived (personal data). Several factors contribute to cell death, including physical strain during injections, inflammation triggered by needle punctures, oxidative stress,[12] apoptosis, ischemia inherent in the poor vascularization of the target post-infarction scars and also probably the loss of the normal interactions between cells and their usual extracellular matrix. This major graft loss is likely to seriously hamper the efficacy of the procedure because of the close relationship, established in a rat model of myocardial infarction, between the number of injected myoblasts and the extent of left ventricular preservation.[13] Indeed, the dose-ranging protocol of our MAGIC trial has been designed to further characterize this dose-effect relationship in a clinical setting.

Intuitively, a first logical means of counteracting this high rate of graft loss is to increase the number of injected myoblasts. This approach, however, has some limitations related to practicality (the duration of cultures should remain within the clinically acceptable time frame of 2 to 3 weeks), cost and safety (the tolerable volume that can be injected intramyocardially should probably not exceed 5-6 mL while multiple passages might favor the emergence of a differentiation-defective population of cells with a subsequent risk of inappropriate graft overgrowth[14]). These limitations emphasize the importance of an alternate approach, which consists of implementing techniques designed at enhancing the survival of the transplanted cells. Currently, anti-inflammatory drugs can already be used to limit injection-induced tissue damage and, in this perspective, we give a perioperative pulse of corticosteroids in our cell transplant patients. In the future, improvements might be provided by delivery devices reducing mechanical cell injury such as pressure-controlled injection pumps, myoblast-seeded biodegradable patches or injection of cells embedded in a protective matrix. However, the importance of the ischemic component of cell death also emphasizes the potential benefits of a concomitant induction of angiogenesis that can be achieved exogenously or endogenously. Exogenous interventions refer to co-injections of angiogenic growth factors, co-transplantation of myoblasts and bone marrow cells[15] or transplantation of transfected myoblasts overexpressing either a given growth factor or, preferably, a master gene like hypoxia-inducible factor (HIF)-1, which regulates the expression of a wide array of genes involved in angiogenesis and therefore allows to hit multiple targets. This approach is supported by our recent findings that co-administration of myoblasts and HIF 1-α increase angiogenesis, myogenic cell engraftment and overall cell survival compared with myoblast transplantation alone, and that these histological patterns correlate with an improvement of left ventricular systolic function (Azarnoush et al., manuscript under review). Endogenous interventions refer to a cytokine-induced mobilization of bone marrow stem cells and are based on the concept that expression by transplanted myoblasts of the potent chemoattractant stroma-derived factor (SDF)-1[16] could establish an effective signalling pathway for stem cell homing through interaction with the receptor CXCR4 expressed by bone marrow cells. Such a homing would then enhance local angiogenesis in the areas of grafted cells, most likely through the release of angiogenic growth factors. Interestingly, one of them, the vascular endothelial growth factor (VEGF), could increase myoblast survival not only through augmented angiogenesis but also by decreasing apoptosis.[17]

3.3. Mechanisms of Action

So far, the precise mechanism of action of engrafted myoblasts remains elusive. The strongest hypotheses include a scaffolding of the infarct area limiting its expansion and/or release of cell-secreted mediators that could paracrinally effect protective effects through changes in extracellular matrix composition,[18] rescue of hibernating cardiomyocytes or recruitment of locally resident cardiac stem cells. At first glance, a direct contribution to pump function is less likely because of the lack of electromechanical connections between engrafted myoblasts and host cardiomyocytes. However, because engrafted cells retain their excitable properties,[9] one cannot totally exclude that field effects may occur in areas of close physical contact between donor and recipient cells and thus allow currents fired by cardiomyocytes to excite neighboring transplanted myotubes directly, i.e., via gap junction-independent pathways. However, this hypothesis is not yet validated by experimental data and it is probably fair to assume that even if the injected cells may occasionally contract, their synchronous contribution to systolic function is likely to be of limited magnitude.

This uncertainty regarding the mechanisms of action have led some investigators to raise the question of the appropriate timing for moving to clinical trials. Here it should be remembered that many drugs have been marketed before their mechanism of action was clarified and that our understanding of their beneficial effects is often provisional. The prerequisite for reasonable and ethically acceptable cell therapy clinical studies is thus to have accumulated enough experimental efficacy and safety data, which was the case when we operated on our first patient with the caveat that the complex clinical setting of ischemic heart failure can never be fully mimicked experimentally, even with the use of large animal models. This limitation is clearly exemplified by the occurrence of ventricular arrhythmias in some patients whereas these complications could not be predicted from preclinical data. Indeed, clinical studies can even, to some extent, contribute to a better understanding of the mechanisms of action. Thus, the echocardiographic observation of changes in left ventricular diastolic dimensions following cell implantation can be taken as a surrogate end point for a limitation of remodelling whereas magnetic resonance imaging provides a reliable means of assessing potential improvements in regional wall kinetics.

4.   Myoblasts in Perspective

While skeletal myoblasts represent the first generation of cells that have been used clinically in patients with ischemic heart failure, it is clear that other cell types will come down the road. Indeed, it is already the case for bone marrow-derived cells. A discussion of the advantages and limitations of these cells is beyond the scope of this chapter as it is addressed in other sections of this book. Our remarks will therefore be confined to the observation that the two face-to-face studies which have compared skeletal myoblasts and either mesenchymal stem cells[19] or hematopoietic progenitors[20] in the chronic setting of postinfarction scars have failed to show any benefit of the bone marrow cells. In fact, a recent study has even reported that acutely administered unselected bone marrow cells derived from clonal expansion could cause significant intramyocardial calcification.[20]

In fact, both skeletal myoblasts and bone marrow cells share a common limitation: they do not convert into cardiomyocytes. This has been demonstrated from the onset with myoblasts[22] whose only milieu-induced phenotypic adaptation consists of the emergence of an increased population of slow-twitch fibers.[3] The issue is more controversial in the case of bone marrow cells, which have been credited for a high plasticity potential. However, this concept is increasingly challenged by studies showing that initially reported transdifferentiation events have been mistakenly interpreted, most likely because of methodologic inaccuracies associated with immunohistochemical methods of cell identification whereas the use of more robust genetic markers now shows that bone marrow cells may eventually fuse with host cells but do not really become "true" cardiomyocytes, at least to a significant extent.[23,24]

Assuming that the two major features of cells intended to repopulate dead areas for re-establishing function are generation of active-force development and electrical coupling with residual host cardiomyocytes, it becomes a matter of clinical good sense to conclude that the most suitable cells are likely to be cardiac cells. Three sources can then be considered. The first could be the recently described resident pool of cardiac stem cells[25] but several issues remain to be clarified, including their occurrence in the human heart, their localization, the means of recruiting them endogenously to such an extent that they become functionally effective or, alternatively, to grow them *ex vivo* before reinjection. Thus, it is quite uncertain that the manipulation of this endogenous pool, although quite exciting, may have clinically relevant applications in a foreseeable future. The second source of cardiac cells is represented by fetal cardiomyocytes, which have actually been those used in the groundbreaking proof-of-principle experiments of cell therapy.[26,27] Nevertheless, the applicability of this approach is seriously hampered by several critical problems like availability, ethics and immunogenicity, which cast equally serious doubts about a clinical applicability. Finally, cardiac cells could be derived from embryonic stem cells following their appropriate programming towards the cardiomyogenic pathway. This approach has already yielded quite encouraging results in that transplantation of embryonic stem cells has been shown, in rodent models of myocardial infarction, to result in differentiation into cardiomyocytes, stable engraftment in infarct areas and improved function.[28] There is no doubt that this path is also plagued with several problems, many of which could be alleviated by xenotransplantation relying on the immune privilege that these cells seem to feature. Our current thinking is that embryonic stem cells may, ultimately, represent the cell line that will truly achieve the regenerating goal that underlies the whole concept of cell therapy.

5.   References

1. Menasché P, Hagege AA., Scorsin M, et al. Myoblast transplantation for heart failure. Lancet 2001 ; 357 : 279–280.
2. Hagège AA, Carrion C, Menasché P, et al. Viability and differentiation of autologous skeletal myoblast grafts in ischaemic cardiomyopathy. Lancet 2003 ; 361 : 491–492.

3. Menasché P, Hagège AA, Vilquin JT, et al. Autologous skeletal myoblast transplantation for severe postinfarction left ventricular dysfunction. J Am Coll Cardiol 2003; 41: 1078–1083.

4. Herreros J, Prosper F, Perez A, et al. Autologous intramyocardial injection of cultured skeletal muscle-derived stem cells in patients with non-acute myocardial infarction. Eur Heart J 2003 ; 24 : 2012–2020.

5. Siminiak T, Kalawski R, Fiszer D, et al. Transplantation of autologous skeletal myoblasts in the treatment of patients with postinfarction heart failure. Early results of phase I clinical trial. Circulation 2002 ; 106 (suppl II) : II-626 (Abstract).

6. Smits PC, Geuns RJM, Poldermans D, et al. Catheter-based intramyocardial injection of autologous skeletal myoblasts as a primary treatment of ischemic heart failure. J Am Coll Cardiol 2003 ; 42 : 2063–2069.

7. Pagani F, DerSimonian R, Zawadska A, et al. Autologous skeletal myoblasts transplanted to ischemia damaged myocardium in humans. J Am Coll Cardiol 2003 ; 41 : 879–888.

8. Makkar RR, Lill M, Chen PS. Stem cell therapy for myocardial repair: Is it arrhythmogenic ? J Am Coll Cardiol 2003 ; 42 : 2070–2072.

9. Leobon B, Garcin I, Menasché P, et al. Myoblasts transplanted into rat infarcted myocardium are functionally isolated from their host. Proc Natl Acad Sci U S A 2003 ; 100 : 7808–7811.

10. Reinecke H, Minami E, Poppa V, Murry C. Evidence for fusion between cardiac and skeletal muscle cells. Circulation 2004 ; 94 : 1–5.

11. Moss AJ, Zareba W, Hall J, et al. Prophylactic implantation of a defibrillator in patients with myocardial infarction and reduced ejection fraction. New Engl J Med 2002 ; 346 : 877–883.

12. Suzuki K, Murtuza B, Beauchamp JR, et al. Dynamics and mediators of acute graft attrition after myoblast transplantation to the heart. FASEB J 2004 ; 18: 1153–1155.

13. Tambara K, Sakakibara Y, Sakaguchi G, et al. Transplanted skeletal myoblasts can fully replace the infracted myocardium when they survive in the host in large numbers. Circulation 2003 ; 108 (suppl II) : II 259–263.

14. Reinecke H, Murry CE. Transmural replacement of myocardium after skeletal myoblast grafting into the heart. Too much of a good thing ? Cardiovasc Pathol. 2000 ; 9 : 337–344.

15. Ott HC, Bonaros N, Marksteiner R, et al. Combined transplantation of skeletal myoblasts and bone marrow stem cells for myocardial repair in rats. Eur J Cardiothorac Surg 2004 ; 25 : 627–634.

16. Askari AT, Unzek S, Popovic ZB, et al. Effect of stromal-cell-drived factor 1 on stem-cell homing and tissue regeneration in ischemic cardiomyopathy. Lancet 2003 ; 362 : 697–703.

17. Germani A, Di Carlo A, Mangoni A, et al. Vascular endothelial growth factor modulates skeletal myoblast function. Am J Pathol 2003 ; 163 : 1417–1428.

18. Murtuza B, Suzuki K, Bou-Gharios G, et al. Transplantation of skeletal myoblasts secreting an IL-1 inhibitor modulates adverse remodeling in infarcted murine myocardium. Proc Natl Acad Sci USA 2004 ; 101 : 4216–4221.

19. Thomson RB, Emani SM, Davis BH, et al. Comparison of intracardiac cell transplantation : autologous skeletal myoblasts versus bone marrow cells. Circulation 2003 ; 108 (suppl I) : I 264–271.

20. Agbulut O, Vandervelde S, Al Attar N, et al. Comparison of human skeletal myoblasts and bone marrow-derived CD133+ progenitors for the repair of infarcted myocardium. J Am Coll Cardiol 2004 ; 44 : 458–463.
21. Yoon YS, Park JS, Tkebuchava T, Luedeman C, Losordo DW. Unexpected severe calcification after transplantation of bone marrow cells in acute myocardial infarction. Circulation 2004 ; 109 : 3154–3157.
22. Reinecke H, Poppa V, Murry CE. Skeletal muscle stem cells do not transdifferentiate into cardiomyocytes after cardiac grafting. J Mol Cell Cardiol 2002 ; 34 : 241–249.
23. Murry CE, Soonpa MH, Reinecke H, et al. Haematopoietic stem cells do not transdifferentiate into cardiac myocytes in myocardial infarcts. Nature 2004 ; 428 : 664–668.
24. Nygren JM, Jovinge S, Breitbach M, et al. Bone marrow-derived hematopoietic cells generate cardiomyocytes at a low frequency through cell fusion, but not transdifferentiation. Nat Med 2004 ; 10 : 494–501.
25. Beltrami AP, Barlucchi L, Torella D, et al. Adult cardiac stem cells are multipotent and support myocardial regeneration. Cell 2003 ; 114 : 763–776.
26. Scorsin M, Hagège AA, Marotte F, et al. Does transplantation of cardiomyocytes improve function of infarcted myocardium ? Circulation 1997 ; 96 [Suppl II] : II 188–193.
27. Leor J, Patterson M, Quinones MJ, Kedes LH, Kloner RA. Transplantation of fetal myocardial tissue into the infarcted myocardium of rat. Circulation 1996 ; 94 [Suppl II] : II 332–336.
28. Min JY, Yang Y, Sullivan MF, et al. Long-term improvement of cardiac function in rats after infarction by transplantation of embryonic stem cells. J Thorac Cardiovasc Surg 2003 ; 125 : 361–369.

7
Skeletal Myoblasts: The U.S. Experience

EDWARD B. DIETHRICH[*]

1. Introduction

In spite of aggressive efforts to reduce the incidence of coronary artery disease, myocardial infarction remains the leading cause of death in the United States[1] and most other developed nations. The problem is likely to escalate as the population ages.

Myocardial infarction causes a remodeling process in which scarred tissue is substituted for viable contracting cardiac muscle. In the most extreme cases, a left ventricular aneurysm forms and the heart muscle becomes largely dysfunctional. Eventually, the majority of patients with such damage will suffer from congestive heart failure (CHF). In the United States (US), CHF is a leading cause of hospital admission.[1]

A variety of approaches directed at improving left ventricular function have been tried. Cardiac transplantation remains the ultimate solution, but the volume of patients in need of treatment far exceeds the potential donor population. Although there are other mechanical and operative approaches that may be appropriate in selected cases (e.g., mitral valve replacement, temporary cardiac-assist devices, pacing and defibrillator strategies), their success is often short-lived.

Basic scientific research on cellular transplantation methods has been an important step in cardiac therapy. Replacing damaged myocardial tissue with new muscle has the potential to revitalize the heart's own ability to contract and improve cardiac performance (Figure 1). The transplantation of myoblasts isolated from skeletal muscle into damaged myocardial tissue has been studied in animal[2,3] and human models,[4-7] and it has been shown that these cells engraft, form myotubules, and enhance cardiac function *in vivo*. In this chapter, the results of early clinical study in the US are reviewed.

2. Methods

We have investigated the feasibility and safety of transplanting autologous myoblasts into the infarcted myocardia of patients undergoing coronary

Transverse Section of Skeletal Muscle

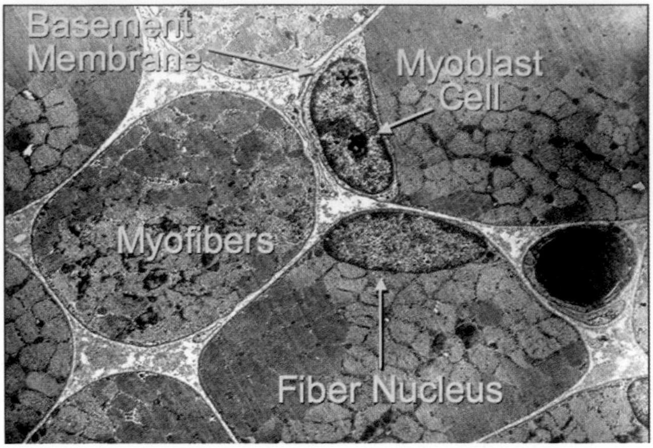

FIGURE 1. Transverse section of skeletal muscle shows myoblast cells, which exist underneath the basement membrane around the myofibers. These cells have the potential to engraft and form myotubes.

artery bypass grafting (CABG) or left ventricular assist device (LVAD) placement. Our protocols for these procedures including patient eligibility criteria, baseline testing requirements, the techniques of myoblast procurement and cell culturing, and the transplantation procedure itself are described.

2.1.   Patient Selection

Autologous skeletal myoblast transplantation is experimental and, as such, it is reserved for patients whose treatment options are limited. Transplantation of myoblasts into the epicardial surface of the infarcted area ideally involves direct visualization of the region—something that is easily achieved during an open procedure such as CABG or LVAD insertion.

Eligibility requirements for elective CABG in our recent evaluation included a previous myocardial infarction (MI) and a left ventricular ejection fraction (LVEF) of less than 40%. The LVAD group (n=6) was included only to establish proof of the engraftment concept. Eligibility for the LVAD procedure required that the device be implanted as a bridge to cardiac transplantation and that the patient was willing to donate his/her heart for histologic evaluation following transplant. In both the CABG and LVAD groups, patients were excluded if they had skeletal muscle disease, active malignancy, recent history of drug or alcohol abuse, were pregnant, or had an active infection.

2.2.   Evaluation

Screening and follow-up evaluations for patients undergoing autologous skeletal muscle transplantation are described in Table 1 and included a physical examination, electrocardiogram, transthoracic echocardiography, 24-hour Holter monitoring, and routine blood testing. Global and regional ventricular wall contractility were measured by two-dimensional echocardiography, and LVEF was calculated by the Simpson rule.

In selected patients, single-photon emission computed tomography (SPECT) was used to assess global left ventricular function, and ischemia and viability of the heart muscle. Magnetic resonance imaging (MRI) and fluorine-18-fluorodeoxyglucose positron emission tomography (FDG PET) were also used to help determine scar segment thickness and myocardial viability in some patients. These tests were not part of the original protocol, but the protocol was amended to allow them in some cases so that we could obtain additional outcome data.

2.3.   Myoblast Procurement

A skeletal muscle biopsy was completed several weeks before the scheduled surgical procedure. The biopsy was performed either in the hospital operating room, or in the outpatient clinic. Strict adherence to sterile technique was used in either locale to avoid contamination.

A local anesthetic (1% xylocaine) was infiltrated into the skin and subcutaneous tissue over an ~6-cm area on the anterior upper thigh. The incision was taken down to the fascia, which was opened to expose the muscle. Fibrous and fatty tissues were excised, and 2-5 grams of skeletal muscle were

TABLE 1. Evaluations

Type of evaluation	Timing of evaluation
Physical exam	Baseline, all visits
Routine blood work	Baseline, all visits
ECG	Baseline, all visits
Urinalysis	Baseline, Weeks 1, 3, 6, 9, 12
	Months 6, 12, 18, 24
Antibody testing	Weeks 1, 3, 12
	Month 6
Echocardiogram	Baseline, Weeks 1, 3, 6, 9, 12
	Months 6, 12, 18, 24
Holter monitoring	Baseline, Weeks 1, 3
	Months 6, 12, 24
PET scan (optional)	Baseline, Week 1
	Months 6, 12, 18, 24
MRI (optional)	Baseline, Week 1
	Months 6, 12, 18, 24

obtained. The tissue was placed into transport medium and transferred to the processing laboratory. The wound was closed, and a compression dressing was applied.

2.4.   Cell Culturing

The biopsies were processed at Diacrin, Inc., Charlestown, MA, according to their standard laboratory procedures. The muscle specimen was minced and dissociated using digestive enzymes. The dissociated tissue was washed several times and filtered into a single-cell suspension. The expansion culture was initiated when the cells were plated into sterile tissue culture flasks in growth media for skeletal muscle myoblasts. The media were changed at regular intervals; the cells were harvested and replated according to cell confluence parameters. Final harvest was done after three to five passages. Myoblasts were identified using an immunohistochemical marker specific for desmin (DAKO) to identify cells committed to a myogenic differentiation. Specific cell lot release specifications (cell viability, cell identity, and sterility tests) were established before the start of the trial.

After a culturing period, the harvested cells were formulated in a specially designed transport/injectate media, transferred into a sterile 30-ml bag, and sent to our hospital packed in frozen gel ice packs (Figures 2 and 3). The method was validated to provide stability over a 96-hour period assuming controlled conditions.

2.5.   Transplantation

The proposed sites for cell transplantation were determined before the procedure by nuclear imaging. Following surgical exposure and direct visualization of the heart, these areas were reviewed and multiple needle insertions were placed.

At the time of the open surgical procedures (CABG or LVAD), cultured myoblasts were warmed to room temperature and injected into the surface of the infarcted area over a period of 15 seconds, using multiple injections at a concentration of 100 million cells per ml via a 30-gauge needle (Figure 4). Cell injections did not overlap and were performed on the beating heart. Patients in the CABG group were first removed from cardiopulmonary bypass, decannulated, and given protamine sulfate, which reduced the potential for epicardial bleeding at the injection sites.

The dosing schedule was proposed by the FDA to establish safety guidelines for cell injections, and was not intended to test the efficacy of the number of cells transplanted (Table 2). There was concern regarding the potential for arrhythmias with large cell doses, therefore an escalating dose schedule was selected. For the LVAD patients, arrhythmia was not as concerning as rhythm disturbances are common following LVAD placement and do not create serious consequences in these patients.

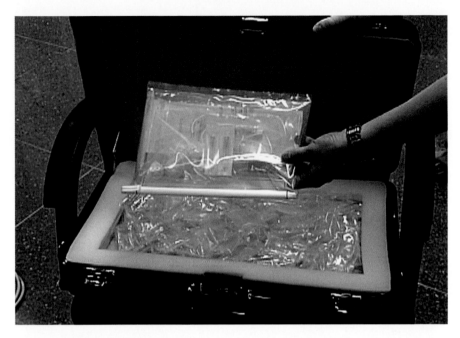

FIGURE 2. Photograph of transport case containing sterile, 30-ml cell bag packed in frozen gel packs.

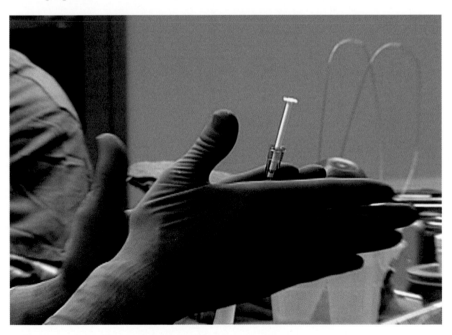

FIGURE 3. The process of thawing cells before transplantation is shown. After a warm cell emulsion is created, the 30-gauge needle is attached to the syringe for injection.

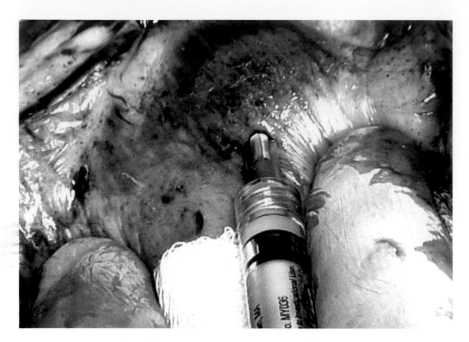

FIGURE 4. Multiple needle injections are performed over the selected areas of the myocardium. Oblique needle insertion creates a long channel for cell delivery.

3.   Results

3.1.   Demographics

We have treated a total of 28 patients using skeletal myoblast cell transplantation techniques during a CABG procedure (n=22) or LVAD procedure (n=6). The baseline demographics of the CABG patients are shown in Table 3. The LVAD group (n=6) was included only to establish proof of the engraftment concept, and demographics for these patients are not included in this chapter.

TABLE 2. Dosing parameters

Subjects	Cell dose
CABG group	
Subjects 1-3	10×10^6
Subjects 4-6	30×10^6
Subjects 7-9	100×10^6
Subjects 10-12	300×10^6
Subjects 13-22	300×10^6
LVAD group	
Subjects 1-6	300×10^6

TABLE 3. Demographics

Parameter	CABG group (n=22)
Age (years)	54.4 ± 11.3
Coronary stenosis (mean vessels)	3
NYHA score (mean)	1.9
Angina	20
Congestive heart failure	13
Hypertension	10
Diabetes	2
Previous percutaneous intervention	7
Previous CABG	2
Ventricular arrhythmia	5
Atrial arrhythmia	4
Existing ICD	1

The skeletal muscle biopsy was successful in all patients; one developed an insignificant hematoma following the procedure.

3.2.   Cell Culturing

Myoblast cultures made between 11 and 13 doublings, with an average doubling time of 24 hours. Analysis of the cultures before they were transplanted showed single cells and no fused multinucleated myoblasts. There was no bacterial or fungal contamination as determined by USP sterility and mycoplasma testing. The target cell dose was achieved in all samples except one—in this case, the patient required emergency LVAD surgery before the culture had adequate time to complete the necessary doublings.

3.3.   Feasibility

We evaluated the following in determining the feasibility of autologous skeletal myoblast transplantation in patients undergoing CABG or LVAD procedures: (1) ability to culture sufficient numbers of myoblasts; (2) ability to deliver myoblasts to the region of myocardial infarct; and (3) ability to demonstrate myoblast engraftment and viability.

As described in Section 3.2, target cell doses of cultured myoblasts were achieved in all but one case. We were able to deliver the myoblasts to the region of the myocardial scar in all patients (range: 3-30 injections), and there were no perioperative complications related to the injection of cells. The 30-gauge needle provided atraumatic entry and easy delivery. ECG monitoring of the injection did not reveal any evidence of rhythm disturbances during the procedure. Systolic blood pressure was, at times, slightly lower than normal (but never below 70mmHg) because injecting the cells in the optimal location sometimes required displacement of the heart. Such pressure changes were transitory.

Myoblast engraftment was demonstrated via histological evaluation of the hearts of three patients who underwent transplantation, and of the hearts of two patients who died (one LVAD patient is awaiting transplant as of this writing). Trichrome staining of the myocardial tissue clearly demonstrated engraftment of striated myotubes containing multiple nuclei developing within the fibrotic tissue; there was no evidence of lymphocyte infiltration. In addition, it did not appear that there was any myoblast migration into normal myocardial tissue. Further evaluation by immunostaining with a skeletal-muscle-reactive antimyosin (MY-32 antibody) confirmed myoblast engraftment (Figure 5).

Comparison of NYHA class at baseline (1.9) and 3 months (1.3) revealed significant improvement (p<0.01). The mean LVEF (via echocardiography) was 24.8 at baseline and 33.6 at 12 months (p<0.003). LV dimension (n=11) was 6.4 at baseline compared with 5.9 at 3 months (p=0.01). PET scanning

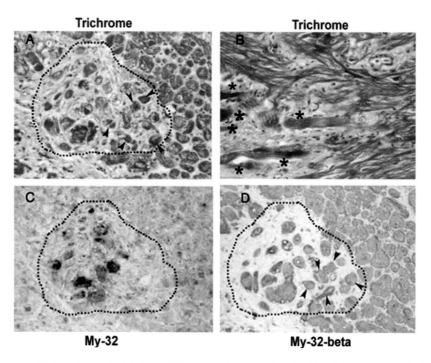

FIGURE 5. Surviving skeletal myofibers are shown stained with trichrome (panels A and B). Skeletal-specific fast myosin MY-32 is shown in panel C, and myosin heavy chain beta slow is shown in panel D. Panels A, C, and D show adjacent sections from the same graft site, and B shows a different graft site from the same patient; the myofibers can be seen in a longitudinal profile. The alignment between grafted myofibers and host myofibers is striking. The area of graft is marked by the dotted line in A, C, and D; individual skeletal myofibers that stained with slow myosin and fast myosin (MY-32, C) are marked by arrowhead.

and SPECT analysis at baseline and 6 months were performed in 7 patients (Figures 6 and 7). Evidence of cell viability in the region of transplantation was seen in three of these patients, and reperfusion was observed in all the CABG patients tested. Cardiac MRI was performed in 4 patients and showed the size of the scar had decreased from baseline (Figure 8).

3.4. Safety

The transplant procedure was well tolerated by patients undergoing CABG and LVAD. No bleeding was encountered except for occasional leakage from a surface vein. Placement of a thrombin-soaked gel-foam pad provided sufficient hemostasis in these cases.

In the CABG group, the average follow-up was 20 months (range 6-40 months). One patient suffered an MI and cardiac arrest at 12 days. He was a 71-year old male with coronary artery disease who had previously undergone a CABG procedure in 1981, a redo in 2003, and was suffering from CHF with a baseline ejection fraction of 35% prior to the third CABG and cell transplantation (dose = 300×10^6 cells).

There were five patients in the CABG group who experienced arrhythmias that were determined to be not related to cell transplant by the safety board. Three of these patients had non-sustained ventricular tachycardia (NSVT) before and following the procedure and were managed medically. One patient who had cardiac resynchronization with an internal cardioverter-defibrillator

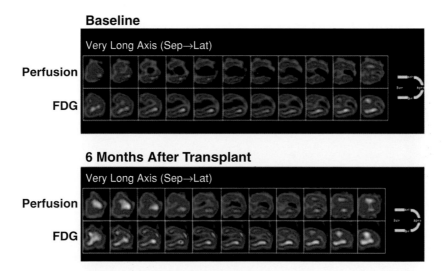

FIGURE 6. Baseline (top) and 6-month follow-up (bottom) showing perfusion and PET scan imaging. There is a matched perfusion defect in the anterior wall, and 6 months following transplantation, there is an FDG uptake increase in the anterior wall.

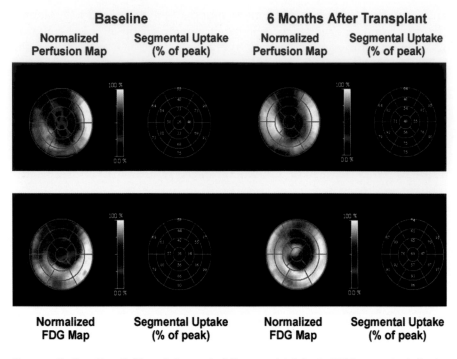

FIGURE 7. Baseline (left) and 6-month follow-up (right) via PET scan. At left, the blue scar is seen in the anterior wall, and there is a decrease in FDG uptake. At right, the size of scar has decreased.

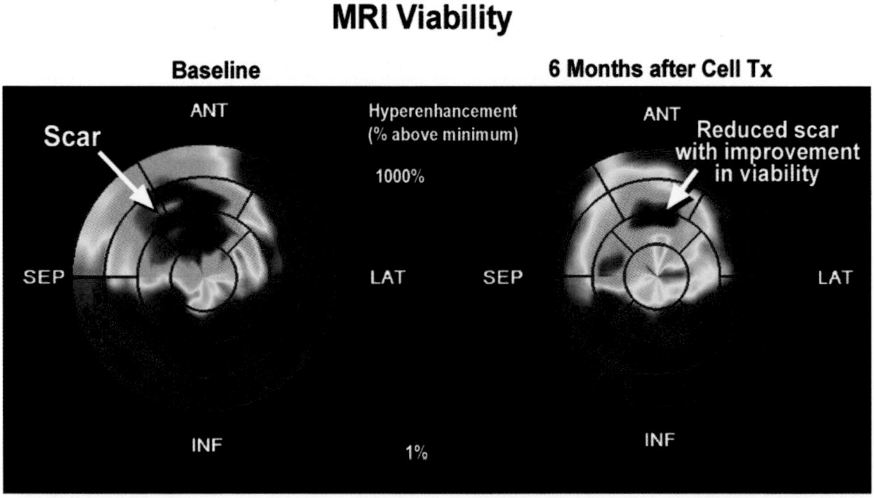

MRI Viability

FIGURE 8. Baseline (left) and 6-month follow-up (right) showing MRI of blue scar in the anterior wall. At 6-months, the size of scar had decreased from baseline.

(ICD) before myoblast transplantation experienced two episodes of ICD firing 9 months after the transplant, and another patient with positive T-wave alterations following cell transplant had demonstrable ischemia in the LIMA graft and received an ICD before discharge. The fifth patient developed NSVT 6 months following the procedure and was managed successfully with amiodarone. Two additional patients experienced arrhythmias that the safety board ruled possibly related to cell transplantation. Both patients had NSVT, one at 7 days and the other at 10 days following CABG and cell transplant. An internal cardioverter-defibrillator was successfully placed in each patient.

   In the LVAD group, one patient had deteriorating cardiac function and required emergency surgery before the cell culture had reached its target cell volume dose. Overall, there were two deaths in the LVAD group, one on day 5 post transplant from complications of an acute right cerebral infarct and thrombus of the LVAD device, and the other from an infection and sepsis (day 68 post transplant). One LVAD patient is still awaiting transplant. The deaths were considered unrelated to the myoblast transplant by the safety board. Although there were instances of arrhythmia noted in patients in the LVAD group, these are an expected consequence of LVAD placement and operation.

4.   Discussion

4.1.   Overview

Congestive heart failure is often difficult to treat effectively, and the patient's condition inevitably deteriorates over time. Successful long-term therapies for this malady have been elusive, and cardiac transplantation is not a viable option for the majority of patients with CHF due to the limited availability of organs. Preclinical success with autologous skeletal myoblast transplantation has encouraged its use in patients with serious myocardial damage, and the early clinical work has been promising.

4.2.   Feasibility and Safety

Our own results suggest that epicardial transplantation of skeletal myoblasts in conjunction with a CABG or LVAD procedure is feasible and safe. The harvesting of skeletal muscle was achieved without incident, and culturing of the cells resulted in large numbers of viable myoblasts. Their subsequent transplantation was achieved without incident, and the procedure was brief, adding only ~20 minutes to the operative time. Bleeding in heparinized patients was not a problem in either the CABG or LVAD groups. Engraftment and viability of the myoblasts were demonstrated in follow-up, and there were no deaths attributed to the procedure. Myoblast cells survived in scar tissue and formed myotubes. More than 60% of the protein expressed by the engrafted tissue showed the fatigue resistant myosin 32-beta (a slow-twitch protein). We interpreted this to mean that the engrafted tissue resembled cardiac tissue.

Although our study population included patients whose myocardial function was severely compromised, non-sustained ventricular tachycardia possibly related to cell transplant was seen in only two patients. The experience of other investigators,[3-5] however, has sensitized researchers to the possibility that serious arrhythmias may be related to myoblast transplantation. Both sustained and non-sustained ventricular tachycardias have been reported, leading some investigators to recommend that ICDs be implanted routinely during the myoblast transplantation procedure.

We were particularly interested in learning more about arrhythmias related to myoblast transplantation as it appears that they may be the only adverse complication of the procedure, at least in the early and/or intermediate recovery stages. Patients suffering from extreme myocardial impairment often experience arrhythmias associated with CABG or LVAD, even in the absence of a cell transplantation procedure. Logically, we might assume a greater propensity for ventricular ectopies and arrhythmias following implantation of new myoblasts, but there is no evidence that the new cell populations have any ability to form Connexin-43 to stimulate arrhythmia. It may also be hypothesized that needle injection and subsequent delivery of non-viable cells could incite an implantation reaction that would precipitate ectopy, but we have no data that support this theory. Indeed, our results suggest that the incidence of ventricular tachycardia following epicardial injection of myoblasts is low.

4.3.   Limitations

The primary purpose of this study was to test feasibility and safety of harvesting techniques, cell culturing procedures, and myoblast transplantation. The trial was not designed or powered to test the efficacy of myoblast transplantation as a treatment for myocardial dysfunction or failure. Although we have reported results of baseline and follow-up evaluations that measure cardiac function, we cannot make any specific conclusions about efficacy, especially regarding patients in the CABG group, as improvement in LV function is well-recognized following revascularization. The LVAD group was included to establish proof of the engraftment concept and, therefore, we have presented only the results of histologic studies confirming engraftment in these patients.

5.   Conclusions

Epicardial transplantation of skeletal myoblasts in conjunction with a CABG or LVAD procedure is feasible and safe, and it does not appear that cell transplantation poses a substantial risk of life-threatening arrhythmia in this small evaluation. Further study of the efficacy of myoblast transplantation is warranted, and we are now involved in investigations of catheter-based delivery systems and imaging protocols that support percutaneous skeletal myoblast transplantation (as described in "Percutaneous Myoblast Transplantation", chapter 14 of this text).

6. References

1. American Heart Association. AHA Heart and Stroke Statistics-2004 Update.
2. Taylor DA, Atkins BZ, Hungspreugs P, et al. Regenerating functional myocardium: improved performance after skeletal myoblast transplantation, *Nat. Med.* 4, 929–1033 (1998).
3. Dib N, Diethrich EB, Campbell A, et al. Endoventricular transplantation of allogenic skeletal myoblasts in a porcine model of myocardial infarction, *J. Endovasc. Ther.* 9, 313–19 (2002).
4. Menasche P, Hagege AA, Scorsin M, et al. Myoblast transplantation for heart failure, *Lancet* 357, 279–80 (2001).
5. Menasche P, Hagege AA, Vilquin JT, et al. Autologous skeletal myoblast transplantation for severe postinfarction left ventricular dysfunction, *J. Am. Coll. Cardiol.* 41, 1078–83 (2003).
6. Herreros J, Prosper F, Perez A, et al. Autologous intramyocardial injection of cultured skeletal-muscle-derived stem cells in patients with non-acute myocardial infarction, *E. Heart J.* 24, 2012–20 (2003).
7. Smits PC, van Geuns RJM, Poldermans D, et al. Catheter-based intramyocardial injection of autologous skeletal myoblasts as a primary treatment of ischemic heart failure, *J. Am. Coll. Cardiol.* 42, 2063–69 (2003).

Progenitor Cells

8
Progenitor Cells for Cardiac Regeneration

ANA SÁNCHEZ AND JAVIER GARCÍA-SANCHO[1]

1. Introduction: Different Choices Of Stem Cells

Regenerative Medicine uses the body's own stem cells and growth factors to re-generate damaged tissues or organs. Because of the relative simplicity of heart organization and function, this organ is a most adequate target for cell therapy. Preliminary results have been promising, so that the idea has become increasingly popular. The purpose of this review is to provide the background regarding the use of different stem cell types for cardiac regeneration. For other aspects, the reader is referred to excellent recent reviews.[1-3]

Stem cells are cells able to divide and self-perpetuate and to differentiate to specialized cells. They do so by a process of asymmetric division, in which one of the daughter cells remains undifferentiated and maintains the stem cell pool whereas the other one differentiates (Figure. 1A). Cells obtained from the fertilized oocyte before the first two divisions are totipotent (able to generate a full embryo). After about 4 days, the blastocyst forms. Then, the cells from the inner cell mass (ICM, which is to become the embryo) begin to specialize to form 3 different layers: ectoderm, endoderm and mesoderm (Figure. 1B). Embryonic stem (ES) cells obtained from the ICM are pluripotent, able to differentiate into almost any cell of the three germ layers. Once the three layers have formed, stem cells in each layer are multipotential: they can produce a limited range of differentiated cell lineages appropriate to their location (for example, haematopoietic stem cells from the bone marrow can generate all the blood cell types). Finally, many adult tissues possess unipotential stem cells, capable of generating only one cell type (for example skin epidermis, intestinal mucosa, liver, skeletal muscle). In the adult organism the stem cells are often clustered in niches with a peculiar microenvironment that governs their behavior. The orthodox view establishes that the daughter cells undergo differentiation to a mature cell lineage of the same germ layer (Figure. 1B). However, on

---

1 Instituto de Biología y Genética Molecular (IBGM), Universidad de Valladolid y CSIC, Departamento de Fisiología, Facultad de Medicina, E-47005 Valladolid, Spain.

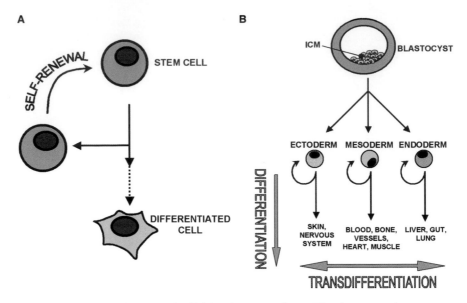

FIGURE 1. **A.** Asymmetric division in stem cells. **B.** The three germ layers.

the basis of recent observations, it has been proposed that, under the pressure of an unusual microenvironment (for example, tissue damage), stem cells from a given germ layer could somehow produce mature cells corresponding to another layer, a process called transdifferentiation. This is a very controversial issue, as others defend that the phenotypic changes attributed to "transdifferentiation" are actually due to fusion of the nuclei of the stem cell and a differentiated cell of a different layer.

When trying to regenerate damaged tissue, we have three different choices for stem cells:

Resident stem (RS) cells. Some tissues such as skin, intestinal mucosa or liver easily regenerate by this mechanism. If we could find a way to stimulate this mechanism in other tissues, for example using the adequate trophic factors, this one would be a most convenient method for regenerative medicine. It was thought that some tissues had no resident stem cells, but this is proving false.

Embryonic stem (ES) cells. Since ES cells are pluripotent this approach would be most versatile, as the same cells and procedures could be used for different tissues. The main practical problem is immunogenecity and rejection, as allogenic (from one person to another) transplantations should be done in most of the cases.

Multipotential adult stem (AS) cells are an excellent option when possible. For example, bone marrow transplantation for regeneration of blood cells is a well-established treatment for leukemia. Recent reports suggest that plasticity of adult stem cells is wider than previously thought, and that they can generate cells of lineages not corresponding to their organ of origin. With AS cells, autologous (patient's own cells) transplantation protocols are possible, thus circumventing immunological problems.

2.   Resident Stem Cells are Present in Heart

It is generally accepted that myocytes of the adult heart are terminally differentiated and unable to divide, and that the myocardium lacks a stem cell population able to generate new myocytes. Recent data suggest, on the contrary, that myocyte death and regeneration are part of the normal homeostasis of the heart.[4,5] A study of chimerism in males transplanted with female hearts showed that more than 10% of the cells displayed the Y chromosome,[6] suggesting a substantial rate of renewal of the cardiac tissue. Measurements of the rates of mitotic division and death in normal mouse heart suggested that the whole ventricular mass was renewed in 4-12 months. Recently, similar measurements have been performed in the male heart, suggesting that the whole ventricular mass is renewed within about 10 years in the normal heart and less than 6 months after myocardial infarction.[4] The presence of dividing cells in heart and its increase (×50) after myocardial infarction has been documented in man and mouse.[7,8]

Very recently, Anversa and colleagues have identified cells with the properties of cardiac stem cells. They were self-renewing, clonogenic, and multipotent, giving rise to myocytes, smooth muscle, and endothelial cells.[9] These cells expressed stem cell markers and telomerase, and accumulated in clusters in which different degrees of transition towards myocytes could be documented. The number of these stem-like cells increased more than 10 times in patients with aortic stenosis, suggesting that they are related to the cardiac hyperplasia that accompanies this disease.[10] The presence of cells expressing stem cell markers (c-kit, MDR1, sca-1) has also been detected in the normal heart.[4] It is not clear at present whether these cardiac stem-like cells are a resident population of embryonic origin or if they come from blood and colonize the cardiac tissue (Figure 2; see below)[1] Understanding the regulation of cardiac renewal will provide not only a better understanding of cardiac homeostasis but will also open new pathways for therapeutic intervention.

3.   Embryonic Stem Cells

ES cells are pluripotent and have the highest differentiation potential. Other advantages of these cells are that they are easy to obtain and can be frozen for storage and expanded *in vitro*. Since telomerase activity is preserved, ES cells can proliferate indefinitely. The normal karyotype is usually preserved, although some cases of genomic instability have been reported.[1,3] The knowledge on the mechanisms of growing and differentiation is very poor, but this also applies to the other stem cell types. The very scarce clinical experience

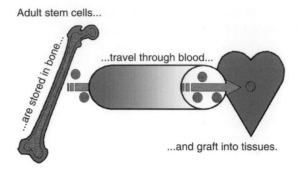

FIGURE 2. Bone marrow could act as a systemic supplier of progenitor cells.

and the potential to form teratomas *in vivo* is a major concern, and the ethical and legal uncertainties may pose many practical problems. Due to these shortcomings the use of ES cells in patients may take longer than other alternatives. On the other hand, the use of allogenic (from a different person) ES cells, which will apply for most of the cases, may occasionally be rejected because of the expression of MHC proteins differing from the host ones. This immunological disparity can be overcome by using the technique of nuclear transfer (NT). The technique requires the injection of a nucleus obtained from a host's cell into an enucleated oocyte to generate an embryo with the same genetic load as the host (except for mitochondrial DNA). This elegant strategy could be used for derivation of isogenic or 'tailor-made' hES cells.[11] Although preparation of NT embryos has been successful in animals, additional complications could be found in primates.[12]

It has been reported that about 10% of spheres derived from human ES cells differentiate towards cardiomyocyte spontaneously.[13] Similarly, co-culture of hES cells with endoderm promotes cardiac differentiation.[14] Both mouse and rat ES cells and fetal cells have been tested *in vivo* in nude rats with ischemic heart lesions. This treatment prevented dilatation, and improved coronary flow and cardiac function,[15-18] but hES cells have not been tested in human patients yet. Successful use of mice stem cells derived by nuclear transplantation to heal experimental myocardial infarction has been published recently.[19] These mouse NT-ES cells formed both muscle and vessels, and coupled electrically and mechanically to the surrounding tissue. Cardiac regeneration (as much as 38% of the scar at 1 month) resulted in an improvement of ventricular hemodynamics and in a reduction of diastolic wall stress.

4.   Adult Stem Cells

The idea that bone marrow progenitors could generate cells of nonlymphohematopoitec lineages came from elegant genetic studies of sex-mismatched bone marrow transplants. These studies evidenced that cells bearing Y chromosome were present in liver, brain, heart and other tissues after male-into-female bone marrow transplantation.[1,20-22] Consistently, in male patients who had received a heart from a female donor, Y chromosome could be detected in a up to 10% of the cells (cardiomyocytes, smooth muscle or endothelial[6]; although there were discrepancies among different laboratories on the frequency of Y chromosome expression.[23,24] The simplest interpretation of these data is that bone marrow progenitors are able to transdifferentiate into terminally differentiated cells ascribed to a different germ layer (Figure. 1B). In the same line of thinking, the ability of bone marrow cells (BMC) to regenerate the myocardium lost during a ischemic accident was demonstrated by Orlic et al.[25] in the mouse, where purified hematopietic stem cells (Lin-, $ckit^{POS}$) grafted in the damaged tissue, transformed into both myocytes and vessels and partly restored function. Consistent results have been attained in other animal studies with different BMC fractions,[26-28] other haematopoietic cells fractions[29] or endothelial cell fractions obtained from peripheral blood.[30-32] Thus it would seem that both haematopietic and endothelial stem cell lineages can evolve towards cardiac phenotypes. Differentiation to cardiomyocytes "in vitro" has been reported to happen from endothelial precursors,[33] from peripheral blood,[34] monocytes[35] mesenchimal stem cells obtained from bone marrow[36,37] or from adipose tissue.[38-42] Conflicting results have been obtained in several studies. Particularly, Murry et al.[43] were unable to find differentiation of haematopoietic stem cells towards cardiomyocytes in the infarcted mouse heart, instead they evolved towards traditional haematopoietic fates.[44]

5.   Transdifferentiation *Vs.* Fusion

The validity of stem-cell plasticity as a mechanism for generating differentiated cells has been questioned. It has been suggested that previously overlooked cell fusion may explain the findings interpreted as transdifferentiation.[45,46] Fusion was documented *in vitro*[47,48] and *in vivo* in studies of mice with a deficit of fumaryl-acetoacetate hydrolase (FAH), a fatal metabolic liver disease.[49,50] Most of the "fused" cells had tetraploid or hexaploid DNA content. Cytogenetic analysis of tetraploid hepatocytes obtained from male recipients transplanted with female donor mice showed XXXY karyotypes, indicative of fusion between donor (XX) and host (XY) cells.[49] It has been claimed, however, that at least part of the genomic instability may be due to the FAH deficit itself rather than to the fusion process.[51] On the other hand, transformation persisted, but no fusion could be documented, when using a more purified fraction of heamatopietic stem cells (HSCs), suggesting that the target for fusion could be another cell, not responsible for the transformation process.[52] In these experiments, the HSCs were separated from the possible fusion targets by a membrane that did not allow cell passage. In addition, FISH analysis of tetraploid cells of female receptors that had received male HSCs showed XYXY karyotype, which is not compatible with fusion. Finally, the transformation rates observed (3-7%)

are much larger than the fusion rates reported (0.001-0.01%).[52] It has been reported that in the heart most of the newly formed myocytes have a diploid DNA content and a cell volume much smaller than the host myocytes.[4]

Using sensitive genetic procedures for detecting fusion events (for example, Cre/lox recombination) low-frequency fusions with bone marrow cells have been demonstrated in the liver, heart and central nervous system.[53-55] However, using similar procedures, other authors found stem cell transformations that could not be attributed to cell fusion.[52,56-59] There is also a discrepancy in the transformation frequencies. Whereas defenders of "transdifferentiation" generally find transformation frequencies close to 1 %, "fusion" is reported to be much rarer (0.01% or less). This could have tremendous importance to determine the practical efficacy of a putative therapeutic procedure, because the hybrid cells resulting from fusion have limited potential for multiplication.[5]

Is there a way to reconcile these diverging views? The different outcomes could be made compatible if the rate of "transdifferentiation" was extremely variable depending on the circumstances: for example, practically non-existent in the normal condition and very much stimulated by the peculiar microenvironment generated near damaged tissue. Should this hypothesis apply, some researchers could see exclusively cell fusion in studies done in the normal condition[53] or with "lesions" that somehow do not fulfill the requisites required to promote "transdifferentiation". On the contrary, for other researchers "fusion" would be hidden by the much more frequent "transdifferentiation" generated by tissue damage. Consistently with this interpretation, it has been shown that hematopoietic stem cells (from transgenic mice expressing β-galactosidase) massively differentiate to renal tubular cells in host mouse kidney subjected to a ischemia-reperfusion lesion. Up to 8% of the cells expressed donor marker in the damaged kidney. In contrast, labeling of the contralateral kidney was extremely low.[60] It has also been reported in humans that labeling with Ki-67 (a marker of cell mitosis) in cardiomyocytes increases more than 50 times (reaching up to 4% of all the cells) in the area close to a myocardial infarction.[7]

6.   Clinical Trials

The reports of improvement of cardiac function in animal studies led to several trials in patients with either acute myocardial infarction or chronic ischemic heart disease (Table 1). Most of the studies have used complete bone marrow fractions containing all the mononuclear bone marrow cells, which contain both hematopoietic and stromal progenitors. In one case, endothelial cell progenitors (AC133+) were selected.[61] In a few cases progenitors were obtained from peripheral blood during apheresis.[62,63] The origin of the cells, either bone marrow or peripheral blood, did not seem to make any difference in the output.[62] The end-point of follow up varied between 3 and 18 months.

TABLE 1. Clinical trials of cardiac regeneration.

STUDY	Stem cell source & (Administration pathway)	(n)	Perfusion/ metabolism	Ejection fraction	Wall thickness	Restenosis
Acute Myocardial Infarction						
Strauer et al. (2002)[67]	BMCs (IC)	10	+	+	n.d.	n.d.
Assmus et al. (2002)[62]	9 BMCs (IC) and 11 PB (IC)	20	+	+	n.d.	n.d.
Stamm et al. (2003)[61]	BMCs AC133+ (IM-S)	6	+	+	n.d.	n.d.
Wollert et al. (2004)[64]	BMCs (IC)	30	+	+	n.d.	Normal
Fernández -Avilés et al. (2004)[65]	BMCs (IC)	20	+	+	+	Normal
Kang et al. (2004)[63]	PB & G-CSF (IC)	10	+	+	n.d.	Increased
Chronic Ischemic Heart Disease						
Hamano et al. (2001)[68]	BMCs (IM-S)	5	+	n.d.	n.d.	n.d.
Tse et al. (2003)[66]	BMCs (IM-PC)	8	+	n.d.	+	n.d.
Perin et al. (2003)[69]	BMCs (IM-PC)	11	+	+	n.d.	n.d.
Fuch et al. (2003)[70]	BMCs (IM-PC)	10	+	n.d.	n.d.	n.d.

BMCs, Blood Marrow Cells; PB, Peripheral Blood; G-CSF, Granulocyte-Colony Stimulating Factor; IC, Intracoronary; IM, Intramyocardial; S, surgical; PC, percutaneous; n.d., not determined

Importantly, no adverse effects were reported in most of the studies, except for an increase of the rate of in-stent restenosis in a series of patients treated with blood-derived progenitors mobilized with Granulocyte-Colony-Stimulating Factor (G-CSF).[63] In contrast, in another two studies using BMCs obtained without G-CSF priming, the rate of restenosis was the same as in the control patients receiving standard therapy.[64,65] In all the cases, there was indication of improvement of heart perfusion and/or metabolism and indexes of ventricular function, such as the ejection fraction or wall motion, were also improved. In a few studies the thickness of the ventricular wall was followed by magnetic resonance imaging measurements and found to increase significantly 3 to 12 months after BMC treatment.[65,66] In the patients with acute myocardial infarction the mode of administration has been mainly by intracoronary delivery to the culprit region during catheterization. Percutaneous intramyocardial or surgical intramyocardial delivery at the time of coronary artery bypass grafting were the preferred procedures in patients with chronic ischemic heart disease (Table 1).

Skeletal myoblasts have shown their ability to improve cardiac function in animal models of ischemic heart failure.[71,72] For assays in humans, autologous satellite cells prepared from a muscular biopsy were expanded *in vitro* and implanted during bypass surgery. It has been reported that the areas of heart that received the myoblasts regained part of the functional capacity.[73] A major caveat is the lack of electrical connections between skeletal muscle cells and cardiac myocytes, and this could favor arrhythmia,[74] however, a recent trial did not find this secondary effect.[75]

7.   Future Prospectives

Autologous bone marrow transplantation has been revealed as a feasible and safe procedure to improve cardiac function after acute myocardial infarction. The final decision on efficacy should be based on the results of randomized, controlled and double-blind clinical trials. Probably, the most generalized protocol (mononuclear fraction of BMCs given by cardiac catheterization) should be used for these studies. In the mean time, the cell process and the delivery method should be simplified.

BMCs and peripheral blood fractions obtained by apheresis have been tested extensively in many thousands of patients for treatment of hematological diseases with little secondary effects. It is clear, for example that BMC transplantation alone does not significantly increase the risk of cancer.[76,77] Alternative sources such as umbilical cord blood or lipoaspirates are highly promising, but will require extensive animal study before use in humans.

Regarding the administration pathway, intracoronary delivery to the culprit area by catheterization seems to be the procedure of choice for acute myocardial infarction, whereas transendocardial injection into ischemic areas after electromechanical mapping of the ventricle[69] seems most adequate for chronic ischemic heart disease. Endovenous administration of progenitors would be much simpler, but the efficacy of this procedure has not been tested. Mobilization and/or priming of stem cells by cytokines[78] is a most promising field for basic research, but present knowledge is not adequate to test it in clinical trials.

Embryonic stem cells are still far from clinical assays, but deserve extensive animal research as this is the stem cell type with higher differentiation potential. Nuclear transfer techniques, once technical problems are solved, will provide a convenient route for the creation of immunologically compatible stem cells from adult somatic cells.[79] Preliminary animal data are encouraging,[19] but extensive research will be required before tested in humans.

A new concept that deserves much attention is one of nuclear reprogramming.[80] All the genetic information necessary for the phenotypic change of "transdifferentiation" is already present in the DNA of all cells. A most elegant procedure would be to "reprogram" the nucleus to express the proteins of the required tissue by adding the adequate transcriptional regulators.

Preliminary results suggest that nuclear reprogramming of adult stem cells[81] or even of somatic cells[82] is possible.

8.   Acknowledgements

Financial support from Instituto de Salud Carlos III, Junta de Castilla y León and Fundación de Investigación Médica Mutua Madrileña Automovilista is gratefully acknowledged.

9.   References

1. Körbling, M., and Estrov, Z. (2003) Adult Stem Cells for Tissue Repair—A New Therapeutic Concept?, *N Engl J Med* 349:570–82.
2. Strauer BE, Kornowski R (2003) Stem Cell Therapy in Perspective. *Circulation* 107:929–934
3. Mathur A, Martin JF. (2004) Stem cells and repair of the heart. *Lancet* 364:183–92.
4. Nadal-Ginard B, Kajstura J, Leri A, Anversa P. (2003) Myocyte death, growth, and regeneration in cardiac hypertrophy and failure. *Circ Res.* 92:139–150.
5. Anversa P, Sussman MA, Bolli R. (2004) Molecular genetic advances in cardiovascular medicine: focus on the myocyte. *Circulation* 109:2832–8.
6. Quaini F, Urbanek K, Beltrami AP, Finato N, Beltrami CA, Nadal-Ginard B, Kajstura J, Leri A, Anversa P. (2002) Chimerism of the transplanted heart. *New Engl J Med.* 346:5–15.
7. Beltrami AP, Urbanek K, Kajstura J, Yan SM, Finato N, Bussani R, Nadal-Ginard B, Silvestri F, Leri A, Beltrami A, Anversa P. (2001) Evidence that human cardiac myocytes divide after myocardial infarction. *N Engl J Med.* 344: 1750–1757.
8. Anversa P, Nadal-Ginard B. (2002) Myocyte renewal and ventricular remodeling. *Nature* 415:240–243.
9. Beltrami AP, Barlucchi L, Torella D, Baker M, Limana F, Chimenti S, Kasahara H, Rota M, Musso E, Urbanek K, Leri A, Kajstura J, Nadal-Ginard B, Anversa P. (2003) Adult cardiac stem cells are multipotent and support myocardial regeneration. *Cell* 114: 763–776.
10. Urbanek K, Quaini F, Tasca G, Torella D, Castaldo C, Nadal-Ginard B, Leri A, Kajstura J, Quaini E, Anversa P. (2003) Intense myocyte formation from cardiac stem cells in human cardiac hypertrophy. *Proc Natl Acad Sci U S A.* 100:10440–5.
11. Rhind SM, Taylor JE, De Sousa PA, King TJ, McGarry M & Wilmut I (2003) Human cloning: can it be made safe? *Nature Review Genetics* 4:855–864.
12. Simerly C, Dominko T, Navara C, Payne C, Capuano S, Gosman G, Chong KY, Takahashi D, Chace C, Compton D, Hewitson L, Schatten G. (2003) Molecular correlates of primate nuclear transfer failures. *Science* 300:297.
13. Kehat I, Kenyagin-Karsenti D, Snir M, Segev H, Amit M, Gepstein A, Livne E, Binah O, Itskovitz-Eldor J, Gepstein L. (2001) Human embryonic stem cells can differentiate into myocytes with structural and functional properties of cardiomyocytes. *J Clin Invest.* 108:407–414.
14. Mummery C, Ward-van Oostwaard D, Doevendans P, Spijker R, van den Brink S, Hassink R, van der Heyden M, Opthof T, Pera M, de la Riviere AB, Passier R,

Tertoolen L. (2002) Differentiation of human embryonic stem cells to cardiomyocytes: role of coculture with visceral endoderm-like cells. *Circulation* 107:2733–40.

15. Sakai T, Li RK, Weisel RD, Mickle DA, Jia ZQ, Tomita S, Kim EJ, Yau TM. (1999) Fetal cell transplantation: a comparison of three cell types. *J Thorac Cardiovasc Surg.* 118:715–24

16. Li RK, Mickle DA, Weisel RD, Rao V, Jia ZQ (2001) Optimal time for cardiomyocyte transplantation to maximize myocardial function after left ventricular injury. *Ann Thorac Surg.* 72:1957–63

17. Min JY, Yang Y, Sullivan MF, Ke Q, Converso KL, Chen Y, Morgan JP, Xiao YF. (2003) Long-term improvement of cardiac function in rats after infarction by transplantation of embryonic stem cells. *J Thorac Cardiovasc Surg.* 125:361–9

18. Kehat I, Gepstein L. (2003) Human embryonic stem cells for myocardial regeneration. *Heart Fail Rev.*8:229–36

19. Lanza R, Moore MA, Wakayama T, Perry AC, Shieh JH, Hendrikx J, Leri A, Chimenti S, Monsen A, Nurzynska D, West MD, Kajstura J, Anversa P. (2004) Regeneration of the infarcted heart with stem cells derived by nuclear transplantation. *Circ Res.* 94:820–7.

20. Körbling M, Katz R, Khanna A, Ruifrok AC, Rondon G, Albitar M, Champlin RE, Estrov Z. (2002) Hepatocytes and epithelial cells of donor origin in recipients of peripheral blood stem cells. *N Engl J Med.* 346:738–746.

21. Mezey E, Key S, Vogelsang G, Szalayova I, Lange GD, Crain B. (2003) Transplanted bone marrow generates new neurons in human brains. *Proc Natl Acad Sci USA* 100:1364–9.

22. Weimann JM, Johansson CB, Trejo A, Blau HM. (2003b) Stable reprogrammed heterokaryons form spontaneously in Purkinje neurons after bone marrow transplant *Nature Cell Biol.* 5:959–966.

23. Laflamme MA, Myerson D, Saffitz JE, Murry CE. (2002) Evidence for cardiomyocyte repopulation by extracardiac progenitors in transplanted human hearts. *Circ Res.* 90:634–640

24. Taylor, DA, Hruban R, Rodriguez, ER, Goldschmidt-Clermont PJ. (2002) Cardiac chimerism as a mechanism for self-repair: does it happen and if so to what degree? *Circulation* 106:2–4.

25. Orlic D, Kajstura J, Chimenti S, Jakoniuk I, Anderson SM, Li B, Pickel J, McKay R, Nadal-Ginard B, Bodine DM, Leri A, Anversa P. (2001a) Bone marrow cells regenerate infarcted myocardium. *Nature* 410:701–705.

26. Tomita S, Mickle DA, Weisel RD, Jia ZQ, Tumiati LC, Allidina Y, Liu P, Li RK. (2002) Improved heart function with myogenesis and angiogenesis after autologous porcine bone marrow stromal cell transplantation. *J Thorac Cardiovasc Surg.* 123:1132–1140.

27. Toma C, Pittenger MF, Cahill KS. (2002) Human mesenchymal stem cells differentiate to a cardiomyocyte phenotype in the adult murine heart. *Circulation* 105:93–98

28. Mangi AA, Noiseux N, Kong K, He H, Rezvani N, Ingwall JS, Dzau VJ. (2003) Mesenchymal stem cells modified with Akt prevent remodeling and restore performance of infracted hearts. Nat Med. 9:1195–1201.

29. Jackson KA, Majka SM, Wang H, Pocius J, Hartley CJ, Majesky MW, Entman ML, Michael LH, Hirschi KK, Goodell MA. (2001) Regeneration of ischemic cardiac muscle and vascular endothelium by adult stem cells. *J Clin Invest.* 107:1395–402.

30. Yeh ET, Zhang S, Wu HD, Körbling M, Willerson JT, Estrov Z (2003) Transdifferentiation of human peripheral blood CD34+-enriched cell population into cardiomyocytes, endothelial cells, and smooth muscle cells in vivo. *Circulation* 108:2070–3.
31. Kawamoto A, Tkebuchava T, Yamaguchi J, Nishimura H, Yoon YS, Milliken C, Uchida S, Masuo O, Iwaguro H, Ma H, Hanley A, Silver M, Kearney M, Losordo DW, Isner JM, Asahara T. (2003) Intramyocardial transplantation of autologous endothelial progenitor cells for therapeutic neovascularization of myocardial ischemia. *Circulation* 107:461–8.
32. Szmitko PE, Fedak PW, Weisel RD, Stewart DJ, Kutryk MJ, Verma S. (2003) Endothelial progenitor cells: new hope for a broken heart. Circulation. 107:3093–100.
33. Condorelli G, Borello U, De Angelis L, Latronico M, Sirabella D, Coletta M, Galli R, Balconi G, Follenzi A, Frati G, Cusella De Angelis MG, Gioglio L, Amuchastegui S, Adorini L, Naldini L, Vescovi A, Dejana E, Cossu G. (2001) Cardiomyocytes induce endothelial cells to trans-differentiate into cardiac muscle: implications for myocardium regeneration. *Proc Natl Acad Sci U S A.* 98:10733–10738.
34. Badorff C, Brandes RP, Popp R, Rupp S, Urbich C, Aicher A, Fleming I, Busse R, Zeiher AM, Dimmeler S. (2003). Transdifferentiation of blood-derived human adult endothelial progenitor cells into functionally active cardiomyocytes. *Circulation* 107:1024–1032
35. Zhao Y, Glesne D, Huberman E. (2003) A human peripheral blood monocyte-derived subset acts as pluripotent stem cells. *Proc Natl Acad Sci USA.* 100:2426–31.
36. Rangappa S, Entwistle JW, Wechsler AS, Kresh JY. (2003a) Cardiomyocyte-mediated contact programs human mesenchymal stem cells to express cardiogenic phenotype. *J Thorac Cardiovasc Surg.* 126:124–32.
37. Pittenger MF, Martin BJ. (2004) Mesenchymal stem cells and their potential as cardiac therapeutics. *Circ Res.* 95:9–20.
38. Zuk PA, Zhu M, Ashjian P, De Ugarte DA, Huang JI, Mizuno H, Alfonso ZC, Fraser JK, Benhaim P, Hedrick MH. (2002) Human adipose tissue is a source of multipotent stem cells. *Mol Biol Cell.* 13:4279–95
39. Rangappa S, Fen C, Lee EH, Bongso A, Wei EK. (2003b) Transformation of adult mesenchymal stem cells isolated from the fatty tissue into cardiomyocytes. *Ann Thorac Surg* 75:775–9.
40. De Ugarte DA, Morizono K, Elbarbary A, Alfonso Z, Zuk PA, Zhu M, Dragoo JL, Ashjian P, Thomas B, Benhaim P, Chen I, Fraser J, Hedrick MH. (2003) Comparison of multi-lineage cells from human adipose tissue and bone marrow. *Cells Tissues Organs.* 174:101–109.
41. Planat-Benard V, Menard C, Andre M, Puceat M, Perez A, Garcia-Verdugo JM, Penicaud L, Casteilla L. (2004) Spontaneous cardiomyocyte differentiation from adipose tissue stroma cells. *Circ Res.* 94:223–9.
42. Xu, W., Zhang, X., Qian, H., Zhu, W., Sun, X., Hu, J., Zhou, H., & Chen, Y. (2004). Mesenchymal stem cells from adult human bone marrow differentiate into a cardiomyocyte phenotype in vitro. *Exp. Biol. Med.* 229:623–631.
43. Murry CE, Soonpaa MH, Reinecke H, Nakajima H, Nakajima HO, Rubart M, Pasumarthi KB, Virag JI, Bartelmez SH, Poppa V, Bradford G, Dowell D, Williams DA, Field LJ. (2004) Haematopoietic stem cells do not transdifferentiate into cardiac myocytes in myocardial Infarcts. *Nature* 428:664–668

44. Balsam LB, Wagers AJ, Christensen JL, Kofidis T, Weissman IL, Robbins RC. (2004) Haematopoietic stem cells adopt mature haematopoietic fates in ischaemic myocardium. *Nature* 428:668–673.
45. Wagers AJ, Sherwood RI, Christensen JL, Weissman IL. (2002) Little evidence for developmental plasticity of adult hematopoietic stem cells. *Science* 297:2256–9
46. Wagers AJ, Weissman IL. (2004) Plasticity of adult stem cells. *Cell* 116:639–4862. Assmus B, Schächinger V, Teupe C, Britten M, Lehmann R, Döbert N, , Grunwald F, Aicher A, Urbich C, Martin H, Hoelzer D, Dimmeler S, Zeiher AM. (2002) Transplantation of progenitor cells and regeneration enhancement in acute myocardial infarction (TOPCARE-AMI). *Circulation* 106:3009–3017.
47. Terada N, Hamazaki T, Oka M, Hoki M, Mastalerz DM, Nakano Y, Meyer EM, Morel L, Petersen BE, Scott EW. (2002) Bone marrow cells adopt the phenotype of other cells by spontaneous cell fusion. *Nature* 416: 542–545.
48. Ying, QL, Nichols J, Evans EP, Smith AG. (2002) Changing potency by spontaneous fusion. *Nature* 416:545–548.
49. Wang X, Willenbring H, Akkari Y, Torimaru Y, Foster M, Al-Dhalimy M, Lagasse E, Finegold M, Olson S, Grompe M. (2003) Cell fusion is the principal source of bone-marrow-derived hepatocytes. *Nature* 422:897–901.
50. Vassilopoulos G, Wang PR, Russell DW. (2003) Transplanted bone marrow regenerates liver by cell fusion. *Nature.* 422:901–4
51. Jorquera, R., Tanguay, R. M. (2001) Fumarylacetoacetate, the metabolite accumulating in hereditary tyrosinemia, activates the ERK pathway and induces mitotic abnormalities and genomic instability. *Hum. Mol. Genet.* 10:1741–1752
52. Jang Y-Y, Collector MI, Baylin SB, Diehl AM, Sharkis SJ. (2004) Hematopoietic stem cells convert into liver cells within days without fusion. *Nature Cell Biol.* 6:532–539.
53. Alvarez-Dolado, M., Pardal, R., Garcia-Verdugo, J.M., Fike, J.R., Lee, H.O., Pfeffer, K., Lois, C., Morrison, S,J., and Alvarez-Buylla, A. (2003) Fusion of bone-marrow-derived cells with Purkinje neurons, cardiomyocytes and hepatocytes, *Nature* 425:968–73.
54. Weimann JM, Charlton GA, Brazelton TR, Hackman RC, Blau H. (2003a) Contribution of transplanted bone marrow cells to Purkinje neurons in human adult brains. *Proc Natl Acad Sci U S A* 100:2088–93.
55. Nygren JM, Jovinge S, Breitbach M, Sawen P, Roll W, Hescheler J, Taneera J, Fleischmann BK, Jacobsen SE. (2004) Bone marrow-derived hematopoietic cells generate cardiomyocytes at a low frequency through cell fusion, but not transdifferentiation. *Nat Med.* 10:494–501.
56. Ianus A, Holz GG, Theise ND, Hussain MA. (2003) In vivo derivation of glucose-competent pancreatic endocrine cells from bone marrow without evidence of cell fusion. *J. Clin. Invest.* 111:843–850.
57. Newsome PN, Johannessen I, Boyle S, Dalakas E, McAulay KA, Samuel K, Rae F, Forrester L, Turner ML, Hayes PC, Harrison DJ, Bickmore WA, Plevris JN. (2003) Human cord blood-derived cells can differentiate into hepatocytes in the mouse liver with no evidence of cellular fusion. *Gastroenterology* 124:1891–1900.
58. Harris RG, Herzog EL, Bruscia EM, Grove JE, Van Arnam JS, Krause DS. (2004) Lack of a fusion requirement for development of bone marrow-derived epithelia. *Science* 305:90–3.
59. Wurmser AE, Nakashima K, Summers RG, Toni N, D'Amour KA, Lie DC, Gage FH. (2004) Cell fusion-independent differentiation of neural stem cells to the endothelial lineage. *Nature.* 430:350–6.

60. Lin F, Cordes K, Li L, Hood L, Couser WG, Shankland SJ, Igarashi P. (2003). Hematopoietic stem cells contribute to the regeneration of renal tubules after renal ischemia-reperfusion injury in mice. *J. Am. Soc. Nephrol.* 14:1188–1199.

61. Stamm C, Westphal B, Kleine HD, Petzsch M, Kittner C, Klinge H, Schümichen C, Nienaber CA, Freund M, Steinhoff G. (2003) Autologous bone-marrow stem-cell transplantation for myocardial regeneration. *Lancet* 361:45–46.

62. Assmus B, Schachinger V, Teupe C, Britten M, Lehmann R, Dobert N, Grunwald F, Aicher A, Urbich C, Martin H, Hoelzer D, Dimmeler S, Zeiher AM. (2002) Transplantation of progenitor cells and regeneration enhancement in acute myocardial infarction (TOPCARE-AMI). *Circulation*: 106: 3009–3017.

63. Kang HJ, Kim HS, Zhang SY, Park KW, Cho HJ, Koo BK, Kim YJ, Lee DS, Sohn DW, Han KS, Oh BH, Lee MM, Park YB. (2004) Effects of intracoronary infusion of peripheral blood stem-cells mobilized with granulocyte-colony stimulating factor on left ventricular systolic function and restenosis after coronary stenting in myocardial infarction: the MAGIC cell randomized clinical trial. *Lancet* 363:751–56

64. Wollert KC, Meyer GP, Lotz J, Ringes-Lichtenberg S, Lippolt P, Breidenbach C, Fichtner S, Korte T, Horning B, Messinger D, Arseniev L, Hertenstein B, Ganser A, Drexler H. (2004) Intracoronary autologous bone-marrow cell transfer after myocardial infarction: the BOOST randomized controlled clinical trial. *Lancet* 364:141–148.

65. Fernández-Avilés F, San Román JA, García-Frade J, Fernández ME, Peñarrubia MJ, de la Fuente L, Bueno M, Cantalapiedra A, Fernández J, Gutierrez O, Sánchez P, Hernández C, Sanz R, García-Sancho J, Sánchez A. (2004) Experimental and clinical regenerative capability of human bone marrow cells after myocardial infarction. *Circ Res.*, in press.

66. Tse HF, Kwong YL, Chan JK, Lo G, Ho CL, Lau CP. (2003) Angiogenesis in ischaemic myocardium by intramyocardial autologous bone marrow mononuclear cell implantation. *Lancet* 361:47–49.

67. Strauer BE, Brehm M, Zeus T, Köstering M, Hernandez A, Sorg RV, Kogler G, Wernet P. (2002) Repair of infarcted myocardium by autologous intracoronary mononuclear bone marrow cell transplantation in humans. *Circulation* 106:1913–1918.

68. Hamano K, Nishida M, Hirata K, Mikamo A, Li TS, Harada M, Miura T, Matsuzaki M, Esato K, (2001) Local implantation of autologous bone marrow for therapeutic angiogenesis in patients with ischemic heart disease: clinical trial and preliminary results. *Jpn Circ J.* 65: 845–847.

69. Perin EC, Dohmann HF, Borojevic R, Silva SA, Sousa AL, Mesquita CT, Rossi MI, Carvalho AC, Dutra HS, Dohmann HJ, Silva GV, Belém L, Vivacqua R, Rancel FO, Esporcatte R, Geng YJ, Vaughn WK, Assad JA, Mesquita ET, Wilerson JT. (2003) Transendocardial, autologous bone marrow cell transplantation for severe, chronic ischemic heart failure. *Circulation.* 107:2294–2302.

70. Fuchs S, Satler LF, Kornowski R, Okubagzi P, Weisz G, Baffour R, Waksman R, Weissman NJ, Cerqueira M, Leon MB, Epstein SE. (2003) Catheter-based autologous bone marrow myocardial injection in no-option patients with advanced coronary artery disease. A feasibility study. *J Am Coll Cardiol.* 41:1721–1724.

71. Taylor DA, Atkins BZ, Hungspreugs P, Jones TR, Reedy MC, Hutcheson KA, Glower DD, Kraus WE. (1998) Regenerating functional myocardium: improved performance after skeletal myoblast transplantation. *Nat Med.* 4:929–33.

72. Thompson RB, Emani SM, Davis BH, van den Bos EJ, Morimoto Y, Craig D, Glower D, Taylor DA. (2003) Comparison of intracardiac cell transplantation:

autologous skeletal myoblasts versus bone marrow cells. *Circulation* 108 Suppl 1:II264–71.

73. Menasche P. (2004) Cellular transplantation: hurdles remaining before widespread clinical use. *Curr Opin Cardiol*.19:154–61.
74. Menasche P, Hagege AA, Vilquin JT, Desnos M, Abergel E, Pouzet B, Bel A, Sarateanu S, Scorsin M, Schwartz K, Bruneval P, Benbunan M, Marolleau JP, Duboc (2003) Autologous skeletal myoblast transplantation for severe postinfarction left ventricular dysfunction. *J Am Coll Cardiol*. 41:1078–83.
75. Herreros J, Prosper F, Perez A, Gavira JJ, Garcia-Velloso MJ, Barba J, Sanchez PL, Canizo C, Rabago G, Marti-Climent JM, Hernandez M, Lopez-Holgado N, Gonzalez-Santos JM, Martin-Luengo C, Alegria E. (2003) Autologous intramyocardial injection of cultured skeletal muscle-derived stem cells in patients with non-acute myocardial infarction. *Eur Heart J*. 24:2012–2
76. Curtis RE, Rowlings PA, Deeg HJ, Shriner DA, Socie G, Travis LB, Horowitz MM, Witherspoon RP, Hoover RN, Sobocinski KA, Fraumeni JF, Boice JD (1997) Solid cancers after bone marrow transplantation. *New England J. Med.* 336:897–904
77. Baker KS, DeFor TE, Burns LJ, Ramsay NKC, Neglia JP, Robison LL (2003) New malignancies after blood or marrow stem-cell transplantation in children and adults: incidence and risk factors. *J. Clin Oncol* 21: 1352–1358
78. Orlic D, Kajstura J, Chimenti S, Limana F, Jakoniuk I, Quaini F, Nadal-Ginard B, Bodine DM, Leri A, Anversa P. (2001b) Mobilized bone marrow cells repair the infarcted heart, improving function and survival. *Proc Natl Acad Sci. USA* 98:10344–10349.
79. Gurdon, J. B., Byrne, J. A., & Simonsson, S. (2003). Nuclear reprogramming and stem cell creation. *Proc.Natl.Acad.Sci.U.S.A* 100 Suppl 1:11819–11822.
80. Collas P. (2003) Nuclear reprogramming in cell-free extracts. *Philos Trans R Soc Lond B Biol Sci*. 358:1389–1395.
81. Gaustad KG, Boquest AC, Anderson BE, Gerdes AM, Collas P. (2004) Differentiation of human adipose tissue stem cells using extracts of rat cardiomyocytes. *Biochem Biophys Res Commun*. 314:420–7.
82. Hakelien AM, Gaustad KG, Collas P. (2004) Transient alteration of cell fate using a nuclear and cytoplasmic extract of an insulinoma cell line. *Biochem Biophys Res Commun*. 316:834–41

Bone Marrow

9
Bone Marrow-Derived Stem Cell for Myocardial Regeneration: Preclinical Experience

BRADLEY J. MARTIN AND MARK F. PITTENGER[*]

1.   Introduction to Mesenchymal Stem Cells

In an effort to replace cardiomyocytes lost subsequent to ischemia, cellular transplantation has been investigated as a potential therapy for myocardial infarction.[1] Termed cellular cardiomyoplasty, the approach has gone from an interesting research novelty to clinical reality. Adult cardiomyocytes have essentially no regenerative capacity, and while a cardiac stem cell has recently been described,[2] its physiologic role in repair following infarction appears minimal and functionally inadequate. Therefore, the implantation of exogenous cells may allow for meaningful replacement of damaged cardiac cells.

Various types of isolated cells have been delivered to the heart including fetal cardiomyocytes,[3-5] skeletal myoblasts[6-8] and more recently, progenitor or stem cells such as those of the endothelial[9] or mesenchymal lineages.[10-14] Studies evaluating these cell types have repeatedly documented that exogenous cells can engraft in adult myocardium and, in some cases, have a measurable functional impact on damaged myocardium, although the degree of improvement is not yet enough to qualify as a therapy. Additionally, studies with these cell types have addressed fundamental questions that must be considered when evaluating mesenchymal stem cells (MSC) for cardiac cell therapy. For example, issues involving delivery strategies and the spatial placement of the cell graft, the ideal temporal relationships between cell delivery and cardiac injury and the electromechanical properties of cell grafts have been addressed with fetal cardiomyocyte and skeletal myoblast grafts. Research with fetal cardiomyocyte grafts has been curtailed due to the improbable likelihood of procuring sufficient amounts of fetal cardiomyocytes thought to be necessary for the damaged adult heart.

*Osiris Therapeutics Inc., Baltimore, MD

There is great interest in using stem cells to treat the cardiovascular system that has been damaged by advancing age, infarction, injury or disease. Enthusiasm for cell therapy for the injured heart has already reached the clinical setting, with physicians in several countries involved in clinical trials. Encouraging results from these early reports suggest new therapies will come from the use of progenitor cells such as myoblasts[15] or the stem cells found in bone marrow.[16,17] Researchers are also seeking a more fundamental understanding of the mechanisms by which cells in bone marrow may enhance cardiac repair. Recognizing there are different stem and progenitor cells in marrow including the MSC, the hematopoietic stem cell (HSC), as well as those of the endothelial system,[9] it will be necessary to sort out the relative contributions of different cell types. Purified MSCs have tested well in animal cardiac models and are now being readied to be evaluated clinically. Many more advances will occur to optimize MSC therapy for heart failure yet the early work is very encouraging.

In this chapter, we have focused on the human mesenchymal stem cell (MSC) isolated from adult bone marrow. These multipotential stem cells offer a very useful compromise among the many different stem cells now described in terms of the ease of accessibility, handling and lineage potentials. MSCs can be utilized allogeneically, delivered systemically, and differentiate into a cardiomyocyte-like phenotype when implanted in healthy myocardium.[11,18] Furthermore, MSCs can be readily transduced by a variety of vectors, and maintain transgene expression following *in vivo* differentiation.[11,19]

Transgene expression by MSCs may ultimately be utilized to augment cell engraftment and myogenic differentiation. While the current knowledge of MSCs will further evolve, it is possible to move forward and use these isolated multipotential cells to ask important questions that could not be addressed previously. These are still the early days of stem cell biology, and as the number of researchers increases and their investigations become more sophisticated, an important understanding of the role of adult MSCs in many aspects of human biology will emerge.

2.   Expansion and Characterization of MSCs

2.1.   MSC Expansion

The isolation of the human MSC was undertaken by Caplan and colleagues in the late 1980s and involved a rethinking of the isolation procedures and means to assay for the presence of the rare MSCs in small aspirates of bone marrow. An important contribution was the use of an osteoconductive ceramic matrix for implantations studies that would faithfully reveal the cell osteo-chondral potential of the human cells cultured *ex vivo* when implanted in immunocompromised mice. This *in vivo* assay allowed them to select appropriate culture conditions for isolation and expansion of the human

MSCs from bone marrow. Of particular importance was attention to the lot of fetal bovine serum selected for MSC growth.[20] While there is indication that addition of basic fibroblast growth factor (FGF-2) to serum is sufficient for supporting hMSC expansion in culture, this is not optimal in our hands.[21] Because we do not understand the full growth requirements of human MSCs (or other stem cells), a serum-free medium with defined growth factor composition has not yet been fully developed.

Researchers have not yet found conditions that allow continuous, indefinite growth of MSCs, yet it is possible to produce billions of MSCs *in vitro* for cell therapy from a modest bone marrow sample drawn through the skin. The MSCs need to be expanded *ex vivo*, as they apparently are very contact inhibited and do not appear to expand *in vivo*. For comparison, the HSC, another well-studied stem cell, requires a feeder layers (such as MSCs) for *ex vivo* growth and such conditions allow only limited expansion of HSCs after many years of experimentation. However, HSCs can be transplanted, to expand *in vivo* and provide life sustaining cell lineages. The current work with embryonic stem cells and neural stem cells encounter great difficulties in producing enough cells in a reproducible manner to contemplate therapeutic development. The human MSCs, with their attributes of ease of isolation, high expansion potential, genetic stability, reproducible attributes from isolate to isolate, reproducible characteristics in widely dispersed laboratories, compatibility with tissue engineering principles, and potential to enhance repair in many vital tissues, may be the preferred stem cell model for the development of cellular therapeutics.

2.2. MSC Characterization

The fibroblastic cells from bone marrow are sometimes generically termed bone marrow stromal cells, but not all stromal cells from bone marrow are multipotent.[18,22,23] Researchers have described a variety of multipotential cells from bone marrow and given them different names, and at times a particular laboratory changes names to refer to the same cells, so the literature nomenclature may be confusing to the reader. Whether the cells described by different labs are truly different cells is not clear, as they have been studied in separate labs, sometimes from different species, and by somewhat different methods. Nevertheless, the different approaches continue to contribute to our understanding of MSCs.

The MSCs in adult bone marrow are thought to be largely quiescent, and the extent to which they proliferate *in vivo* is unknown as mentioned. The initial attachment of cells from bone marrow to a substrate is followed by a stationary phase that may last several days before the cells divide and expand. The initial expansion process is due to those colony forming units (CFU) – the single cells that continue to divide to form clonal cell colonies. Although perhaps quiescent, the MSCs from bone marrow can rapidly divide once cell division begins and this is seen best at very dilute plating density. While differences in cell morphology and characteristics may initially exist, the MSC population becomes very homogeneous with time in culture, and remains so for many passages. Even the very late, passaged cultures of MSCs are very uniform but some senescent cells appear (but do not further contribute to future cell generations). Figure 1 illustrates the process from which a light density fraction bone marrow sample is expanded in culture and passaged, resulting in a homogeneous MSC preparation.

Cell populations are often characterized by analyzing their gene expression of surface molecules by fluorescence activated flow cytometry. The expressed genes that appear on the hMSC surface include receptors for growth factors, matrix molecules and other cells, and indicate how the hMSC will interact with its environment. The flow cytometry analysis also indicates the homogeneity of the hMSC population or whether it is a mixture of different cell

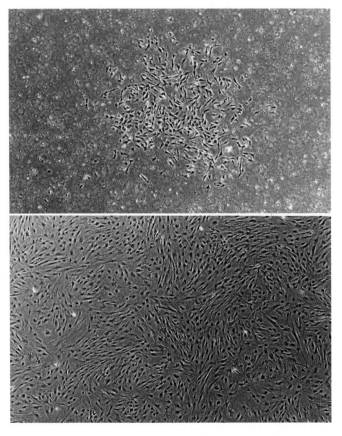

FIGURE 1. Illustration of the process from which a light density fraction bone marrow sample is expanded in culture and passaged, resulting in a homogeneous MSC preparation.

types. An extensive, yet incomplete, list of the surface molecules on hMSCs is provided in Table 1.

It is possible to isolate MSCs, or very similar cells from different mesenchymal tissues, that can be expanded to a homogeneous population capable of differentiating to several mesenchymal lineages. It was recognized early that bone-related tissues (bone, bone marrow, periosteum) could yield cultured cells that produced bone-forming cells. Recently, it was shown that fibroblastic cells from adipose differentiate to mesenchymal lineages and their characteristics and behavior are virtually indistinguishable from bone marrow-derived MSCs.[24-26]

It is not possible to directly extrapolate the identity of stem cells from species to species based on a surface marker, partly because not all antibodies are cross-reactive across species. There have been recognized differences between stem cells found in different species such as different *in vitro* requirements to culture MSCs from mouse and man.[27,28] These types of species differences are similarly found for hematopoetic or embryonic stem cells, where, for the later LIF is required for mouse ES cells but not for human. Similarly, MSCs can be isolated by a number of methods from different tissue sources but their stem cell nature cannot be assured; it must be tested or assayed. Most surface markers have been found inadequate as a means to identify stem cells, as the putative marker(s) may also be found on non-stem cells, or a particular marker may only be expressed on a stem cell at a certain stage or under certain conditions, such as with CD34 marker on HSCs. Nevertheless, surface markers or other attributes are useful in characterizing the stem cell as isolated or cultured, and as a means to begin to understand its potential interactions with neighboring cells and the cell environment. Recently, Simmons and colleagues[29,30] reported a much more extensive characterization of

TABLE 1. Mesenchymal stem cell markers

	Positive	Negative
Surface antigens	CD13, CD29, CD44, CD49b (Integrin α2), CD49b (Integrin α5), CD54 (ICAM1), CD71 (Transferrin Rec), CD73(SH-3), CD90 (Thy-1), CD105 (Endoglin, SH-2), CD106 (VCAM), CD166 (ALCAM)	CD3, CD4, CD6, CD9, CD10, CD11a,b, CD14, CD15, CD18 (Integrin β2), CD31 (PECAM), CD34, CD45, CD49d (Integrin α4), CD50 (ICAM3), CD62E (E-Selectin), CD117, CD133
Growth factor and cytokine receptors	IL-1, IL-3, IL-4, IL-6, IL-7, Interferon Gamma, TNF-a, FGF, PDGRF, LIF, CxCR4	IL-2 HLA DR (inducible), B7 co-stimulatory, SSEA-1,
Others	B2 microglobulin, Nestin, P75, HLA (A,B and C), SSEA-4, TRK (ABC)	c-kit, Sca-1
In vitro differentiation	Adipo, Osteo, Chrondo, Endothelial, Neural, Stromal	

a subpopulation of marrow stromal cells selected by an antibody to an unknown surface marker, STRO-1. The selected cells from bone marrow had many of the attributes of MSCs.[31]

2.3. Immunology of MSCs

Several laboratories have begun to characterize the interactions between MSCs and cells of the immune system. Human MSCs have a number of surface molecules that would predict interaction with T cells. Major histocompatibility complex I (MHC class I), vascular cell adhesion molecule (VCAM), intracellular adhesion molecule 1 (ICAM-1) and ICAM–2, activated leukocyte cell adhesion molecule (ALCAM), lymphocyte functional antigen-3 (LFA-3) and integrins α1-3, α5-6, β1, β3-4 are surface molecules expressed on hMSCs that have cognate ligands on T cells.[18,22,32,33] Intuitively, one might expect allogeneic MSCs would stimulate T cell proliferation, and that donor MSCs would be recognized by responder T cells and likely rejected by a recipient host. However, experimental evidence indicates this may not be the case. hMSCs lack the B7 co-stimulatory molecules CD80 and CD86 required for T-cell activation.[34,35] MSCs have been shown to inhibit T cell proliferation in several laboratories.[34-37]

Perhaps the most compelling data supporting the immune-privileged status of MSCs comes from the several studies that have utilized allogeneic MSCs *in vivo*.[34,38,39] These data indicate that allo MSCs are not rejected (cells have been identified in tissues for as long as 1 year), engraft, and may have positive effects on engraftment of third party cells or tissue.[38] As will be discussed later in this chapter, MSC may even be applicable in the xenogeneic setting.[40]

Collectively, the current studies on the interactions between MSCs and T cells, support the potential use of allogeneic MSCs in cell therapy. Along with studies of allogeneic MSCs introduced into the infarcted heart models and encouraging early clinical results, we conclude the future use of allo-MSCs has significant clinical potential.

3.   Preclinical Use of Mscs

3.1.   Cell Labeling

One of the problems inherent to the study of cellular cardiomyoplasty, is the difficulty in tracking the movement and/or fate of implanted cells. The inability to definitively identify individual cells of interest makes conclusions regarding their fate following implantation impossible. While investigators have utilized a number of method to identify delivered cells, all have their shortcomings and the ideal technique remains elusive.

The prolonged length of many in-vivo cardiomyoplasty studies requires that the label be long lasting. Maximal cellular differentiation of cardiac functional benefits may take as long as six months to manifest in a large animal model and it is critical that one still be able to identify the implanted cells. Additionally, any label utilized must not interfere with normal cellular growth kinetics, differentiation or functionality. Lastly the truly ideal label would be quantifiable, allowing the investigator to determine (with a degree of certainty) the number of cells of interest in a tissue section. Quantitative labels are particularly problematic, and many investigators have opted to sacrifice quantitation in lieu of long lasting labels that are relatively benign to cellular function. In the following sections, the advantages and disadvantages of several labels commonly used to track cell persistence and fate in in-vivo studies will be discussed.

3.1.1.   Fluorescent Labels

One of the most commonly used methods of labeling exogenously delivered cells, and tracking their movements, is through the use of fluorescent dyes. These labels have the advantage of being easy to use, fairly long lasting and, facilitate the identification of cells with simple fluorescent microscopy.

The commercially available compound Cell Tracker CM-DiI (Molecular Probes, Eugene OR) is a fluorescent label that has been used extensively this investigator and others. It is a nonspecific lipophilic compound that effectively labels the plasma membrane of cells in culture, and emits a bright orange fluorescence when viewed with fluorescent microscopy. CellTracker CM-DiI contains a thiol-reactive chloromethyl moiety that allows the dye to covalently bind to cellular thiols. Thus, unlike other membrane stains, the label is well retained in some cells throughout fixation and permeabilization steps. In the case of MSCs, we have demonstrated that CM-DiI does not effect cell growth or differentiation potential and we have been able to identify labeled cells in the rat heart as long as one year after implantation. One of the primary difficulties in the in-vivo application of CM-DiI is that upon stimulation it emits an orange fluorescence that can be confused with the autofluorescence of macrophages. In order to avoid this confusion, we have taken the approach of double labeling MSC with both CM-DiI and the nuclear stain dapi. This process can be completed during the final day of culture, prior to cell harvest and cryopreservation. The blue nuclear staining of DAPI, when combined with the orange plasma membrane labeling of CM-DiI, makes for a cell label that is unique and very conclusive during histology. An example of this double labeling technique can be seen in Figure 2A.

3.1.2.   Genetic Labeling of MSCs

MSCs can be readily transduced by a variety of vectors, and maintain transgene expression following *in vivo* differentiation.[11,19] MSCs can be efficiently transduced (gene modified) by several different methods to produce cells that overproduce a particular gene of interest. Introduction of exogenous genes into MSCs can be accomplished by all transduction methods including calcium phosphate, electroporation, retrovirus, adenovirus, lentivirus, lipofectamine etc. Such gene tagging can be used to label and track MSCs that are then introduced into animal models as well as to provide therapeutic proteins.

Introduction of genes into MSCs varies from 20-80%, but can be easily optimized, or selection methods, such as including the neomycin resistance gene and selection with G418, can be used to assure all MSCs are transduced.[41] Such important therapeutic molecules as human growth hormone and factor IX have been produced by transfected MSCs in animal models.[42] Moreover, differentiation of MSCs to several lineages has not prevented the expression of marker genes such as green fluorescence protein (GFP) or LacZ.[43] An example of MSCs transduced via a retroviral vector to express Lac-Z can be found in Figure 2B.

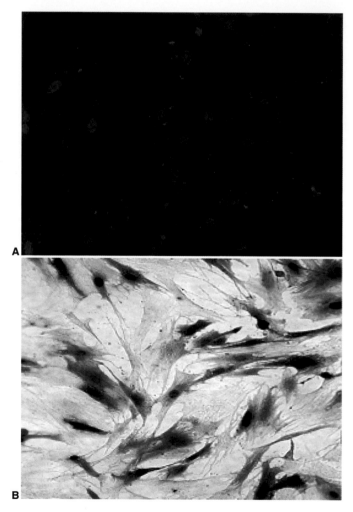

FIGURE 2. A. (top) Example of double labeling technique; B. (bottom) MSCs transduced via a retroviral vector to express Lac-Z.

Gene-transduced MSCs have been introduced into hearts in several animal models. Adenovirus has been utilized to introduce the LacZ gene into MSCs to provide a label that can be followed by immunofluorescence or biochemical means, and it does not appear to interfere with differentiation of MSCs in the heart.[11]

While MSCs appear to be a useful treatment for heart therapy, researchers are already using gene transduction to improve the MSC potential. In the rat infarct model, Dzau and colleagues have used retroviral transduction to introduce the Akt gene into rat MSCs to provide an improved survival mechanism for the cells. When introduced into the infarcts of recipient rats, the transduced MSCs provided benefits that limited collagen deposition and prevented deleterious remodeling, resulting in improved function at 2 weeks after injection.[44]

4.   *In Vivo* MSC Cardiomyoplasty

Interest in MSCs in general, and as a cardiac therapy in particular, has increased exponentially over the last ten years. Compared to other cells types considered for cardiomyoplasty, MSCs appear to possess unique properties that may allow for convenient and highly-effective cell therapy. MSCs can be utilized allogenically (see immunology section), delivered systemically, and differentiate into a cardiomyocyte-like phenotype when implanted in healthy myocardium.[11,18]

The first use of marrow-derived MSCs as a cell for cardiomyoplasty was reported in 1999 by the laboratories of Weisel and Lee at the University of Toronto.[12] In this study, autologous bone marrow cells were implanted in the left ventricle of rats by direct injection three weeks after cryoinjury. Transplanted marrow cells could be identified in all animals eight weeks after injury and were found to express muscle specific proteins not present prior to implantation. Furthermore, improved systolic and diastolic function was observed in animals that received cells pretreated with the DNA demethylating agent 5-azacytidine, which has been reported to enhance myogenic differentiation of pluripotent cells.

As opposed to the muscle precursor cells (which must be used autologously), MSCs have the ability to be used immediately following acute injury.[45] The ability to treat myocardial infarction patients with allogeneic MSCs in an emergent setting at the time of coronary reperfusion may constitute a distinct clinical advantage over autologous cellular cardiomyoplasty. Furthermore, MSCs appear to have the ability to home to the site of myocardial injury when administered intravenously following acute infarction (see below).

Orlic et al.[46] demonstrated myocytic differentiation with intracellular connections between myocytes after injecting mouse bone marrow cells into viable murine myocardium surrounding an infarct. The transplanted cells likely migrated into the injured myocardium through local cell signaling mechanisms. Neovascularization, *de novo* regeneration of myocardium, and improved left ventricular end-diastolic pressure were evident in the treatment group. Stamm et al.[47] demonstrated the clinical utility of this approach, reporting a marked improvement in global cardiac function in patients following injection of whole, unselected bone marrow cells.

Our lab and others have demonstrated that after injection into infarcted myocardium, engrafted MSCs differentiate towards a myogenic lineage as evidenced by the expression of muscle specific proteins including α-actinin, troponin-T, tropomyosin, myosin heavy chain-MHC, phospholamban, and other muscle-specific proteins.[48] Additionally, the presence of connexin-43, a protein responsible for intracellular connection and electrical coupling between cells, further suggests cardiomyocyte differentiation. However, complete myogenic differentiation with mature sarcomeric organization, intercalated discs etc., has not been observed following implantation of MSCs in infarcted myocardium. This is in contrast with our experience regarding injection of MSCs into viable, non-infarcted murine myocardium where evidence of a contractile apparatus and extensive myogenic differentiation have been observed.[11] The lack of extensive myocytic differentiation in the infarcted heart likely speaks to the importance of the local extracellular milieu in driving differentiation of MSCs (Figure 3).

However, even without appropriate differentiation within infarcted tissue, MSC cardiomyoplasty has been associated with a number of significant functional improvements in the post-infarcted heart. Previously described benefits of engrafted stem cells include prevention of pathologic wall thinning and improved post-infarction hemodynamics.[48] Significantly lower end-diastolic pressures in MSC-treated animals suggests improved diastolic relaxation and decreased wall stress that are likely attributable to favorable ventricular remodeling.[49] The absence of improvement in systolic function may be considered somewhat expected in light of the absence of sarcomeric

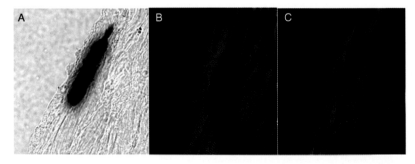

FIGURE 3. The lack of extensive myocytic differentiation in the infarcted heart likely speaks to the importance of the local extracellular milieu in driving differentiation of MSCs.

organization in the implanted MSCs. Taken together these data suggest that the implantation of MSCs results in a more compliant, less stiff ventricle with improved diastolic filling properties. How implantation of MSCs improves diastolic function mechanistically is not yet clear but, early evidence suggests that improved pathological remodeling, specifically alterations in tissue cellularity and extracellular matrix remodeling, may be involved. Although patients with isolated left ventricular diastolic dysfunction have relatively low mortality compared to those with systolic dysfunction, significant morbidities are common including symptoms of congestive failure and recurrent chest pain. As a result, the diastolic benefits of MSC cardiomyoplasty may play an important role in the treatment of ischemic heart disease.

4.1.   Allogeneic MSC Implantation

As described earlier, MSCs from human and other species have a cell surface phenotype that is of low immunogenicity.[22,32,50] In 2000, data from several research groups at Osiris demonstrated long-term allogeneic MSCs engraftment in a variety of non-cardiac tissues in the absence of immunosupression.[34,38,39,49] Based on these observations, we began to investigate the ability of allogeneic MSCs to engraft in infarcted myocardium. Initially in rats, and later in swine, allogeneic MSC were found to readily engraft in necrotic myocardium and favorably alter ventricular function following infarction. Furthermore, engraftment of allogeneic MSCs in the myocardium occurs without evidence of immunologic rejection or lymphocytic infiltration, even in the absence of immunosuppressive therapy. Our results utilizing allogeneic MSCs further emphasize some of the apparent advantages of mesenchymal stem cells over other cell populations for cellular cardiomyoplasty. These unique characteristics of MSCs may allow for enhanced clinical applicability, as allogeneic MSCs can be readily available and administered without concern for immunologic compatibility.

The immunologically privileged status of MSCs may even extend to the xenogeneic setting. In a recent study from Saito et al,[40] MSCs obtained from C57Bl/6 mice were intravenously injected into immunocompetent adult Lewis rats. Labeled mouse cells engrafted into the bone marrow for at least 12 weeks without immunosuppression. When these animals were later subjected to myocardial infarctions, murine MSCs could be identified in the region of necrosis, and these cells expressed muscle-specific proteins not present prior to coronary ligation. Xenogeneic MSC engraftment was not associated with immunologic activation or rejection, but rather appeared to form a stable cardiac chimera.

4.2.   Tracking and Quantification of MSCs

Recently Barbash et al.[51] have utilized gamma camera imaging of technetium 99m labeled MSCs to determine their distribution following intravenous or intraventricular injection in a rat MI model. They reported that four hours after intravenous injection, a significant number of MSC were trapped in the lungs, with lesser numbers in the heart and other organs. Cardiac engraftment was significantly augmented (and pulmonary plugging attenuated) with intraventricular administration. MRI imaging of iron labeled cells is another technique that has recently been utilized to track the distribution of MSCs *in vivo*.[52,53] Hill et al.[53] have demonstrated that iron labeling does not alter MSC multipotentiality, and that imaging in a standard 1.5 Tesla magnet is feasible, and provides excellent spatial resolution in the beating heart. Furthermore, the iron label can be conjugated to a fluorescent particle to aid in histologic identification of MSCs.

The localization of MSCs *in vivo* with either MRI or gamma imaging is of tremendous value to those attempting to demonstrate the biodistribution or persistence of MSCs following cardiomyoplasty. However, the techniques inability to accurately quantify the number of MSCs is troubling to those seeking to optimize the therapeutic utility of MSCs. When attempting to calculate dose/response relationships in such studies, it is the number of cells engrafting that is of concern, as opposed to the number administered. Accurate quantification of cell engraftment has been elusive regardless of cell type examined. Some investigators have attempted to generate indexes of engraftment by simply counting the number of labeled cells in a representative sampling of high-powered fields. This methodology is hindered by the possibility of counting multiple cell layers or fractions of cells and, therefore, is far from exact. We have attempted to quantify MSC engraftment utilizing RT-PCR amplification of transgene expression. While theoretically sound, in our experience PCR-based quantification of transduced MSCs was determined to lack the sensitivity required for accurate quantification.

A method found to provide a more accurate quantification of MSC engraftment is radiolabeling of MSCs with tritiated-thymidine (^{3}H-thymidine). Following implantation, the degree of radioactivity in a tissue can be correlated to MSC engraftment in a linear fashion. While PCR techniques would allow for the detection of 50,000 cells in a rat heart, tritium labeling has a 10-fold lower threshold of detection (5,000 cells), greatly improving the accuracy of measurements as well as our ability to detect modest numbers of cells in the heart.

Using these types of techniques has allowed investigators to quantify the degree of MSC engraftment in the heart following delivery. While the exact numbers vary, it can be said that in all cases the extent of engraftment is modest. Our experiments have indicated that fewer than 3% of MSCs administered by direct injection persist at two weeks. Administration of higher numbers of cells resulted in only modest augmentation of long term engraftment. Engraftment efficiency in the heart with IV delivery is even lower, with under 1% of injected cells present two weeks post-MI (unpublished Osiris data). However, the efficiency of IV delivery is likely to be highly dependent upon the time of delivery relative to the time of injury. Cardiac engraftment is below detection limits when IV MSC delivery is delayed until two weeks post-MI. In other words, the degree of cardiac "homing" appears to be significantly attenuated by delayed MSC administration. This finding suggests that whatever the mechanism of this injury-specific homing, it has significantly subsided by two weeks post-reperfusion. This timecourse is consistent with the hypothesis that an inflammatory mediator, similar to those that recruit macrophage and lymphocytes to damaged tissue, may be responsible for MSC cytotaxis.

4.3. MSC-Induced Angiogenesis

Because cardiac function depends critically on myocardial perfusion, restoration of cardiac function after myocardial infarction must require not only replacement of lost cardiomyocytes, but also revascularization of the injured region. There is evidence from ischemic hind limb models that circulating stem cells are incorporated into newly forming blood vessels[54,55] and contribute to increased capillary density and enhanced tissue perfusion.[54,56] In damaged myocardium, endogenous increases in capillary density have also been reported.[12,57,58]

Recent studies have also shown that stem cells isolated from adult tissues have the potential for enhancing neovascularization and regenerating infarcted myocardium.[9,12,46,54,58-63] Myocardial perfusion is characterized by close matching of blood flow to myocardial demand. Therefore, it will be important to examine not only maximal blood flow (indicative of total vascularity) but also the responsiveness of coronary flow to changes in myocardial demand, and the distribution of myocardial perfusion.

Experiments to evaluate the effect of MSC therapy on myocardial perfusion are ongoing. However, evidence for MSC involvement in vascular repair or regeneration can be found in Figure 4.

The image was obtained from a pig eight weeks following catheter-based endocardial delivery of MSCs. The H&E images in the upper panels clearly illustrate the presence of blood vessel within a region of generalized myocardial necrosis. Prior to implantation MSCs were labeled with the nuclear stain DAPI, which emits a strong blue fluorescence and aids in the identification of implanted cells within the tissue. In the confocal images of serial sections (bottom panels), DAPI labeled cells can be seen throughout the section. However, a localization of implanted MSCs can be readily identified surrounding, and associated with, these blood vessels. Green fluorescence represents a FITC-labeled monoclonal antibody directed against smooth muscle actin. One can see that the DAPI-labeled MSC's (blue) are localized within, and intimately associated with, the smooth muscle layer of the vessel. In addition to actin, implanted MSCs have been demonstrated to express the Von Willebrands factor, VEG-F and other proteins indicative of angiogenesis. It should again be noted that these protein are not found in cultured MSCs, but rather are expressed only after several weeks in the cardiac environment.

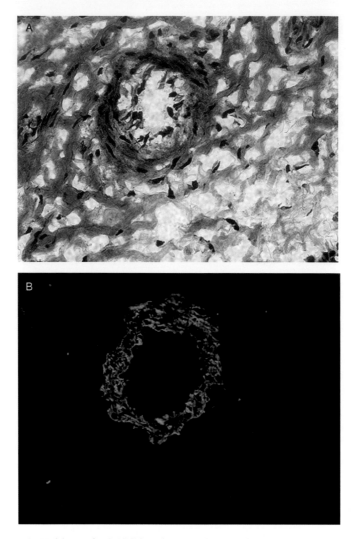

FIGURE 4. Evidence for MSC involvement in vascular repair or regeneration

These findings are consistent with the recent results of Kinnaird et al.[64] These authors reported that human MSCs constitutively express a wide array of arteriogeneic cytokine genes, and that several more were significantly upregulated by hypoxic stress. Furthermore, it was observed that culture media exposed to MSCs (termed MSC-conditioned media), promoted endothelial cells migration and proliferation consistent with the hypothesis that MSCs produce a number of angiogenic proteins when implanted *in-vivo*.[64]

4.4.   Cardiac Homing of MSCs to Sites of Infarction

Perhaps the most unique characteristic of MSCs is their ability to home to sites of tissue damage or inflammation.[65] While the cytotactic factors responsible for injury-specific MSC migration and its physiologic consequences have yet to be fully elucidated, it is postulated that MSC migrate to participate in wound repair. This extraordinary ability of MSCs to home to sites of acute tissue injury has been demonstrated in the setting of bone fracture[19,65,66] and cerebral ischemia,[67] as well as the infarcted heart.[40,68]

Chui et al.[40] were the first to demonstrate that MSCs administered intravenously engraft within regions of myocardial infarction. Mouse MSCs were transduced with a LacZ reporter gene and injected intravenously to rats (in the absence of immunosuppression). In healthy (non-injured) animals, IV delivered MSCs preferentially engraft in the marrow cavity. However, when these rats were subsequently subjected to a cycle of ischemia/reperfusion, significant numbers of labeled cells could be identified in the circulation and subsequently the infarcted heart. The majority of engrafting MSCs were found to be positive for cardiomyocyte-specific proteins, while a distinct subpopulation were determined to participate in angiogenesis.

Our lab has utilized a similar model in an attempt to characterize the movements of MSCs following intravenous adminstration. MSCs obtained from ACI rats were transduced with a retroviral vector encoding for β-gal expression. Labeled MSCs were identified within the bone morrow of Fisher rats 10 days following intravenous injection. MSCs were not detected in the heart or lungs at that time. When rats with β-gal labeled cells in their marrow were then submitted to a 45 minute cycle of LAD occlusion and reperfusion, a significant number of β -gal positive MSCs were detected within the region of infarction. This engraftment was highly specific in that labeled cells were not detected in non-cardiac tissues or the viable myocardium of the right ventricle, atria of LV posterior wall.[69]

While these data shed some light on the physiology of MSCs in wound repair, the question remained as to whether MSCs administered intravenously after infarction could similarly home to, and possibly aid in the repair of, damaged myocardium. Indeed, when administered during the acute reperfusion period, MSCs will home to the myocardium in significant numbers.[69,70] In a rat infarct model, the administration of 5 million MSCs IV at 10 minutes of reperfusion resulted in significant and sustained cardiac engraftment. This engraftment was specific to the region of necrosis with no significant numbers of MSCs being detected in normal myocardium or non-cardiac tissues at four weeks post-administration.[69] However, the "window" of MSC homing is limited. If MSC administration was delayed until two weeks post-infarction, no significant cardiac engraftment was observed with most cells returning to the bone marrow. The remarkable specificity with which MSCs home to regions of injury following systemic delivery, with essentially no engraftment in normal tissue is illustrated in Figure 5. While the factors responsible for MSC

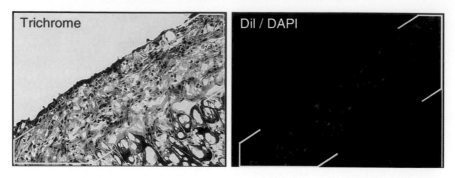

FIGURE 5. MSCs home to regions of injury following systemic delivery, with essentially no engraftment in normal tissue

migration have not yet been clearly defined, the transient nature of the phenomenon is consistent with the involvement of an inflammatory mediator similar to those responsible for macrophage and neutrophil infiltration in tissue injury. Further complexity is added by a recent report suggesting that expansion of murine MSCs in culture may diminish the efficacy of injury-induced homing.[71] The degree to which species differences may account for these varying results requires further investigation.

5.   Summary

Adult stem cells are found in many tissues and participate in adult growth as well as repair and regeneration of damaged tissue. Adult stem cells such as MSCs may be the cell of choice for tissue repair because the cellular and tissue environment in the adult is likely very different from the early embryo conditions that produce embryonic stem cells. Bone marrow provides an accessible and renewable source of adult mesenchymal stem cells that can be greatly expanded in culture and characterized. Culture-expanded and characterized MSCs have been tested for their ability to differentiate into several lineages *in vitro* and also tested in animal models for their ability to enhance tissue repair and undergo *in vitro* differentiation. One of their greatest attributes is their potential to supply growth factors and cytokines to repairing tissue. MSCs do not appear to be rejected by the immune system, allowing for large scale production, appropriate charaterization and testing, and the subsequent ready availability of allogeneic tissue repair enhancing cellular therapeutics. This provides for the further development of this new field and paves the way for the use of yet other stem cells. The potential to use MSCs to repair damaged cardiovascular tissue is very promising and moving forward quickly. The current results from many labs and early cardiac clinical studies suggest important therapeutic approaches will be forthcoming through the use of MSCs. Perhaps most importantly, the understanding of adult stem cells such as the MSCs will provide us with greater understanding of the role they play in human biology in the developing and aging man.

6.   References

1. Kao RL, Chiu RC. *Cellular Cardiomyoplasty: Myocardial Repair with Cell Implantation.* Austin, TX: Landes Bioscience; 1997.
2. Anversa P, Nadal-Ginard B. Myocyte renewal and ventricular remodelling. *Nature.* 2002;415:240–3.
3. Kessler PD, Byrne BJ. Myoblast cell grafting into heart muscle: cellular biology and potential applications. *Annu Rev Physiol.* 1999;61:219–42.
4. Scorsin M, Hagege A, Vilquin JT, Fiszman M, Marotte F, Samuel JL, Rappaport L, Schwartz K, Menasche P. Comparison of the effects of fetal cardiomyocyte and skeletal myoblast transplantation on postinfarction left ventricular function. *J Thorac Cardiovasc Surg.* 2000;119:1169–75.
5. Soonpaa MH, Koh GY, Klug MG, Field LJ. Formation of nascent intercalated disks between grafted fetal cardiomyocytes and host myocardium. *Science.* 1994;264:98–101.
6. Murry CE, Wiseman RW, Schwartz SM, Hauschka SD. Skeletal myoblast transplantation for repair of myocardial necrosis. *J Clin Invest.* 1996;98:2512–23.
7. Taylor DA, Atkins BZ, Hungspreugs P, Jones TR, Reedy MC, Hutcheson KA, Glower DD, Kraus WE. Regenerating functional myocardium: improved performance after skeletal myoblast transplantation. *Nat Med.* 1998;4:929–33.
8. Taylor DA. Cellular cardiomyoplasty with autologous skeletal myoblasts for ischemic heart disease and heart failure. *Curr Control Trials Cardiovasc Med.* 2001;2:208–210.
9. Fuchs S, Baffour R, Zhou YF, Shou M, Pierre A, Tio FO, Weissman NJ, Leon MB, Epstein SE, Kornowski R. Transendocardial delivery of autologous bone marrow enhances collateral perfusion and regional function in pigs with chronic experimental myocardial ischemia. *J Am Coll Cardiol.* 2001;37:1726–32.
10. Orlic D, Kajstura J, Chimenti S, Limana F, Jakoniuk I, Quaini F, Nadal-Ginard B, Bodine DM, Leri A, Anversa P. Mobilized bone marrow cells repair the infarcted heart, improving function and survival. *Proc Natl Acad Sci U S A.* 2001;98:10344–9.
11. Toma C, Pittenger MF, Cahill KS, Byrne BJ, Kessler PD. Human mesenchymal stem cells differentiate to a cardiomyocyte phenotype in the adult murine heart. *Circulation.* 2002;105:93–8.
12. Tomita S, Li RK, Weisel RD, Mickle DA, Kim EJ, Sakai T, Jia ZQ. Autologous transplantation of bone marrow cells improves damaged heart function. *Circulation.* 1999;100:II247–56.
13. Fukuda K. Development of regenerative cardiomyocytes from mesenchymal stem cells cardiovascular tissue engineering. *Artif Organs.* 2001;25:187–93.
14. Ferrari G, Cusella-De Angelis G, Coletta M, Paolucci E, Stornaiuolo A, Cossu G, Mavilio F. Muscle regeneration by bone marrow-derived myogenic progenitors. *Science.* 1998;279:1528–30.
15. Menasche P, Hagege AA, Vilquin JT, Desnos M, Abergel E, Pouzet B, Bel A, Sarateanu S, Scorsin M, Schwartz K, Bruneval P, Benbunan M, Marolleau JP,

Duboc D. Autologous skeletal myoblast transplantation for severe postinfarction left ventricular dysfunction. *J Am Coll Cardiol*. 2003;41:1078–83.

16. Perin EC, Dohmann HF, Borojevic R, Silva SA, Sousa AL, Mesquita CT, Rossi MI, Carvalho AC, Dutra HS, Dohmann HJ, Silva GV, Belem L, Vivacqua R, Rangel FO, Esporcatte R, Geng YJ, Vaughn WK, Assad JA, Mesquita ET, Willerson JT. Transendocardial, autologous bone marrow cell transplantation for severe, chronic ischemic heart failure. *Circulation*. 2003;107:2294–302.

17. Strauer BE, Brehm M, Zeus T, Kostering M, Hernandez A, Sorg RV, Kogler G, Wernet P. Repair of infarcted myocardium by autologous intracoronary mononuclear bone marrow cell transplantation in humans. *Circulation*. 2002;106:1913–8.

18. Pittenger MF, Mosca JD, McIntosh KR. Human mesenchymal stem cells: progenitor cells for cartilage, bone, fat and stroma. *Curr Top Microbiol Immunol*. 2000;251:3–11.

19. Mosca JD, Hendricks JK, Buyaner D, Davis-Sproul J, Chuang LC, Majumdar MK, Chopra R, Barry F, Murphy M, Thiede MA, Junker U, Rigg RJ, Forestell SP, Bohnlein E, Storb R, Sandmaier BM. Mesenchymal stem cells as vehicles for gene delivery. *Clin Orthop*. 2000:S71–90.

20. Lennon DP, Haynesworth SE, Young RG, Dennis JE, Caplan AI. A chemically defined medium supports in vitro proliferation and maintains the osteochondral potential of rat marrow-derived mesenchymal stem cells. *Exp Cell Res*. 1995;219:211–22.

21. Martin I, Muraglia A, Campanile G, Cancedda R, Quarto R. Fibroblast growth factor-2 supports ex vivo expansion and maintenance of osteogenic precursors from human bone marrow. *Endocrinology*. 1997;138:4456–62.

22. Pittenger MF, Mackay AM, Beck SC, Jaiswal RK, Douglas R, Mosca JD, Moorman MA, Simonetti DW, Craig S, Marshak DR. Multilineage potential of adult human mesenchymal stem cells. *Science*. 1999;284:143–7.

23. Pittenger MF, Mackay AM. Multipotential Human Mesenchymal Stem Cells. *Graft*. 2000;3:288–294.

24. Halvorsen YC, Wilkison WO, Gimble JM. Adipose-derived stromal cells–their utility and potential in bone formation. *Int J Obes Relat Metab Disord*. 2000;24:S41–4.

25. Zuk PA, Zhu M, Ashjian P, De Ugarte DA, Huang JI, Mizuno H, Alfonso ZC, Fraser JK, Benhaim P, Hedrick MH. Human adipose tissue is a source of multipotent stem cells. *Mol Biol Cell*. 2002;13:4279–95.

26. Zuk PA, Zhu M, Mizuno H, Huang J, Futrell JW, Katz AJ, Benhaim P, Lorenz HP, Hedrick MH. Multilineage cells from human adipose tissue: implications for cell-based therapies. *Tissue Eng*. 2001;7:211–28.

27. Phinney DG, Kopen G, Isaacson RL, Prockop DJ. Plastic adherent stromal cells from the bone marrow of commonly used strains of inbred mice: variations in yield, growth, and differentiation. *J Cell Biochem*. 1999;72:570–85.

28. Phinney DG, Kopen G, Righter W, Webster S, Tremain N, Prockop DJ. Donor variation in the growth properties and osteogenic potential of human marrow stromal cells. *J Cell Biochem*. 1999;75:424–36.

29. Simmons PJ, Torok-Storb B. CD34 expression by stromal precursors in normal human adult bone marrow. *Blood*. 1991;78:2848–53.

30. Simmons PJ, Torok-Storb B. Identification of stromal cell precursors in human bone marrow by a novel monoclonal antibody, STRO-1. *Blood*. 1991;78:55–62.

31. Gronthos S, Zannettino AC, Hay SJ, Shi S, Graves SE, Kortesidis A, Simmons PJ. Molecular and cellular characterisation of highly purified stromal stem cells derived from human bone marrow. *J Cell Sci*. 2003;116:1827–35.

32. Majumdar MK, Keane-Moore M, Buyaner D, Hardy WB, Moorman MA, McIntosh KR, Mosca JD. Characterization and functionality of cell surface molecules on human mesenchymal stem cells. *J Biomed Sci.* 2003;10:228–41.
33. Majumdar MK, Thiede MA, Mosca JD, Moorman M, Gerson SL. Phenotypic and functional comparison of cultures of marrow-derived mesenchymal stem cells (MSCs) and stromal cells. *J Cell Physiol.* 1998;176:57–66.
34. McIntosh KR, Bartholomew A. Stromal cell modulation of the immune system: A potential role for mesenchymal stem cells. *Graft.* 2000;3:324–328.
35. Tse WT, Pendleton JD, Beyer WM, Egalka MC, Guinan EC. Suppression of allogeneic T-cell proliferation by human marrow stromal cells: implications in transplantation. *Transplantation.* 2003;75:389–97.
36. Di Nicola M, Carlo-Stella C, Magni M, Milanesi M, Longoni PD, Matteucci P, Grisanti S, Gianni AM. Human bone marrow stromal cells suppress T-lymphocyte proliferation induced by cellular or nonspecific mitogenic stimuli. *Blood.* 2002;99:3838–43.
37. Le Blanc K, Tammik L, Sundberg B, Haynesworth SE, Ringden O. Mesenchymal stem cells inhibit and stimulate mixed lymphocyte cultures and mitogenic responses independently of the major histocompatibility complex. *Scand J Immunol.* 2003;57:11–20.
38. Bartholomew A, Patil S, Mackay A, Nelson M, Buyaner D, Hardy W, Mosca J, Sturgeon C, Siatskas M, Mahmud N, Ferrer K, Deans R, Moseley A, Hoffman R, Devine SM. Baboon mesenchymal stem cells can be genetically modified to secrete human erythropoietin in vivo. *Hum Gene Ther.* 2001;12:1527–41.
39. Liechty KW, MacKenzie TC, Shaaban AF, Radu A, Moseley AM, Deans R, Marshak DR, Flake AW. Human mesenchymal stem cells engraft and demonstrate site-specific differentiation after in utero transplantation in sheep. *Nat Med.* 2000;6:1282–6.
40. Saito T, Kuang JQ, Bittira B, Al-Khaldi A, Chiu RC. Xenotransplant cardiac chimera: immune tolerance of adult stem cells. *Ann Thorac Surg.* 2002;74:19–24; discussion 24.
41. Allay JA, Dennis JE, Haynesworth SE, Majumdar MK, Clapp DW, Shultz LD, Caplan AI, Gerson SL. LacZ and interleukin-3 expression in vivo after retroviral transduction of marrow-derived human osteogenic mesenchymal progenitors. *Hum Gene Ther.* 1997;8:1417–27.
42. Hurwitz DR, Kirchgesser M, Merrill W, Galanopoulos T, McGrath CA, Emani S, Hansen M, Cherington V, Appel J, Bizinkauskas CB, Brackmann HH, Levine PH, Greenberger JS. Systemic delivery of human growth hormone or human factor IX in dogs by reintroduced genetically modified autologous bone marrow stromal cells. *Human Gene Therapy.* 1997;8:137–156.
43. Lee K, Majumdar MK, Buyaner D, Hendricks JK, Pittenger MF, Mosca JD. Human mesenchymal stem cells maintain transgene expression during expansion and differentiation. *Mol Ther.* 2001;3:857–66.
44. Mangi AA, Noiseux N, Kong D, He H, Rezvani M, Ingwall JS, Dzau VJ. Mesenchymal stem cells modified with Akt prevent remodeling and restore performance of infarcted hearts. *Nat Med.* 2003;10:10.
45. Koc ON, Peters C, Aubourg P, Raghavan S, Dyhouse S, DeGasperi R, Kolodny EH, Yoseph YB, Gerson SL, Lazarus HM, Caplan AI, Watkins PA, Krivit W. Bone marrow-derived mesenchymal stem cells remain host-derived despite successful hematopoietic engraftment after allogeneic transplantation

in patients with lysosomal and peroxisomal storage diseases. *Exp Hematol.* 1999;27:1675–81.

46. Orlic D, Kajstura J, Chimenti S, Jakoniuk I, Anderson SM, Li B, Pickel J, McKay R, Nadal-Ginard B, Bodine DM, Leri A, Anversa P. Bone marrow cells regenerate infarcted myocardium. *Nature.* 2001;410:701–5.

47. Stamm C, Westphal B, Kleine HD, Petzsch M, Kittner C, Klinge H, Schumichen C, Nienaber CA, Freund M, Steinhoff G. Autologous bone-marrow stem-cell transplantation for myocardial regeneration. *Lancet.* 2003;361:45–6.

48. Shake JG, Gruber PJ, Baumgartner WA, Senechal G, Meyers J, Redmond JM, Pittenger MF, Martin BJ. Mesenchymal stem cell implantation in a swine myocardial infarct model: engraftment and functional effects. *Ann Thorac Surg.* 2002;73: 1919–26.

49. Caparrelli DJ, Cattaneo SM, Shake JG, Flynn EC, Meyers J, Baumgartner WA, Martin BJ. Cellular myoplasty with mesenchymal stem cells results in improved cardiac performance in a swine model of myocardial infarction. *Circulation.* 2001;104:II–599.

50. Devine SM, Peter S, Martin BJ, Barry F, McIntosh KR. Mesenchymal stem cells: stealth and suppression. *Cancer J.* 2001;7:S76–82.

51. Barbash IM, Chouraqui P, Baron J, Feinberg MS, Etzion S, Tessone A, Miller L, Guetta E, Zipori D, Kedes LH, Kloner RA, Leor J. Systemic delivery of bone marrow-derived mesenchymal stem cells to the infarcted myocardium: feasibility, cell migration, and body distribution. *Circulation.* 2003;108:863–8.

52. Kraitchman DL, Heldman AW, Atalar E, Amado LC, Martin BJ, Pittenger MF, Hare JM, Bulte JW. In vivo magnetic resonance imaging of mesenchymal stem cells in myocardial infarction. *Circulation.* 2003;107:2290–3.

53. Hill JM, Dick AJ, Raman VK, Thompson RB, Yu ZX, Hinds KA, Pessanha BS, Guttman MA, Varney TR, Martin BJ, Dunbar CE, McVeigh ER, Lederman RJ. Serial Cardiac Magnetic Resonance Imaging of Injected Mesenchymal Stem Cells. *Circulation.* 2003;11:11.

54. Asahara T, Murohara T, Sullivan A, Silver M, van der Zee R, Li T, Witzenbichler B, Schatteman G, Isner JM. Isolation of putative progenitor endothelial cells for angiogenesis. *Science.* 1997;275:964–7.

55. Asahara T, Masuda H, Takahashi T, Kalka C, Pastore C, Silver M, Kearne M, Magner M, Isner JM. Bone marrow origin of endothelial progenitor cells responsible for postnatal vasculogenesis in physiological and pathological neovascularization. *Circ Res.* 1999;85:221–8.

56. Kalka C, Masuda H, Takahashi T, Kalka-Moll WM, Silver M, Kearney M, Li T, Isner JM, Asahara T. Transplantation of ex vivo expanded endothelial progenitor cells for therapeutic neovascularization. *Proc Natl Acad Sci U S A.* 2000;97: 3422–7.

57. Kawamoto A, Gwon HC, Iwaguro H, Yamaguchi JI, Uchida S, Masuda H, Silver M, Ma H, Kearney M, Isner JM, Asahara T. Therapeutic potential of ex vivo expanded endothelial progenitor cells for myocardial ischemia. *Circulation.* 2001;103:634–7.

58. Kocher AA, Schuster MD, Szabolcs MJ, Takuma S, Burkhoff D, Wang J, Homma S, Edwards NM, Itescu S. Neovascularization of ischemic myocardium by human bone-marrow-derived angioblasts prevents cardiomyocyte apoptosis, reduces remodeling and improves cardiac function. *Nat Med.* 2001;7:430–6.

59. Al-Khaldi A, Al-Sabti H, Galipeau J, Lachapelle K. Therapeutic angiogenesis using autologous bone marrow stromal cells: improved blood flow in a chronic limb ischemia model. *Ann Thorac Surg*. 2003;75:204–9.
60. Fedak PW, Verma S, Weisel RD, Mickle DA, Li RK. Angiogenesis: protein, gene, or cell therapy? *Heart Surg Forum*. 2001;4:301–4.
61. Kobayashi T, Hamano K, Li TS, Katoh T, Kobayashi S, Matsuzaki M, Esato K. Enhancement of angiogenesis by the implantation of self bone marrow cells in a rat ischemic heart model. *J Surg Res*. 2000;89:189–95.
62. Reinlib L, Field L. Cell transplantation as future therapy for cardiovascular disease?: A workshop of the National Heart, Lung, and Blood Institute. *Circulation*. 2000;101:E182–7.
63. Jackson KA, Majka SM, Wang H, Pocius J, Hartley CJ, Majesky MW, Entman ML, Michael LH, Hirschi KK, Goodell MA. Regeneration of ischemic cardiac muscle and vascular endothelium by adult stem cells. *J Clin Invest*. 2001;107:1395–402.
64. Kinnaird T, Stabile E, Burnett MS, Lee CW, Barr S, Fuchs S, Epstein SE. Marrow-derived stromal cells express genes encoding a broad spectrum of arteriogenic cytokines and promote in vitro and in vivo arteriogenesis through paracrine mechanisms. *Circ Res*. 2004;94:678–85. Epub 2004 Jan 22.
65. Devine SM, Bartholomew AM, Mahmud N, Nelson M, Patil S, Hardy W, Sturgeon C, Hewett T, Chung T, Stock W, Sher D, Weissman S, Ferrer K, Mosca J, Deans R, Moseley A, Hoffman R. Mesenchymal stem cells are capable of homing to the bone marrow of non-human primates following systemic infusion. *Exp Hematol*. 2001;29:244–55.
66. Devine MJ, Mierisch CM, Jang E, Anderson PC, Balian G. Transplanted bone marrow cells localize to fracture callus in a mouse model. *J Orthop Res*. 2002;20:1232–9.
67. Wang L, Li Y, Chen J, Gautam SC, Zhang Z, Lu M, Chopp M. Ischemic cerebral tissue and MCP-1 enhance rat bone marrow stromal cell migration in interface culture. *Exp Hematol*. 2002;30:831–6.
68. Price MJ, Frantzen M, Kar S, McClean D, Gou G, Shah PK, Martin BJ, Makkar RR. Intravenous allogeneic mesenchymal stem cells home to myocardial injury and reduce left ventricular remodeling in a porcine balloon occlusion-reperfusion model of myocardial infarction. *J. Am. Coll. Card*. 2003;41:269A.
69. Martin BJ, Meyers J, Kuang J-K, Smith A. Allogeneic mesenchymal stem cell engraftment in the infarcted rat myocardium: timing and delivery route. *Bone Marrow Trans*. 2002;29:S144–P577.
70. Sorger JM, Despres D, Hill J, Schimel D, Martin BJ, McVeigh ER. MRI tracking of intravenous magnetically-labeled mesenchymal stem cells following myocardial infarction in rats. *Circulation*. 2002;106:II–16.
71. Rombouts WJ, Ploemacher RE. Primary murine MSC show highly efficient homing to the bone marrow but lose homing ability following culture. *Leukemia*. 2003;17:160–70.ABSTRACT

10
Bone Marrow Derived Stem Cells for Myocardial Regeneration: Clinical Experience, Surgical Delivery

Manuel Galiñanes[*]

1. Introduction

Heart failure is one of the commonest causes of death in the world. Despite advances in medical treatment, the management of the patient with end-stage heart failure is based on the replacement of the heart by transplantation of a new organ, but this has been restricted by the shortage of donors. The replacement of the heart by a total artificial heart is a procedure that still remains experimental. An alternative strategy to restore cardiac function can be the regeneration of the diseased myocardium by transplantation of cell lines that can differentiate into muscle. In this regard, it has been demonstrated in animal models of heart failure that a diverse range of cell types such as skeletal myoblasts,[1] bone marrow,[2] fetal and neonatal cardiomyocytes,[3,4] and even autologous heart cells[5] can improve cardiac function. There is now considerable experimental evidence that transplantation of bone marrow cells into the heart induces angiogenesis and improves contractility[6-9] but little is known of its effects in man.

The use of the patient's own cells for the regeneration of cardiac muscle has the advantages that it is ethically acceptable and immunosupression is unnecessary. The use of unmanipulated bone marrow cells as opposed to myoblasts and other cell types has the additional benefit of ready availability, without the need for *in vitro* cell culture preparation. In this chapter, the results of a phase I, non-randomized study performed by my group in which unmanipulated autologous bone marrow cells were injected into the scarred myocardium of patients undergoing coronary bypass surgery are presented. This study shows that the procedure is safe and improves myocardial contractility, a benefit that is maintained for at least the first 2 years following

---

[*]Integrative Human Cardiovascular Physiology and Cardiac Surgery Group, Department of Cardiovascular Sciences, University of Leicester, The Glenfield Hospital, Clinical Sciences, Leicester LE3 9QP, U.K.

treatment. The results of transplantation of bone marrow cells in the acute phase of a myocardial infarction are discussed in other chapters of this book, however the issues of the ideal autologous cell type for myocardial repair, the best mode of cell delivery and the potential mechanism of myocardial repair are addressed in this chapter.

2.   Effect of Autologous Bone Marrow Transplantation into Scarred Myocardium

2.1.   Experimental Studies

Bone marrow has been shown to have multipotential progenitor cells that can differentiate into muscle, cartilage, bone, fat and tendon.[10] In agreement with this thesis, experimental studies have reported that the injection of autologous bone marrow cells into ventricular scar tissue in the rat induces angiogenesis and improves myocardial function[6] and that the injection into the infarcted mouse heart of bone marrow-derived cells expressing the receptor for stem-cell factor *c-kit* but not expressing differentiation markers (*lin-*) reduces the infarct area and improves cardiac function.[2] Using immunofluorescence techniques, the same authors suggested that derived bone marrow cells differentiate into cardiomyocytes.[2] However, more recently, other researchers have shown using genetic markers that bone marrow-derived cells do not transdifferentiate into cardiomyocytes and that the fate of these cells is mainly to differentiate along the hematopoietic lineage.[11] Therefore, at present, it remains unclear whether the observed beneficial effect of bone marrow transplants is caused by differentiation of the marrow-derived cells into cardiac tissue, by stimulation of intra-cardiac progenitor cells, or by some other mechanism (see below).

2.2.   Clinical Studies

The only reported study at this writing[13] on the effect of direct injection of bone marrow cells into scarred myocardium at the time of coronary bypass graft surgery has involved 14 patients with one or more previous myocardial infarctions sustained more than 3 months before the treatment. In this study, all the patients were diagnosed with triple vessel coronary artery disease and had impaired global left ventricular function. The bone marrow was injected into the scarred areas of the left ventricle (250μl/injection 1cm apart) at the end of the revascularization procedure.

In this phase I, non-randomized study, the myocardial injections did not cause myocardial damage as suggested by the electrocardiographic and cardiac enzymes (CK, troponin T) changes and there were no perioperative complications attributable to the injections. As shown in Figures 1a and 1b, during the first 2 years of follow-up all patients improved clinically in terms of angina and dyspnea class, and there were no deaths, new myocardial infarctions or other cardiac events. These results demonstrate that transplantation of unmanipulated autologous bone marrow by intramyocardial injections during heart surgery is safe and that it is not associated with perioperative complications or detrimental medium-term effects. The absence of ventricular arrhythmias provides reassurance in the light of *in vitro* evidence that stem cell-derived cardiomyocytes have the potential to generate arrhythmias.[14]

The analysis of the contractile status of the scarred myocardium showed that following treatment there was a partial but significant recovery of function. Some of the infarcted segments, such as those in the intraventricular septum, were not accessible for injection, and other injected segments could not be revascularized due to the presence of small epicardial coronary arteries that were ungraftable. Because of this, the 34 infarcted segments in the 14 study patients were divided into 3 groups according to the treatment applied: (1) bone marrow injection alone (n=11 segments), (2) bypass graft alone (n=13 segments), and (3) bone marrow injection and bypass graft in combination (n=10 segments). Figure 2 shows that whereas bone marrow transplantation and bypass graft alone did not ameliorate segmental wall motion stress index (WMSI), the combination of the two treatment modalities resulted in statistically significant improvement of the scores at low (10μg/kg/min) and peak dobutamine stress (maximum dobutamine dose of 40μg/kg/min) at 6 weeks, 10 months and 2 years after surgery, which may indicate an increase in contractile tissue in these segments.

The number of mononuclear cells and dual staining $CD34^+/CD117^+$ (*c-kit^{pos}*) injected per each treated segment was $31.5\pm3.5 \times 10^6$ and $0.61\pm0.1 \times 10^6$, respectively, and they were not correlated with the improvement in

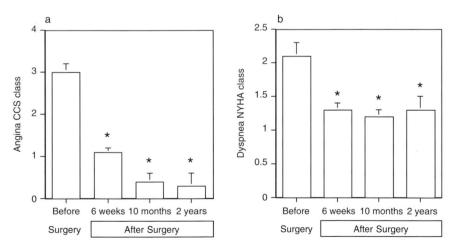

FIGURE 1. Angina and dyspnea class before surgery and 6 weeks, 10 months and 2 years after surgery. *p<0.05 versus the mean values before surgery.

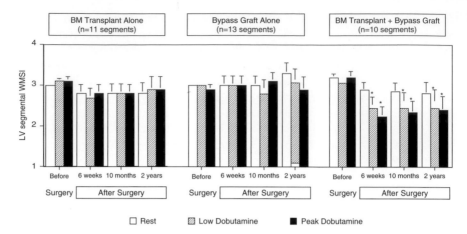

FIGURE 2. Left ventricle (LV) segmental wall motion score index (WMSI) before surgery and 6 weeks, 10 months and 2 years after surgery at rest and at low and peak dobutamine stress of infarcted segments that received injection of bone marrow alone (n= 11 segments), bypass graft alone (n= 13 segments), or bone marrow and bypass graft in combination (n= 10 segments). *p<0.05 versus the corresponding mean values before surgery.

contractility. Previous studies have demonstrated that the putative pluripotential stem cell is Lin⁻-*c-kit^pos* in murine models of cardiac regeneration.[2] These cells exist at a low level within the bone marrow somewhere between 1 in 10,000 to 100,000 cells and it is reasonable to assume that only a relatively small number of true pluripotent stem cells were transplanted at each injection site in this study.

3.   Identifying a Bone Marrow Cell Type Specifically Suited for Myocardial Repair

The unfractionated bone marrow contains a mixture of hemopoeitic and mesenchymal stem cells and other undefined stem cells. Both hemopoeitic and mesenchymal stem cells have now been shown to have significant capacity to differentiate into a variety of cell types[15-19]; however, it has been recently suggested that hemopoeitic stem cell transdifferentiation into non-hemopoeitic cell lines is not common in the steady state,[20] although the response in the setting of selective tissue, whether this is normal or injured, is unknown. Therefore, the debate over the specific capacity of hemopoeitic stem cells to transdifferentiate remains to be resolved.

Human mesenchymal stem cells were first isolated and shown to have multiple differentiation potential by Haynesworth et al.[21] Thereafter, the multilineage potential of human mesenchymal cells was demonstrated by *in vitro* methods[22] and also that these cells can differentiate into cardiomyocytes when injected in the left ventricle of the adult murine heart.[23] All the evidence suggests that bone marrow is a potential inexhaustible source of pluripotential cells that can differentiate into a variety of cell types dependent on local environmental cues, although, as discussed above, recent reports have challenged this thesis.[11,12]

Despite the intense on-going investigation, the origin (hemopoeitic stem cell, mesenchymal stem cells or other undefined cells) and the mechanism responsible for the reconstitution of heart tissue by bone marrow cells remain unclear. Therefore, at present is not possible to recommend the use of a specific marrow-derived cell type for clinical use. The results of our study in patients undergoing cardiac surgery[13] suggest that, while these questions are addressed, there is no obvious impediment to proceed with further studies in human beings in order to refine the treatment and to identify the group of patients who may benefit from this therapy before a wider clinical application is considered.

It is important to emphasize that the growth of bone marrow cells in *in vitro* culture conditions is slow and labor-intensive and that it may cause some loss of the multilineage potential originally present in these cells. Therefore, from a practical point of view, it may be better to transplant the unfractionated bone marrow rather than to separate and grow the cells before their administration even if a specific cell type is identified as cardiac progenitor. However, the report that direct transplantation of unselected bone marrow cells into the acutely infarcted rat myocardium may induce significant intramyocardial calcification[24] would raise a word of caution.

4. Route of Delivery of Bone Marrow Cells

The route of administration of bone marrow cells probably plays an important role on the success of the treatment but the optimal mode of cell delivery is currently unknown. The administration of bone marrow during cardiac surgery by injection into the selected myocardial areas may appear the preferred route because of direct vision of the scar tissue. However this modality, that seems to be safe and easily applied to the target areas, may be an inefficient and impractical route of cell delivery since the injected cells will be localized to a few points of the heart and the majority of the myocardium would not be in contact or in the vicinity of the transplanted cells. A variation of the direct injection through the epicardium is the catheter-based transendocardial transplantation via the arterial system, which has also been shown to be safe in subjects with advanced coronary artery disease[25] and with chronic ischemic heart failure.[26] The concomitant use of electromagnetic mapping to generate

3-dimensional left ventricular reconstruction helps to identify the target areas with this approach, however the intraventricular catheter manipulation has the potential to injure the myocardium and to induce ventricular arrhythmias.

The preferred route of delivery of bone marrow cells in cardiology patients has been the intracoronary administration that again has been reported to be safe and effective in the context of acute myocardial infarction.[27] The theoretical advantages of this approach are that the entire target area would be exposed to the transplanted cells during the immediate first passage and that the procedure can be repeated without the need for general anesthetic agents. However, preliminary results from my group obtained from patients undergoing coronary bypass graft surgery are suggesting that both routes, intracoronary and intramyocardial, are equally safe and effective (Galiñanes et al. 2004, unpublished data). The easiest route of cell delivery is the intravenous administration, but the main disadvantage of this approach is that only a small fraction of the injected cells will flow through the heart and the lungs may retain many of these cells during the first passage, thus reducing the number of cells that could populate the target areas. In the future, detailed studies should be carried out to elucidate which cell delivery route is the safest and most effective.

5. Potential Mechanism of Myocardial Repair by Bone Marrow Cells

Very little is known on how transplanted bone marrow cells improve cardiac function. The pluripotential properties of bone marrow cells may lead to the assumption that the heart is repaired by differentiation of these cells into myocardial tissue structures (e.g., myocytes, endothelium, smooth muscle, fibroblasts). There is experimental evidence that this may be the case but, as discussed above, this hypothesis has been recently disputed.[11,12] The realization that the myocardium, as many other tissues, may possess resident stem cells[28,29] offers the possibility that the transplantation of bone marrow cells may in fact act as a trigger for the division and differentiation of local progenitor cells. This possibility would be supported by the observation that the beneficial action of implanted bone marrow cells may be mediated through the production of cytokines such as VEGF and bFGF[8,30] that, in turn, could stimulate resident progenitor cells. Growth factors have cardioprotective properties[31-33] and yet another possibility could be that the production of these factors by bone marrow cells may result in a reduction in myocardial cell death, which is a salient feature of heart failure.[34,35] A reduction in cardiomyocyte apoptosis in the peri-infarct region with long-term salvage and survival of viable myocardium has been seen in a rat model of ischemic myocardium when human bone marrow cells were injected intravenously.[36] The debate is further complicated by the concept of cell fusion of bone marrow cells with native cells that offers an explanation for the presumed transdifferentiation, but its relevance as a potential mechanism of myocardial repair is under considerable dispute.[37] Tissue repair with stem cells is a new emerging field, and it is clear that more research is needed to elucidate the mechanism by which contractility of the scarred myocardium is improved.

6.   Summary

The studies reviewed herein suggest that transplantation of unmanipulated autologous bone marrow may provide a novel and promising means of reversing post-infarction left ventricular dysfunction caused by scarred tissue, and may have important clinical implications for improving the long-term prognosis of these patients and possibly the prevention of the occurrence of heart failure. The intramyocardial injection of marrow cells during coronary bypass graft surgery seems to be safe and the beneficial effect in contractile function, that requires revascularization of the scarred areas at the same time, is maintained for at least the first 2 years after its application. The use of bone marrow avoids the complexity of cell-culture techniques and the concerns that repeated *in vitro* passaging of primary cells like myoblasts may alter their ability to fuse and differentiate.[38] Furthermore, in comparison to transplanted allogenic and xenogenic cells, the use of autologous bone marrow does not pose a risk of rejection, does not require immunosuppressant drugs and has no ethical constraints.

It is important to note that the beneficial effect of autologous bone marrow transplantation on contractility was only partial, but it is unknown whether repeated injections of bone marrow cells or the use of genetic modification to prolong their survival may result in a full restitution of function. Thus, studies in the rat suggest that overexpression of the prosurvival gene Akt1 (encoding the Akt protein) in mesenchymal stem cells injected in the border zone of the ischemic left ventricle inhibits remodeling, regenerates most of the lost myocardial volume and normalizes cardiac function.[39] There is an urgent need for more research on the underlying mechanism of recovery of cardiac function by transplantation of bone marrow to optimize this therapy.

7.   Acknowledgments

The author greatly appreciates the support of the British Heart Foundation (project grant No. PG/04/050) and the assistance of Nicola Harris in preparing this chapter.

8.   References

1. Taylor, D.A.; Atkins, B.Z.; Hungspreugs, P.; et al. Regenerating functional myocardium: improved performance after skeletal myoblast transplantation. Nat Med. 4:929–933; 1998.
2. Orlic, D.; Kajstura, J.; Chimenti, S.; et al. Bone marrow cells regenerate infarcted myocardium. Nature. 410:701–705; 2001.
3. Soonpaa, M.H.; Koh, G.Y.; Klug, M.G.; Field, L.J. Formation of nascent inter-calated disks between grafted fetal cardiomyocytes and host myocardium. Science. 264: 98–101; 1994.
4. Muller-Ehmsen, J.; Peterson, K.L.; Kedes, L.; et al. Rebuilding a damaged heart: long-term survival of transplanted neonatal rat cardiomyocytes after myocardial infarction and effect on cardiac function. Circulation. 105:1720–1726; 2002.
5. Li, R.K.; Weisel, R.D.; Mickle, D.A.; et al. Autologous porcine heart cell trans-plantation improved heart function after a myocardial infarction. J Thorac Car-diovasc Surg. 119:62–68; 2000.
6. Tomita, S.; Li, R.K.; Weisel, R.D.; et al. Autologous transplantation of bone mar-row cells improves damaged heart function. Circulation. 100(Suppl):II247–II256; 1999.
7. Fuchs, S.; Baffour, R.; Zhou, Y.F.; et al. Transendocardial delivery of autologous bone marrow enhances collateral perfusion and regional function in pigs with chronic experimental myocardial ischemia. J Am Coll Cardiol 37:1726–1732; 2001.
8. Kamihata, H.; Matsubara, H.; Nishiue, T.; et al. Implantation of bone marrow mononuclear cells into ischemic myocardium enhances collateral perfusion and regional function via side supply of angioblasts, angiogenic ligands, and cytokines. Circulation. 104:1046–1052; 2001.
9. Tomita, S.; Mickle, D.A.; Weisel, R.D.; et al. Improved heart function with myo-genesis and angiogenesis after autologous porcine bone marrow stromal cell transplantation. J Thorac Cardiovasc Surg. 123:1132–1140; 2002.
10. Saito, T.; Dennis, J.E.; Lennon, D.P.; Young, R.G.; Caplan, A.I. Myogenic expres-sion of mesenchymal stem cells within myotubes of mdx mice in vitro and in vivo. Tissue Eng. 1:327–343; 1995.
11. Murry, C.E.; Soonpaa, M.H.; Reinecke, H.; et al. Haematopoietic stem cells do not transdifferentiate into cardiac myocytes in myocardial infarcts. Nature. 428:664–668; 2004.
12. Balsam, L.B.; Wagers, A.J.; Christensen, J.L.; Kofidis T.; Weissman, I.L.; Robbins, R.C. Haematopoietic stem cells adopt mature haematopoietic fates in ischaemic myocardium. Nature. 428:668–673; 2004.
13. Galiñanes, M.; Loubani, M.; Davies, J.; Chin, D.; Pasi, J.; Bell, P.R. Autotrans-plantation of unmanipulated bone marrow into scarred myocardium is safe and enhances cardiac function in humans. Cell Transpl. 13:7–13; 2004.
14. Zhang, Y.M.; Hartzell, C.; Narlow, M.; Dudley, S.C. Stem cell-derived cardiomy-ocytes demonstrate arrhythmic potential. Circulation. 106:1294–1299; 2002.
15. Petersen, B.E.; Bowen, W.C.; Patrene, K.D.; et al. Bone marrow as a potential source of hepatic oval cells. Science. 284:1168–1170; 1999.
16. Ferrari, G.; Cusella-De Angelis, G.; Coletta, M.; et al. Muscle regeneration by bone marrow-derived myogenic progenitors. Science. 279:1528–1530; 1998.

17. Kopen, G.C.; Prockop, D.J.; Phinney, D.G. Marrow stromal cells migrate through-out forebrain and cerebellum, and they differentiate into astrocytes after injection into neonatal mouse brains. Proc Natl Acad Sci USA. 96:10711–10716; 2000.
18. Reyes, M.; Dudek, A.; Jahagindar, B.; Koodie, L.; Marker, P.H.; Verfaillie, C. Origin of endothelial progenitors in human postnatal bone marrow. J Clin Invest. 109:337–346; 2002.
19. Krause, D.S.; Theise, N.D.; Collector, M.I.; et al. Multi-organ, multi-lineage engraftment by a single bone marrow-derived stem cell. Cell. 105:369–377; 2001.
20. Wagers, A.J.; Sherwood, R.I.; Christensen, J.L.; Weissman, I.L. Little evidence for developmental plasticity of adult hematopoietic stem cells. Science. 297:2256–2259; 2002.
21. Haynesworth, S.E.; Goshima, J.; Goldberg, V.M.; Caplan, A.I. Characterization of cells with osteogenic potential from human marrow. Bone. 13:81–88; 1992. 28. Beltrami, A.P.; Barlucchi, L.; Torella, D.; et al. Adult cardiac stem cells are multi-potent and support support myocardial regeneration. Cell. 114:763–776; 2003.
22. Pittenger, M.F.; Mackay, A.M.; Beck, S.C.; et al. Multilineage potential of adult human mesenchymal stem cells. Science. 284:143–147; 1999.
23. Toma, C.; Pittenger, M.F.; Cahill, K.S.; Byrne, B.J.; Kessler, P.D. Human mesenchymal stem cells differentiate to a cardiomyocyte phenotype in the adult murine heart. Circulation. 105:93–98; 2002.
24. Yoon, Y.-S.; Park, J.-S; Tkebuchava, T.; Luedeman, C.; Losordo, D.W. Unexpected severe calcification after transplantation of bone marrow cells in acute myocardial infarction. Circulation. 109:3154–3157; 2004.
25. Fuchs, S.; Satler, L.F.; Kornowski, R.; et al. Catheter-based autologous bone marrow myocardial injection in no-option patients with advanced coronary artery disease. J Am Coll Cardiol. 41:1721–1724; 2003.
26. Perin, E.C.; Dohmann, H.F.R.; Borojevic, R.; et al. Transendocardial autologous bone marrow cell transplantation for severe, chronic ischemic heart failure. Circulation. 107:2294–2302; 2003.
27. Strauer, B.E.; Brehm, M.; Zeus, T.; et al. Repair of infarcted myocardium by autologous intracoronary mononuclear bone marrow cell transplantation in humans. Circulation. 106:1913–1918; 2002.
28. Beltrami, A.P.; Barlucchi, L.; Torella, D.; et al. Adult cardiac stem cells are multi-potent and support myocardial regeneration. Cell. 114: 763–776; 2003.
29. Oh, H.; Bradfute, S.B.; Gallardo, T.D.; et al. Cardiac progenitor cells from adult myocardium: homing, differentiation, and fusion after infarction. PNAS. 100:12313–12318; 2003.
30. Kinnaird, T.; Stabile, E.; Burnett, M.S.; et al. Marrow-derived stromal cells express genes encoding a broad spectrum of arteriogenic cytokines and promote in vitro and in vivo arteriogenesis through paracrine mechanisms. Circ Res. 94:678–685; 2004.
31. Spyridopoulos, I.; Brogi, E.; Kearny, M.; et al. Vascular endothelial growth factor inhibits endothelial cell apoptosis induced by tumor necrosis factor-alpha: balance between growth and death signals. J Mol Cell Cardiol. 29:1321–1330; 1997.
32. Kim, I.; Moon, S.O.; Han, C.Y.; et al. The angiopoietin-tie2 system in coronary artery endothelium prevents oxidized low-density lipoprotein-induced apoptosis. Cardiovasc Res. 49:872–881; 2001.

33. Edelberg, J.M.; Lee, S.H.; Kaur, M.; et al. Platelet-derived growth factor-AB limits the extent of myocardial infarction in a rat model: feasibility of restoring impaired angiogenic capacity in the aging heart. Circulation. 105:608–613; 2002.
34. Narula, J.; Haider, N.; Virmani, R.; et al. Apoptosis in myocytes in end-stage heart failure. N Engl J Med. 335:1182–1189; 1996.
35. Olivetti, G.; Abbi, R.; Quaini, F.; et al. Apoptosis in the failing human heart. N Engl J Med. 336:1131–1141; 1997.
36. Kocher, A.A.; Schuster, M.D.; Szabolcs, M.J.; et al. Neovascularization of ischemic myocardium by human bone-marrow-derived angioblasts prevents cardiomyocyte apoptosis, reduces remodeling and improves cardiac function. Nat Med. 7:430–436; 2001.
37. Mathur, A.; Martin, J.F. Stem cells and repair of the heart. Lancet 364:183–192; 2004.
38. Rosenblatt, J.D.; Lunt, A.I.; Parry, D.J.; Partridge, T.A. Culturing satellite cells from living single muscle fiber explants. In Vitro Cell Dev Biol Anim. 31:773–779; 1995.
39. Mangi, A.A.; Noiseux, N.; Kong, D.; et al. Mesenchymal stem cells modified with Akt prevent remodeling and restore performance of infarcted hearts. Nat Med. 9:1195–1201; 2003.

11
Autologous Mononuclear Bone Marrow Cell Transplantion for Myocardial Infarction: The German Experience

MICHAEL BREHM, TOBIAS ZEUS AND BODO E. STRAUER[*]

1. Introduction

Ischemic heart disease accounts for approximately 50% of all cardiovascular deaths and is the leading cause of congestive heart failure.[1] With 1.1 million myocardial infarctions and more than 400.000 new cases of congestive heart failure each year in the United States, cardiovascular disease severely impacts men and women. For patients diagnosed with congestive heart failure, a consequence of chronic heart failure, the one-year mortality rate is 20%. Myocardial necrosis is due to myocardial infarction and is, by nature, an irreversible injury.[2] After 15 to 20 minutes of coronary artery occlusion the cardiomyocytes are destroyed irreversible.[3] The extent of the infarction, respectively the loss of cardiomyocytes, depends on the duration and severity of perfusion defect.[4] However, the extent of infarction is also modulated by a number of factors including collateral blood supply, medications, and ischemic preconditioning.[5] Beyond contraction and fibrosis of myocardial scar, progressive ventricular remodeling of nonischemic myocardium can further reduce cardiac function in the weeks to months after the initial event.[6] Many of the therapies, available to clinicians today, can significantly improve the prognosis of patients with acute myocardial infarction.[7] Although angioplasty and thrombolytic agents can relieve the cause of the infarction by prompt reperfusion of the occluded artery, the time from onset of occlusion to reperfusion determines the degree of irreversible myocardial injury.[8] However, postinfarction heart failure remains a major challenge, resulting from ventricular remodeling processes, characterized by progressive expansion of the infarct area and dilatation of the left ventricular (LV) cavity.[9]

[*]Michael Brehm and Bodo Strauer, Dept. of Internal Medicine, Div. of Cardiology, Pneumology and Angiology, Heinrich-Heine-University, Moorestr. 5, 40225 Düsseldorf, Germany; e-mail: brehmic@aol.com, strauer@med.uni-duesseldorf.de.

The major goal to reverse LV remodeling would be the enhancement of regeneration of cardiac myocytes as well as the stimulation of neovascularization within the infarct area, by repopulation of the injured myocardium with healthy autologous cells or by induced proliferation of endogenous resident cardiac stem cells.[10-14] Experimental studies suggested that bone marrow-derived or blood-derived progenitor cells may contribute to the regeneration of the infarcted myocardium[15] and enhance neovascularization ischemic myocardium.[16-18] Indeed, either intravenous infusion or intramyocardial injection of adult progenitor cells resulted in sustained improvement of cardiac function after experimentally induced myocardial infarction.[19,20] Therefore, clinical studies were performed to investigate the feasibility, safety and initial clinical outcome of transplantation of autologous progenitor cells in patients with acute myocardial infarction or ischemic left ventricular impairment (Figure 1, 2).

2.   Physiological Cell Regeneration After Myocardial Infarction

Until very recently, there was widespread consensus that proliferation of cardiac myocytes ceases permanently soon after birth and that there is no replacement with new cardiomyocyts either physiologically or after damage. Although cardiomyocytes do arise by nuclear division, cytokinesis appears to be blocked in humans. This block of cellular proliferation occurs as a specific event in human cardiac muscle, as human skeletal myocytes and cardiac cell

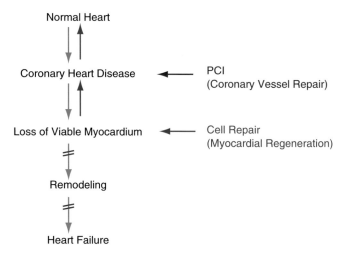

FIGURE 1. Development of heart failure after myocardial infarction and therapeutical interventions for prevention.

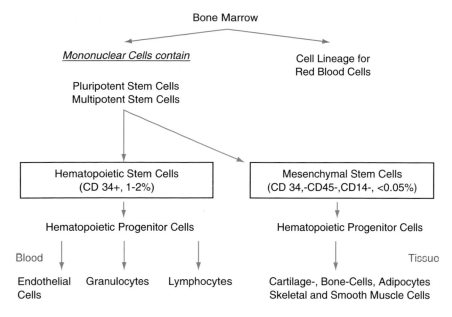

FIGURE 2. Components of bone marrow cells and their differentiation pathway.

in other species seem to be endowed with considerably greater mitotic potential.[21,22] New data suggest, however, that there is a low level of myocyte proliferation also in the human postnatal heart, amounting to approximately 14 cells per million in normal heart, which is increased tenfold in heart disease. Since there is also a progressive loss of cardiomyocytes, calculated at 6×10^6 cardiomyocytes per year, it now appears that there indeed may be a slow turnover of cardiac myocytes throughout life.[23,24] Understanding cell cycle control of human cardiomyocytes has become an area of intensive scientific research, but the master regulators of postnatal cardiomyocyte mitosis are currently still largely unclear.[25]

The traditional understanding implicates that cardiomyocytes are unable to undergo mitosis and proliferation, however they are limited to hypertrophy in order to compensate the loss of functional tissue after myocardial infarction. So the dogma that the heart is a terminally differentiated postmitotic organ incapable of self-renewal has recently been changed.[26-28,57]

Proliferative repair mechanisms were thought to be restricted to vascular cells in the way of angiogenesis and arteriogenesis for the formation of collateral vessels and also fibroblasts, replacing cardiac muscle with connective tissue (scar formation). recently A notable study has extended the findings on myocardial cell proliferation described above to the immediate postinfarction period.[29] Analyzing cardiac tissue samples from the border of the infarct zone and from areas distant form the infarct for the expression of a nuclear proliferation marker, they demonstrated a reentry into the cell cycle in about 0.08% of myocytes in the infarct zone and in 0.03% in the distant area, both significant elevations over the levels found in control hearts. Of course their ability to minimize the deleterious effects of remodeling and recovery of cardiac function is limited. In addition, events characteristic of cell division – the formation of mitotic spindles, karyokinesis and cytokinesis – were identified. Overall, these results raise the probability, that the regeneration of myocytes may, indeed, contribute to a true increase of muscle mass following myocardial infarction. Despite the enormous impact of this report the actual origin of the dividing cells found in the infarcted hearts remains unclear, i.e., whether these were locally resident heart muscle cells reentering a cell-division program or whether circulation cells endowed with a preserved higher mitotic potential had infiltrated the infarct area and other parts of the functionally impaired heart. This question becomes even more intriguing when viewed in the context of another seminal study, investigating the contribution of bone marrow-derived stem cells to repair mechanisms operative in ischemically damaged heart muscle in an animal model.[30] A certain subpopulation of highly enriched hematopoietic stem cells from the bone marrow cells, the so-called side population cells, were transplanted in to lethally irradiated mice. The side population cells were taken from a transgenic mouse strain, expressing a marker antigen in all cells of the body. Ten weeks after the bone marrow transplantation the recipient mice were rendered ischemic by coronary artery occlusion for 60 minutes followed by reperfusion. Subsequent histological examination showed that the engrafted side population cells or their progeny migrated into the ischemic cardiac muscle and blood vessels, differentiated to cardiomyocytes and endothelial cells, and contribute to the formation of functional tissue. Donor-derived cardiomyocytes were found primarily in the perinfarct region at a prevalence of around 0.02%. Endothelial engraftment was found at a prevalence of around 3.3%, primarily in small vessels adjacent to the infarct. These results demonstrate the cardiomyogenic potential of hematopoietic stem cells and suggest a possible alternative explanation for the presence of dividing cells in the infarct area as described above[29] especially as in the study performed in human hearts the presence of stem cell markers have not specifically been investigated. In this regard it is interesting to note that similar infiltration of bone marrow-derived or circulating stem cells or progenitor cells has now been reported by several authors as a (patho-) physiological event after cardiac transplantation,[31,32] a situation in which the presence of non-resident cell in the heart can be demonstrated very easily, because of their different tissue type and gender.

Overall, in contrast to the long-standing dogma, there is now evidence to support some proliferation of postnatal cardiomyocytes in humans, especially after heart damage. The origin of such proliferating cardiomyocytes currently remains enigmatic, but contribution by bone marrow–derived stem cells or circulation progenitor cells appear most likely. Nonetheless, these human data should be interpreted as nothing more than a proof basically for physiological repair mechanisms after myocardial infarction, because the functional relevance of these findings is entirely still unproven. In contrast to some animal data, especially the issues of true myocardial differentiation and the development of intercellular contacts for force transmission and electrical conductance have not been rigorously addressed in these studies. Furthermore, it should not be ignored that these autoreparative processes either through local proliferation or the invasion of stem/progenitor cells are exceedingly infrequent and cannot significantly mitigate the adverse functional consequences of myocardial infarction in animals or humans.[33] The realization that self-healing processes are clearly insufficient to counter the loss of functional tissue after ischemic injury to the heart is of course very much in line with our clinical experience of myocardial infarction under current standard medical care. On the other hand, the increasing understanding of mechanisms of repair and regeneration of the damaged heart forms the indispensable foundation for exciting novel approaches to the treatment of myocardial infarction.

3.   Cellular Cardiomyoplasty

When confronted with the problem of therapy of heart damage after infarction, replacement of myocytes is the only causal and therefore ideal treatment, as only full regeneration of functional cardiac tissue lost through necrosis can avoid the unwanted consequences of cardiac remodeling. Because of the recent data on cardiac autoregeneration and growing list of stimulating animal data, there is increasing interest in cell transplantation as a potential therapy for cardiovascular disease. Independent of the type of cell or tissue used for cellular regeneration therapy, there are some basic principles to be borne in mind when assessing the relative usefulness of such treatment strategies: to be clinically effective, the enhancement of cardiomyocyte proliferation after damage must be rapid if the organism is to survive any acute insult that disrupts heart function through damage to the individual cardiac myocytes. In cases in which there is chronic damage to the heart muscle, the proliferation might need to be sustained to slowly but continually replace myocytes as necessary during the course of disease. Regardless the source of the cells and the use to which they are put, a concurrent revascularization must also keep pace with repopulation of the infarct to ensure viability and survival of the repaired region and prevent further scar tissue formation. Finally, the newly formed myocardium must integrate into the existing myocardial wall if it is to assume the function of the tissue it replaces. All of this must occur while the heart continues to beat and perform the essential work of supplying blood throughout the organism. Furthermore, even small areas of imperfectly integrated tissues are likely to severely alter electrical conduction and syncytial concentration of the heart, with long-term life-threatening consequences.

The ideal cellular source for transplantation and regeneration is currently an issue of intensive scientific debate[25,34,58,59] for both theoretical and practical purpose the following cell types seem to hold some promise for an eventual clinical application in the treatment of acute myocardial infarction: adult stem cells, embryonic stem cells, umbilical cord stem cells and endothelial progenitors cells (Table 1).

4.   Administration of Stem Cells

The appropriate route of cell administration to the damaged organ is an essential prerequisite for the success of organ repair (Figure 3). Large cell concentrations within the area of interest and prevention of homing of transplanted cells into other organs are desirable. Different routes of application may be important for different kinds of heart disease. Therefore, targeted and regional administration and transplantation of cell should be preferred.

In regional heart muscle disease, as in myocardial infarction, selective cell delivery by intracoronary catheterization techniques leads to an effective accumulation and concentration of cells within the infarcted zone, a mechanism which tries to offer the stem cells the best chance to find their niche within the myocardium. This can be realized in humans with bone marrow-derived cells. By the intracoronary administration, all cells must pass the infarct and perinfarct tissue during the immediate first passage. Accordingly, by the intracoronary procedure the infarct tissue can be enriched and infiltrated with the maximum available number of cells at all times.[35]

The second way, the transendocardial and transpericardial administration method has been used in large animal experiments,[36] and was also recently tested in patients.[37-39] Current clinical experience is limited to one injection system, using electromechanical mapping to generate three-dimensional left ventricular reconstruction prior to the injection. Intraventricular catheter

TABLE 1. Different types of cells for therapeutic potentials in cellular cardiomyoplasty after myocardial infarction

	Cell types
Clinical trials	Adult stem cells
	Endothelial progenitor cells
	Angioblasts (AC133+ cells)
	Skeletal myoblasts
Animal models	Embryonic stem cells
	Umbilical cord stem cells
	Neonatal cardiomyocytes
	Adult cardiomyocytes

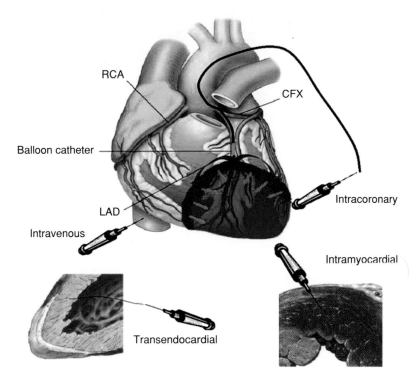

FIGURE 3. Administration pathways for stem cell transfer to the heart. The red colored area represents apical lesion of the left ventricle by myocardial infarction. The
balloon catheter is localized in the infarct related artery and is placed above the border zone of the infarction. Blue and green arrows suggest the possible route of cell
infusion and migration into the infarct. The two small figures depict the transendocardial and intrmyocardial route of administration. RCA, right coronary artery;
LAD, left anterior descending coronary artery; CFX, circumflex artery.

manipulation, however, can injure the myocardium, inducing ventricular premature beats, short runs of ventricular tachycardia and pericardial effusion.[18,40] Future developments with steerable transendocardial injection and
delivery systems with mapping of the injured zone are needed.

The third application route, the <u>intravenous</u> administration is the easiest
way. However, it is disadvantageous that approximately only 3% of normal
cardiac output will flow per minute through the left ventricle and it is also
limited due to transpulmonary first-pass attenuation effect on the cells. Therefore, this administration technique will require many circulation passages to
enable infused cells to come into contact with the infarct-related artery. During that time, homing of infused cells to other organs will considerably reduce
the number of cells that will populate the infarcted area. This homing effect
has been evaluated, demonstration large amount of injected stem cells in

various extracardiac organs as in liver, spleen or in the lungs, but only to a minor proportion in the heart.[41,42] Thus, direct application of cells into the target organ is desirable for example by selective catheterisation techniques to avoid homing to non-desired organs.

The fourth approach, especially in animal experiments, displays the direct intramuscular cell injection which has also been used in open heart surgery[43] for coronary artery bypass grafting (CABG), showing improvement in myocardial perfusion in three of five treated patients. These changes were determined by pre- and postoperative thallium scintigraphy.[44] It may be conceivable that different and individual cell application routes are necessary for specific heart muscle diseases for coronary as well as for valve disease.

5.   Detection of Transplanted Stem Cells

Another experimental and clinical problem will be aimed to identify and localize transplanted autologous stem cells within the injured area of the heart. The transplanted cell or cell population is a single unit in a complex biological network of other cells. Therefore, for both, localization and gate mapping of stem cells within the target organ, specific cell markers are desirable. However, a hallmark of most stem cells is the lack of expression of a specific stem cell marker. Therefore, analysis of stem cell behavior will presume in situ labeling of a single cell or a transplanted population or transplantation of already *in vitro* labeled cells or cell populations.

Myocardial implanted myogenic precursor cells, previously loaded with iron oxide, can be reliably detected *in vivo* in animals by cardiac magnetic resonance imaging (MRI). Seven farm pigs with myocardial infarction were treated with autologous myogenic precursor cells, injected through a percutaneous catheter allowing for left ventricular electromechanical mapping and guided micro-injections into normal and infarcted myocardium. The iron-loaded myogenic precursor cells were detected *in vivo* by cardiac MRI. This ability to identify noninvasively intramyocardial cell implantation by cardiac MRI, may allow analyzing subsequent effects of cell therapy.[45]

For labeling in animal experiments retroviral transduction with a marker gene or labeling thymidine or bromodeoxyuridine (BrdU) have been used. For clinical detection of stem cells, magnetic labeling and *in vivo* tracking of bone marrow cells by the use of magnetodendrimers, iron oxide or radioactive detection methods may be useful. Single photon emission computed tomography (SPECT) and positron emission tomography (PET) imaging can determine myocardial perfusion and viability. Magnetic resonance imaging (MRI) evaluates cardiac anatomy and volumes.[46] Furthermore, iron labeled stem cells[47] may be detected noninvasively with MRI in the healthy and infarcted myocardium.[45,47,48] These methods, however, have not yet been established in humans. Myocardial biopsies hardly will be justifiable under these circumstances. Recently, an autopsy report demonstrated that 17.5 months after transplantation of autologous skeletal myoblast the grafted post-infarction scar showed well developed skeletal myoblasts with a preserved contractile apparatus. The myoblast grafts survived and showed a switch to slow-twitch fibres, which might lead to sustained improvement in cardiac function.[49]

6.   Stem Cells for Cardiac Repair: Clinical Data

6.1.   Endogenous Bone Marrow Cells

Therapeutic transplants of sex-mismatched bone marrow and orthotopic organ transplants in male recipients have been used to study human bone marrow stem cells plasticity. Archival samples of liver and heart, obtained from female recipients of a male bone marrow transplant, and from male patients, who had received a liver or heart transplants from female donors, were positive for Y-chromosome.[50,51] Although differing widely in percentage of Y-positive myocytes detected, several reports[31,32] conclude that recipient cells repopulate the myocardium in transplanted heart.[57] Taken together, these data provide the evidence that circulation human bone marrow stem cells traffic to nonhematopoietic organs, where they give rise to cells of completely different origin and phenotypes.[53]

6.2.   Exogenous Bone Marrow Cells

In March 2001, the first patient was treated with direct administration of autologous mononuclear bone marrow cells.[35] A 46 year-old patient with an acute myocardial anterior wall infarction due to occlusion of the left anterior descending coronary artery was treated with percutaneous transluminal catheter angioplasty and stent placement. Five days later, the patient's own bone marrow cells were harvested from the hip and after one over-night culture 12×10^6 mononuclear bone marrow cells were transplanted at low pressure over catheter injection into the infarct-related artery.

Cells were directly transplanted into the infarcted zone (Figure 4). This was accomplished by the use of a balloon catheter, which was placed within the infarcted-related artery. After exact positioning of the balloon at the site of the former infarct-vessel occlusion, percutaneous coronary intervention (PCI) was performed six to seven times for two to four minutes each. During this time, intracoronary cell transplantation over the balloon catheter was performed, using six to seven fractional high-pressure infusions of 2 to 3ml cell suspension, each of which contained 1.5 to 4 million mononuclear cells. PCI (balloon inflation) thoroughly prevented the backflow of cells and at the same time produced a stop-flow beyond the site of the balloon inflation to

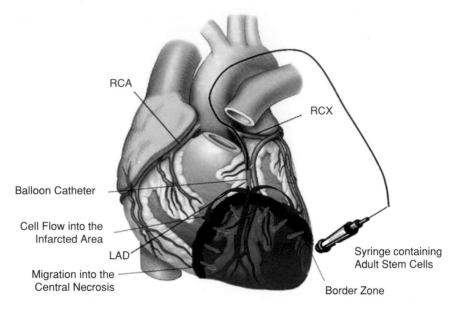

RCA

RCX

Balloon Catheter

Cell Flow into the
Infarcted Area

LAD

Migration into the
Central Necrosis

Syringe containing
Adult Stem Cells

Border Zone

FIGURE 4. Bone marrow cell transplantation into infarcted myocardium in humans. The balloon catheter enters the infarct-related artery and is placed above the border zone of the infarction. It is then inflated and the cell suspension (including the bodies own cytokines) is infused at high pressure under stop-flow conditions. In this way, cells are transplanted into the infarcted zone over the infarct-related vessel system. Cells and cytokines infiltrate the infarcted zone. Blue and green arrows suggest the possible route of cell migration and cytokine infiltration. RCA, right coronary artery; LAD, left anterior descending coronary artery; CFX, circumflex artery.

facilitate high-pressure infusion of cells into the infarcted zone. Thus, prolonged contact time for cellular migration was allowed.

Ten weeks after, the infarcted area had decreased in size from 24.6 to 15.7% of left ventricular circumference, while global ejection fraction, cardiac index and stroke volume increased by 20 to 30%. During exercise, end-diastolic volume and pulmonary capillary wedge pressure (PC) had decreased by 30%. This case report demonstrated for the first time, the potential of autologous stem cell therapy to achieve restoration of cardiac function and improvement in myocardial perfusion after transmural infarction. This patient has been the first in a larger phase I clinical trial with direct intracoronary autologous transplantation of adult stem cells in patients following acute myocardial infarction.[54] Twenty patients participated in this trial. Ten patients were treated by autologous, mononuclear bone marrow cells in addition to standard therapy of infarction. The other ten patients received standard therapy solely, consisting of balloon angioplasty and subsequent stent placement, in parallel a medication consisting of betablocker, angiotensin-converting enzyme inhibitor and statin were given.

After a three month follow-up, the size of the infarct region decreased significantly compared with 10 patients, not given cell therapy. The cell-treated patients showed improved left ventricular end-systolic volume, stroke volume index, contractility and myocardial perfusion of the infarcted region. The therapeutical effect may be attributed to bone marrow cell-associated myocardial regeneration and neovascularization. This is the first report (54) to demonstrate the feasibility and safety of intracoronary administration of bone marrow cells for myocardial repair.

Subsequent clinical trials have now been reported using variations of cell sources, different isolation procedures and different specific cell types. Overall results are in general agreement with the initial findings of Strauer et al.[54]

While the amount of patients per group has been small, the clinical outcome of these studies have been important, because the patients have tolerated the treatment safely, none of the patients had deterioration of regional wall motion and none showed left ventricular end-systolic volume expansion after stem cell therapy. Transplantation of cells either bone marrow cells or other progenitor cells did not induce any inflammatory response.

Recently, B. Meier reported the effects of intracoronary and systemic administration of granulocyte-macrophage colony-stimulating factor (GM-CSF) in patients with coronary artery disease. GM-CSF is a cytokine with effects on bone marrow similar to the more commonly utilized G-CSF, albeit with less potency for bone marrow stem cell mobilization. Twenty-one patients who were not amenable to or refused coronary bypass surgery (CABG) participated in this randomized, double blind, placebo-controlled study. The individuals received GM-CSF via intracoronary infusion into the vessel believed to subserve ischemic myocardium and followed by systemic administration of GM-CSF daily for two weeks. Analysis of mobilization of bone marrow stem cells was not performed in this studydue to the fact that the leukocyte counts were only twice the baseline values, therefore was suggested that only modest bone marrow stem cell mobilization has been achieved.

An invasive measure of collateral artery blood flow (estimated by coronary artery pressure distal to balloon occlusion) before and after administration of GM-CSF or placebo indicated improved collateral flow in the GM-CSF group at two weeks, but not in the placebo group, with reduced ECG signs of myocardial ischemia during coronary balloon occlusion.[55] Because the quantity of bone marrow stem cells mobilized with GM-CSF was probably low, the coronary vascular benefit determined in this study may have resulted from direct effects of this cytokine on angiogenesis or on collateral vascular dilator tone with improved regional blood flow. No clinically relevant end points (e.g., exercise-induced myocardial ischemia or left ventricular contractile response to stress) were assessed in this study.

Patients with severe ischemic heart disease also profit from intramyocardial implantation of bone marrow cells. Eight patients with stable angina refractory to maximum medical therapy and left ventricular ejection fraction above 30% participated in this phase I trial.[37] The individuals received isolated autologous bone marrow mononuclear cells obtained by bone marrow puncture of the iliac crest and administered after non-fluoroscopic left ventricular electromechanical mapping to guide the later injections of bone marrow cells to area of ischemic myocardium, which were documented by stress SPECT-sestamibi investigations. There were no ECG changes or sustained ventricular or atrial arrhythmias as well no increase in concentrations of creatine kinase-MB, echocardiographic evidence of pericardial effusion, and bleeding or excessive pain at the site of harvested of bone marrow cells after the procedure.

Clinically, the angina episodes per week of the patients decline and the consumed number of nitroglycerin tablets per week decrease during the 3 months' follow-up. In magnet resonance imaging (MRI) the radical motion and thickening of the target wall was significantly less than those of the normal wall at baseline during pharmacological stress. Three months after implantation of bone marrow cells, MRI showed an improvement in target wall thickening and in target wall motion. Furthermore, the percentage of hypoperfused myocardium was reduced at three months, by comparison with baseline. Although an improvement in symptoms and myocardial perfusion and function was noted, the study involved only a few patients and the benefits of the procedure may have been the placebo effect or attributable to the variability of MRI.

The results of surgical implantation of bone marrow stem cells in patients with transmural myocardial infarction and undergone coronary artery bypass grafting (CABG) were published recently. Six patients with an transmural myocardial infarction greater than ten days but less then three months participated in this clinical phase I trial to assess safety and feasibility of stem cell transplantation in coronary artery bypass patients.[56] The individuals received isolated autologous bone marrow stem cells obtained by bone marrow puncture of the iliac crest. Purified AC133+ cells have been injected into the circumference of the infarct border after all bypass to coronary artery anastomoses had been completed. Within the AC133+ population the non-hematopoietic (CD34−) subpopulation is included, which has a high potential for multiplication and angiogenetic differentiation. After the procedure some patients developed atrial arrhythmia, pneumonia, bleeding from the left internal mammary artery and pericardial effusion. Up to now no malignant neoplasia, ventricular arrhythmia and ventricular tachycardia occurred.

In echocardiography the left ventricular ejection fraction and diastolic left ventricular dimension (LVEDD) improved definitely during follow up, compared to the baseline. Furthermore, the myocardial perfusion improved in the non-perfused or hypoperfused infarct zone. However, the effectiveness of stem cell transplantation cannot be readily assessed alone, because the cell implantation have been done in association with surgical revascularization.

Recently, Dr. J. Willerson of the Texas Heart Institute reported an ongoing study using autologous mononuclear bone marrow cells.[38] This study examined the safety and efficacy of catheter-based direct intramyocardial injections of these cells for treatment of 20 patients with severe, chronic ischemic heart failure. Fourteen patients were treated with autologous bone marrow cells and seven patients were controls. The safety of the treatment has been proved. After four months an improvement of the cardiac function has been scheduled, and the ejection fraction increased from 20% to 29%. Additional significant mechanical improvement of the injected segments and a reduction in end-systolic volume were registered.

In a concurrent study from Dr. S.E. Epstein, catheter-based transendocardial delivery of autologous bone marrow was also performed in patients with severe symptomatic chronic myocardial ischemia, not amenable to conventional revascularization.[39] Ten patients underwent transendocardial injection of autologous bone marrow cells using left ventricular electromechanical guidance. Three months later Canadian Cardiovascular Society angina score significantly improved and as well stress-induced ischemia, occurring within the injected myocardial territories, improved. However, treadmill exercise duration increased non-significantly. The injection procedure was associated with no serious adverse effects: arrhythmia, evidence of infection, myocardial inflammation or pericardial effusion.

7. Conclusions and Future Perspectives

The exciting clinical potential of the use of stem cells to regenerate infarcted myocardium must be tempered by the reality of its unknown role in the treatment of myocardial infarction. Stem cell transplantation will play a major role in the routine treatment of myocardial infarction. Recent clinical results have shown the feasibility of adult autologous cell therapy in humans after myocardial infarction (Figure 5). However, there are many unresolved questions in experimental and clinical cardiology, especially many basic problems concerning the following issues: (1) The long-term fate of transplanted stem cells in the recipient tissue, (2) the ability of transplanted stem cells to find their optimum myocardial "niche", (3) the variable potency of stem cells to transdifferentiate into heart muscle cells, (4) the optimal angiogenic milieu needed for transplanted cells in hypoperfused tissue, (5) the capability of the recipient tissue to enable an enhanced environment to offer optimum, milieus-dependant differentiation of engrafted cells, (6) specific detection of engrafted cells or cell populations by labeling techniques, (7) the optimal time course of availability and application for stem cell replacement therapy in cardiovascular disease, (8) the arrhythmogenic potential of implanted cells, (9) the specific characterization of the progenitor cells that should be measured to predict therapeutic effect of transplanted cells, (10) development of safe and reproducible catheter-based delivery systems for depositing stem cells to recipient heart muscle and (11) the adequate assessment of myocardial function and viability after cell transplantation.

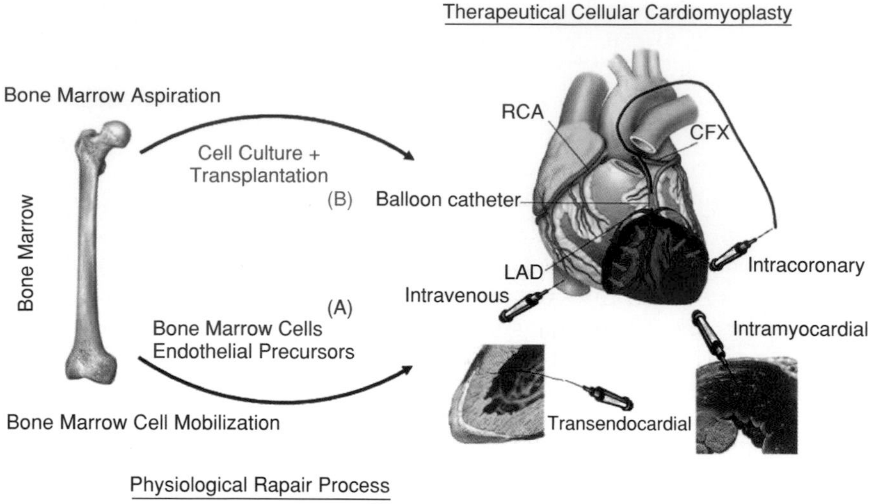

FIGURE 5. Cellular mobilization routes of endogenous cells for physiological regeneration process (A) and various therapeutic administration routes of exogenous autologous cells for cellular repair (B) after myocardial infarction. (A) Bone marrow derived-cells become mobilized from their niches after myocardial infarction and engraft in the infarct zone. (B) Stem cells and precursor cells were collected by bone marrow aspiration and readministered by intracoronary, intramyocardial or transendocardial routes: The red colored area represents apical lesion of the left ventricle by myocardial infarction. The balloon catheter is localized in the infarct-related artery and is placed above the border zone of the infarction area. Blue and green arrows suggest the possible route of cell infusion and migration in the infarct. The other two pictures depict the transendocardial and intramyocardial administration route. RCA, right coronary artery; LAD, left anterior descending coronary artery; CFX, circumflex artery.

The combination of stem cell therapy with other treatments may increase therapeutic options. Nevertheless at present it will serve more as an adjunct to existing therapies rather than a cure. Gene therapy has shown encouraging results in promoting angiogenesis, but the safety of gene delivery by viral vectors is not reliable. Bone marrow cells may serve as new vehicles for transporting genes into the target tissues.

With regard to the clinical practicability, to ethical problems and to hazards of immunogenity, actual and future research will focus preferably on adult stem cells, whereas embryonic and umbilical cord blood stem cells may emerge presumably into comparable clinical relevance in future.

According to our present experience, autologous stem cell transplantation is feasible and has the potential for beneficial effects on ventricular remodeling after myocardial infarction.

Future clinical trials will establish the magnitude of benefit from stem cell therapy.

8.   References

1. American Heart Association. Heart and Stroke Statistical Update. Dallas, Tex: American Heart Association 2001.
2. Ho KK, Anderson KM, Kannel WB, Grossman W, Levy D. Survival after the onset of congestive heart failure in Framingham Heart Study subjects. Circulation 1993; 88:107–115.
3. Heyndrickx GR, Baig H, Nellens P, Leusen I, Fishbein MC, Vatner SF. Depression of regional blood flow and wall thickening after brief coronary occlusions. Am J Physiol 1978; 234:H653–H659.
4. Reimer KA, Lowe JE, Rasmussen MM, Jennings RB. The wavefront phenomenon of ischemic cell death. 1. Myocardial infarct size vs duration of coronary occlusion in dogs. Circulation 1977; 56:786–794.
5. Murry CE, Jennings RB, Reimer KA. Preconditioning with ischemia: a delay of lethal cell injury in ischemic myocardium. Circulation 1986; 74:1124–1136.
6. Pfeffer MA. Left ventricular remodeling after acute myocardial infarction. Annu Rev Med 1995; 46:455–466.
7. Ryan TJ, Antman EM, Brooks NH, Califf RM, Hillis LD, Hiratzka LF et al. 1999 update: ACC/AHA guidelines for the management of patients with acute myocardial infarction. A report of the American College of Cardiology/American Heart Association Task Force on Practice Guidelines (Committee on Management of Acute Myocardial Infarction). J Am Coll Cardiol 1999; 34:890–911.
8. Schwarz F, Schuler G, Katus H, Hofmann M, Manthey J, Tillmanns H et al. Intracoronary thrombolysis in acute myocardial infarction: duration of ischemia as a major determinant of late results after recanalization. Am J Cardiol 1982; 50:933–937.
9. Pfeffer MA, Braunwald E. Ventricular remodeling after myocardial infarction. Experimental observations and clinical implications. Circulation 1990; 81:1161–1172.
10. Blau HM, Brazelton TR, Weimann JM. The evolving concept of a stem cell: entity or function? Cell 2001; 105:829–841.
11. Pittenger MF, Mackay AM, Beck SC, Jaiswal RK, Douglas R, Mosca JD et al. Multilineage potential of adult human mesenchymal stem cells. Science 1999; 284:143–147.
12. Graf T. Differentiation plasticity of hematopoietic cells. Blood 2002; 99:3089–3101.
13. Reyes M, Lund T, Lenvik T, Aguiar D, Koodie L, Verfaillie CM. Purification and ex vivo expansion of postnatal human marrow mesodermal progenitor cells. Blood 2001; 98:2615–2625.
14. Strauer BE, Kornowski R. Stem cell therapy in perspective. Circulation 2003; 107:929–934.
15. Orlic D, Kajstura J, Chimenti S, Jakoniuk I, Anderson SM, Li B et al. Bone marrow cells regenerate infarcted myocardium. Nature 2001; 410:701–705.
16. Kocher AA, Schuster MD, Szabolcs MJ, Takuma S, Burkhoff D, Wang J et al. Neovascularization of ischemic myocardium by human bone-marrow-derived angioblasts prevents cardiomyocyte apoptosis, reduces remodeling and improves cardiac function. Nat Med 2001; 7:430–436.

17. Kawamoto A, Gwon HC, Iwaguro H, Yamaguchi JI, Uchida S, Masuda H et al. Therapeutic potential of ex vivo expanded endothelial progenitor cells for myocardial ischemia. Circulation 2001; 103:634–637.
18. Fuchs S, Baffour R, Zhou YF, Shou M, Pierre A, Tio FO et al. Transendocardial delivery of autologous bone marrow enhances collateral perfusion and regional function in pigs with chronic experimental myocardial ischemia. J Am Coll Cardiol 2001; 37:1726–1732.
19. Asahara T, Masuda H, Takahashi T, Kalka C, Pastore C, Silver M et al. Bone marrow origin of endothelial progenitor cells responsible for postnatal vasculogenesis in physiological and pathological neovascularization. Circ Res 1999; 85: 221–228.
20. Orlic D, Kajstura J, Chimenti S, Limana F, Jakoniuk I, Quaini F et al. Mobilized bone marrow cells repair the infarcted heart, improving function and survival. Proc Natl Acad Sci U S A 2001; 98:10344–10349.
21. Olivetti G, Quaini F, Sala R, Lagrasta C, Corradi D, Bonacina E et al. Acute myocardial infarction in humans is associated with activation of programmed myocyte cell death in the surviving portion of the heart. J Mol Cell Cardiol 1996; 28:2005–2016.
22. Li F, Wang X, Bunger PC, Gerdes AM. Formation of binucleated cardiac myocytes in rat heart: I. Role of actin-myosin contractile ring. J Mol Cell Cardiol 1997; 29:1541–1551.
23. Kajstura J, Leri A, Finato N, Di Loreto C, Beltrami CA, Anversa P. Myocyte proliferation in end-stage cardiac failure in humans. Proc Natl Acad Sci U S A 1998; 95:8801–8805.
24. Soonpaa MH, Field LJ. Survey of studies examining mammalian cardiomyocyte DNA synthesis. Circ Res 1998; 83:15–26.
25. Grounds MD, White JD, Rosenthal N, Bogoyevitch MA. The role of stem cells in skeletal and cardiac muscle repair. J Histochem Cytochem 2002; 50:589–610.
26. Adler CP, Friedburg H, Herget GW, Neuburger M, Schwalb H. Variability of cardiomyocyte DNA content, ploidy level and nuclear number in mammalian hearts. Virchows Arch 1996; 429:159–164.
27. Sun Y, Weber KT. Infarct scar: a dynamic tissue. Cardiovasc Res 2000; 46:250–256.
28. Buschmann I, Schaper W. The pathophysiology of the collateral circulation (arteriogenesis). J Pathol 2000; 190:338–342.
29. Beltrami AP, Urbanek K, Kajstura J, Yan SM, Finato N, Bussani R et al. Evidence that human cardiac myocytes divide after myocardial infarction. N Engl J Med 2001; 344:1750–1757.
30. Jackson KA, Majka SM, Wang H, Pocius J, Hartley CJ, Majesky MW et al. Regeneration of ischemic cardiac muscle and vascular endothelium by adult stem cells. J Clin Invest 2001; 107:1395–1402.
31. Quaini F, Urbanek K, Beltrami AP, Finato N, Beltrami CA, Nadal-Ginard B et al. Chimerism of the transplanted heart. N Engl J Med 2002; 346:5–15.
32. Laflamme MA, Myerson D, Saffitz JE, Murry CE. Evidence for cardiomyocyte repopulation by extracardiac progenitors in transplanted human hearts. Circ Res 2002; 90:634–640.
33. Rosenthal N. High hopes for the heart. N Engl J Med 2001; 344:1785–1787.
34. Goodell MA, Jackson KA, Majka SM, Mi T, Wang H, Pocius J et al. Stem cell plasticity in muscle and bone marrow. Ann N Y Acad Sci 2001; 938:208–218.

35. Strauer BE, Brehm M, Zeus T, Gattermann N, Hernandez A, Sorg RV et al. [Intracoronary, human autologous stem cell transplantation for myocardial regeneration following myocardial infarction]. Dtsch Med Wochenschr 2001; 126:932–938.
36. Kornowski R, Fuchs S, Leon MB, Epstein SE. Delivery strategies to achieve therapeutic myocardial angiogenesis. Circulation 2000; 101:454–458.
37. Tse HF, Kwong YL, Chan JK, Lo G, Ho CL, Lau CP. Angiogenesis in ischaemic myocardium by intramyocardial autologous bone marrow mononuclear cell implantation. Lancet 2003; 361:47–49.
38. Perin EC, Dohmann HF, Borojevic R, Silva SA, Sousa AL, Mesquita CT et al. Transendocardial, autologous bone marrow cell transplantation for severe, chronic ischemic heart failure. Circulation 2003; 107:2294–2302.
39. Fuchs S, Satler LF, Kornowski R, Okubagzi P, Weisz G, Baffour R et al. Catheter-based autologous bone marrow myocardial injection in no-option patients with advanced coronary artery disease. A feasibility study. J Am Coll Cardiol 2003; 41:1721–1724.
40. Losordo DW, Vale PR, Hendel RC, Milliken CE, Fortuin FD, Cummings N et al. Phase 1/2 placebo-controlled, double-blind, dose-escalating trial of myocardial vascular endothelial growth factor 2 gene transfer by catheter delivery in patients with chronic myocardial ischemia. Circulation 2002; 105:2012–2018.
41. Toma C, Pittenger MF, Cahill KS, Byrne BJ, Kessler PD. Human mesenchymal stem cells differentiate to a cardiomyocyte phenotype in the adult murine heart. Circulation 2002; 105:93–98.
42. Aicher A, Brenner W, Zuhayra M, Badorff C, Massoudi S, Assmus B et al. Assessment of the tissue distribution of transplanted human endothelial progenitor cells by radioactive labeling. Circulation 2003; 107:2134–2139.
43. Menasche P, Hagege AA, Scorsin M, Pouzet B, Desnos M, Duboc D et al. Myoblast transplantation for heart failure. Lancet 2001; 357:279–280.
44. Hamano K, Nishida M, Hirata K, Mikamo A, Li TS, Harada M et al. Local implantation of autologous bone marrow cells for therapeutic angiogenesis in patients with ischemic heart disease: clinical trial and preliminary results. Jpn Circ J 2001; 65:845–847.
45. Garot JJ, Unterseeh T, Teiger E, Champagne S, Chazaud BB, Gherardi R et al. Magnetic resonance imaging of targeted catheter-based implantation of myogenic precursor cells into infarcted left ventricular myocardium. J Am Coll Cardiol 2003; 41:1841–1846.
46. Orlic D, Hill JM, Arai AE. Stem cells for myocardial regeneration. Circ Res 2002; 91:1092–1102.
47. Zhao M, Beauregard DA, Loizou L, Davletov B, Brindle KM. Non-invasive detection of apoptosis using magnetic resonance imaging and a targeted contrast agent. Nat Med 2001; 7:1241–1244.
48. Lederman RJ, Guttman MA, Peters DC, Thompson RB, Sorger JM, Dick AJ et al. Catheter-based endomyocardial injection with real-time magnetic resonance imaging. Circulation 2002; 105:1282–1284.
49. Hagege AA, Carrion C, Menasche P, Vilquin JT, Duboc D, Marolleau JP et al. Viability and differentiation of autologous skeletal myoblast grafts in ischaemic cardiomyopathy. Lancet 2003; 361:491–492.
50. Theise ND, Nimmakayalu M, Gardner R, Illei PB, Morgan G, Teperman L et al. Liver from bone marrow in humans. Hepatology 2000; 32:11–16.

51. Korbling M, Katz RL, Khanna A, Ruifrok AC, Rondon G, Albitar M et al. Hepatocytes and epithelial cells of donor origin in recipients of peripheral-blood stem cells. N Engl J Med 2002; 346:738–746.
52. Muller P, Pfeiffer P, Koglin J, Schafers HJ, Seeland U, Janzen I et al. Cardiomyocytes of noncardiac origin in myocardial biopsies of human transplanted hearts. Circulation 2002; 106:31–35.
53. Thiele J, Varus E, Wickenhauser C, Kvasnicka HM, Metz K, Schaefer UW et al. [Chimerism of cardiomyocytes and endothelial cells after allogeneic bone marrow transplantation in chronic myeloid leukemia An autopsy study]. Pathologe 2002; 23:405–410.
54. Strauer BE, Brehm M, Zeus T, Kostering M, Hernandez A, Sorg RV et al. Repair of infarcted myocardium by autologous intracoronary mononuclear bone marrow cell transplantation in humans. Circulation 2002; 106:1913–1918.
55. Seiler C, Pohl T, Wustmann K, Hutter D, Nicolet PA, Windecker S et al. Promotion of collateral growth by granulocyte-macrophage colony-stimulating factor in patients with coronary artery disease: a randomized, double-blind, placebo-controlled study. Circulation 2001; 104:2012–2017.
56. Stamm C, Westphal B, Kleine HD, Petzsch M, Kittner C, Klinge H et al. Autologous bone-marrow stem-cell transplantation for myocardial regeneration. Lancet 2003; 361:45–46.
57. Lee M, Lill M, Makkar R. Stem cell transplantation in myocardial infarction. Rev Cardiovasc Med. 2004; 5(2): 82–98.
58. Mathur A, Martin JF. Stem cells and the repair of the heart. Lancet 2004; 364:183–192.
59. Pittenger MF, Martin BJ. Mesenchymal stem cells and their potential as cardiac therapeutics. Circulation Res. 2004; 95:9–20.

12
Autologous Mononuclear Bone Marrow Transplantation for Myocardial Infarction: The Spanish Experience

FRANCISCO FERNÁNDEZ-AVILÉS, PEDRO L SÁNCHEZ, ALBERTO SAN ROMÁN, LUIS DE LA FUENTE, RICARDO SANZ, CAROLINA HERNÁNDEZ, MANUEL GÓMEZ BUENO, ANA SÁNCHEZ AND JAVIER GARCÍA-FRADE

1. Introduction

Ischemic heart disease is still the biggest killer in developed countries, causing more than 50% of all cardiovascular deaths.[1] Myocardial infarction is the main component of the cardiovascular plague and the leading cause of congestive heart failure, which is associated with a poor prognosis (40% of people diagnosed dying within one year) and accounts for most of the social and economic burden caused by this group of diseases in the Western world.[2] Although modern treatments have improved dramatically the prognosis of patients with acute myocardial infarction -early reperfusion therapies in particular[3] -today less than 50% suffering ongoing myocardial necrosis achieve adequate epicardial and microvascular reperfusion before irreversible damage of the supplied myocardial tissue.[4] Moreover, neither medications nor procedures have so far shown any efficacy in increasing the resistance of the jeopardized myocardium to severe ischemia or in replacing necrosed myocardium with functional contractile tissue.[5] As a result, a high proportion of survivors of myocardial infarction are still at risk of developing heart failure due to left ventricular remodeling, a process characterized by mechanical expansion of the scarred infarcted wall followed by progressive left ventricle dilation and dysfunction.[6]

Since the main underlying cause of postinfarction left ventricle remodeling and dysfunction is irreversible damage to the infarcted wall,[7] the devel-

187

opment of treatments aimed at regenerating its muscular and vascular components is now considered a main therapeutic challenge. The rationale for such an approach includes recent evidence demonstrating the remarkable ability of adult stem cells to produce differentiated cells from embryologically unrelated tissues,[8] as well as convincing data supporting that the heart has a potent intrinsic regenerative capacity.[9] In fact, contrary to traditional thought, evidence has recently demonstrated the existence of cardiac stem cells able to regenerate myocytes and vasculature after ageing or damage.[10-12] In addition, recent data from investigations carried out in sex-mismatched heart transplant patients strongly suggest that dividing cardiac stem cells are myocytes derived from an extracardiac origin,[13,14] such as bone marrow.[15]

On this basis, the hypothesis that the natural capability of the mammalian heart to regenerate infarcted myocardium can be reinforced has lead to several investigations that suggest that adult stem cell-based therapies could prevent postinfarction left ventricular remodeling.[11] Particularly, bone marrow-derived stem cells locally delivered, or mobilized by means of systemic administration of stimulating factors (cytokines, for instance), have been shown to home to the necrotic tissue, engraft in the border zone of the infarct, replicate, induce both myogenesis and angiogenesis, reduce infarct size and ameliorate cardiac function and survival after acute myocardial infarction in mice and pigs.[16-19] In general, these observations have been interpreted as due to metaplasic transformation of bone marrow-derived stem cells into myocytes and vascular cells (transdifferentiation). However, the mechanism through which bone marrow-derived stem cells benefit postinfarction left ventricular remodeling is controversial, and other views include the proposal of cell fusion or paracrine effect as the actual mechanisms of tissue repair.[20-22] In addition, concerns regarding the risk of myocardial damage and progression of restenotic and "de novo" coronary lesions after post-infarction stem cell therapy have arisen recently.[22-26]

In spite of these doubts and concerns, the capability of adult stem cells to prevent postinfarction left ventricular remodeling has been investigated in humans. In this chapter we summarize the available evidence regarding the application of bone-marrow stem cells in patients with ST-segment elevation acute myocardial infarction (STEMI) and describe the intracoronary delivering method already used, discussing the safety and the efficacy of such an approach. The first section includes a comprehensive description of the procedure for the preparation and the intracoronary infusion of bone marrow stem already used in humans. In the second section, the results of the last relevant clinical studies are discussed. In addition, we also speculate on the value of current clinical data to gain an insight into the mechanism of stem cell-based cardiac repair and to design clinical trials in the future.

2.   Intracoronary Bone-Marrow Cell Transfer After Myocardial Infarction: Timing and Method for Transplantation and Follow-up

Different routes of stem cell delivery have been used to repair infarcted myocardium after acute myocardial infarction.[24,27-41] Of these, intracoronary administration of hematopoietic progenitors represents the best tried method for stem cell therapy in patients with acute myocardial infarction, without any existing experience out of this context.[24,37-41]

The procedure described in this chapter is based upon our experience and those previously reported on, which have been empirically designed. It is clear that the procedure herein proposed will partially or fully change in the future as new experimental and clinical evidence emerges. Basically, the entire procedure can be divided into three stages: the standard care of a patient with STEMI; the extraction and management of stem cells; and the infusion of stem cells.

Although the standard optimal management of a patient with STEMI is beyond the scope of this chapter, it should be stressed that a percutaneous coronary intervention of the culprit artery must be undertaken to ensure a vascular access for the stem cells to be infused. Regarding the stem cell transplant procedure itself, timing of percutaneous revascularization therapy (primary, facilitated or delayed) makes no difference provided that the culprit artery is widely opened.

2.1.   Extraction and Management of Bone Marrow Stem Cells

Stem cells can be obtained from bone marrow. In that case, bone marrow is aspirated from the iliac crest under local anesthesia with an aspiration needle. Briefly, 5 cc are obtained in every puncture and the procedure is repeated until 50 cc of bone marrow is obtained. The bone marrow is then filtered and mononuclear cells are isolated by means of Ficoll density ultrafiltration. Then, the erythrocytes are lysed with water. At this time, the cells can be injected,[37,39,40] or cultivated overnight before being infused into the coronary artery.[38,41] It is not known yet whether all mononuclear cells or a specific subpopulation of cells previously selected should be given. The clinical studies available utilized an unselected solution because several different fractions of mononuclear bone marrow cells may differentiate into myocytes and vessels. Therefore, not only hematopoietic and mesenchymal stem cells, but also other mononuclear cells are infused to the necrotic area. Circulating progenitor cells can also serve as a source for stem cells.[37] In that case, peripheral venous blood (250 ml) is collected, mononuclear cells are purified and *ex vivo* cultured for 3 days and then reinfused into the culprit artery.

2.2.   Intracoronary Infusion Procedure

For intracoronary delivery of the cells, an over-the-wire angioplasty balloon is used. After positioning in the infarct-related coronary segment previously stented, the balloon is inflated at 2-4 atmospheres until a complete block of blood flow is achieved to allow a prolonged contact between the stem cells and the microcirculation and to avoid a retrograde flow of the cells. Then, the guide-wire is withdrawn and the central lumen of the balloon is used to infuse the cells. Intracoronary infusion of the cell suspension is carried out, manually or with a pump, alternating periods of occlusion-infusion (2-3 minutes) and reperfusion (1-3 minutes) until the total dose is given (Figure 1). Figure 2 summarizes the entire transplantation procedure.

The timing of infusion of stem cells is an unresolved issue. Theoretically, it could be performed as early as immediately after the percutaneous coronary intervention with a short delay to allow for bone marrow extraction and manipulation and as late as 15-30 days after the acute phase. Although little evidence is available in this regard, several experimental data are worth taking into account. Recently, an injection of fetal cardiomyocytes after 4 weeks of permanent coronary artery ligation in rats failed to reverse left ventricular dilatation, suggesting that it could be too late to have any impact on cardiac remodeling.[42] One animal study aimed at determining the optimum time for cardiomyocyte transplantation to enhance myocardial function after left ventricular injury.[43] Rat hearts were cryoinjured and fetal cardiomyocytes were transplanted immediately, 2 weeks, and 4 weeks afterwards. Histologic studies performed in sacrificed animals showed that the inflammatory reaction was greatest during the first week and that scar size expanded at 4 to 8 weeks. Cardiomyocytes transplanted immediately after cryoinjury were not found at 8 weeks, and scar size and ventricular function were similar in control hearts. On the contrary, cardiomyocytes transplanted 2 and 4 weeks formed cardiac tissue within the scar, limited scar expansion and had a better ventricular function than controls. The authors conclude that cardiomyocyte transplantation was most successful after the inflammatory reaction resolved but before scar expansion. In the clinical setting, it could be assumed that transplantation of stem cells too early or too late might lead them to take part in the inflammatory reaction or in the scar formation process, respectively, instead of forming functional myocytes or vessels. Clinical studies have infused stem cells 4 to 7 days after pain onset.

2.3.   Follow-Up

In the follow-up of patients put under this treatment two main aspects have to be considered: safety and assessment of efficacy.

Bearing in mind that a favorable risk-benefit ratio should be guaranteed before advancing with this therapy in the clinical arena, it is crucial to assess the safety of such a procedure, which implies intracoronary manipulation

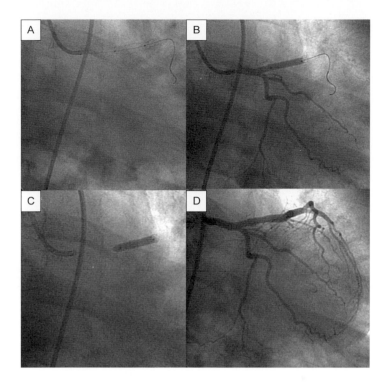

FIGURE 1. Procedure of percutaneous intracoronary transplantation of bone marrow-derived stem cells. For intracoronary delivery of the cells an over-the-wire angioplasty balloon catheter oversized by 0.5 mm is used (Panel A and B). After positioning at the site of the former infarct-related coronary occlusion where the stent had been implanted, the balloon is inflated at low pressure (2-4 atmospheres) to block blood flow (Panel B). Then, the guide-wire is removed and the Bone marrow-derived stem cells suspension is infused through the internal lumen of the balloon under stop-flow conditions (Panel C). Bone marrow-derived stem cells are infused with a pump at 1-2 ml/min during periods of 3 minutes of inflation and cell infusion alternating with 1 minute of de-inflation and reperfusion until the total dose of cells is given to the patient. Integrity of the coronary artery used for transplantation and blood flow perfusion in the supplied myocardial area are checked after the procedure (Panel D).

and block of the coronary flow in patients with recent myocardial infarction. First of all, ischemic complications and myocardial injury secondary to the procedure must be ruled out. Therefore, ECG and myocardial injury markers have to be periodically obtained within 24 hours after stem cell transplantation. Moreover, although arrhythmias have not been reported on with bone marrow or blood-derived stem cells, ECG monitoring for 24 to 48 hours is mandatory as well as ECG Holter monitoring at least 1 and 6 months after discharge. Finally, it is also necessary to investigate whether the mechanical manipulation of the stented segment or a potential proliferative effect of the

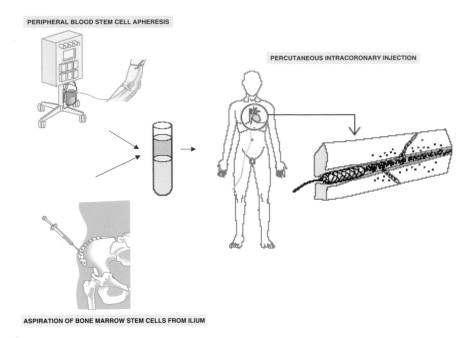

FIGURE 2. Bone marrow stem cell isolation and intracoronary cell transplantation into the infarcted myocardium in humans.

cells could induce higher restenosis or atherosclerosis progression than expected.

To establish the risk-benefit ratio of intracoronary bone marrow stem cells transplantation the assessment of efficacy is equally important. In this regard, the following parameters can be used: global and regional function, viability, infarct size, thickness and thickening of the infarcted wall, contractile reserve, perfusion and coronary reserve. Global and regional function can be calculated with angiography, echocardiography and magnetic resonance. In our opinion, magnetic resonance imaging is the technique of choice to follow these patients. This technique is non-invasive, has high temporal and spatial resolution and, thus, a high reproducibility. What is more, exposure to ionizing radiation is avoided. Finally, given its tomographic nature, it is more accurate than echocardiography or cine-angiography in assessing remodeling because it does not make assumptions regarding ventricular geometry, which is crucial in distorted postinfarction ventricles. When assessing regional function, the wall motion score index must be calculated.[44] Viability is another parameter to be measured, which could be assessed with low-dose dobutamine echocardiography, scintigraphic techniques or with magnetic resonance by means of late hyperenhancement sequences after gadolinium administration. The latter also allows an accurate measurement of infarct size. Several investigations have demonstrated that thickness and thickening of the infarcted wall calculated by magnetic resonance imaging or echocardiography correlate well with viability.[45,46] Contractile reserve defined as the potential of the myocardium to increase its contractility after an inotropic stimulation will be assessed by monitoring the response of the ventricle with echocardiography or magnetic resonance to administration of dobutamine at low doses (from 5 up to 10 or 20 micrograms/kg/min). Positron emission tomography and scintigraphic techniques permit an accurate estimate of myocardial perfusion. Lastly, coronary flow reserve and fractional flow reserve are measured in the infarct and in a noninfarct reference vessel by using an intracoronary Doppler or thermodilution wire and infusing adenosine through the guiding catheter.[47] To demonstrate any benefit of stem cells transplantation, a basal and a follow-up study must be compared (Figure 3). This follow-up examination should not be performed within at least 3 months after the acute event to rule out myocardial stunning which could lead to confusing results.

A practical algorithm for intracoronary stem cell transplantation and follow-up in patients with STEMI is proposed in Table 1.

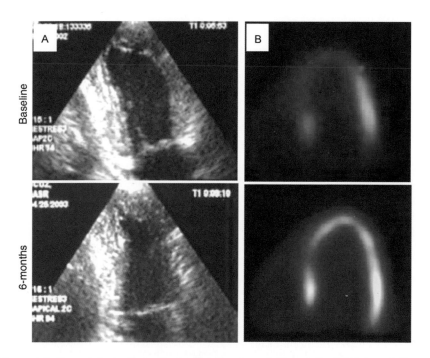

FIGURE 3. Low-dobutamine echocardiogram (panel A) and the PET (panel B) carried 6 months after cell transplantation (bottom) show respectively marked improvement in anterior and apical contractility and metabolism suggesting recovery of viability not seen at baseline studies (top).

TABLE 1. Summary of clinical studies of intracoronary bone marrow stem cell transplantation in patients with STEMI

Author	No. pts.	Follow-up (months)	End point	Results	Complications
Strauer[38]	10	3	Δ LVEF	NS	NO
			LVESV	−15 ml	
			Improvement of myocardial perfusion	YES	
Assmus[37]	19	4	Δ LVEF	8.5%	NO
			LVESV	−13.9 ml	
			Improvement of miocardial viability	YES	
Kang[24]	7	6	Δ LVEF	6.4%	
			Improvement of myocardial perfusion	YES	70% intrastent restenosis
Avilés[39]	20	6	Δ LVEF	5.8%	NO
			LVESV	−9.6 ml	
			Δ Thickness of infarct wall	0.9 mm	
Wollert[40]	30	6	Δ LVEF	6.7%	NO
			LVESV	NS	
Chen[41]	34	6	Δ LVEF	18%	NO
			LVESV	−25 ml	
			Improvement of myocardial perfusion	YES	

G-CSF: Granulocyte-colony stimulating factor; LVEF: Left ventricular ejection fraction; LVESV: Left ventricular end-systolic volume; NS: No significant; Δ: Increment.

3.   Results from Clinical Studies

The evidence that stem cells can reconstitute necrotic myocardium and improve cardiac function in animals has led to an initiation of clinical studies, which have been mainly focused on addressing the feasibility the safety of this therapy. The main differences between these studies were the type of cell employed and the type of patient. The most of the patients suffered from ischemic heart disease in different stages. The method of measurement was different as it has not yet been assured what is the best in these settings. The principal end-point was to assess if stem cell transplantation improved the left ventricular function. In patients with STEMI bone marrow-derived or circulating blood-derived progenitor cells and mobilization with granulocyte-colony stimulating factor (G-CSF) were used.

Assmus et al.[37] randomly allocated 20 patients with reperfused STEMI to receive intracoronary infusion of either bone marrow–derived (n=9) or circulating blood– derived progenitor cells (n=11) into the infarct artery 4.3 ±1.5 days after infarction. There were no differences for any measured parameter between both groups of progenitor cells. Transplantation of progenitor cells was associated with a significant increase in global left ventricular ejection fraction, improved regional wall motion in the infarct zone, and profoundly reduced end-systolic left ventricular volumes at 4-month follow-up. Coronary blood flow reserve was increased in the infarct artery. Quantitative F-18-fluorodeoxyglucose–positron emission tomography analysis revealed an increase in myocardial viability in the infarct zone.

Strauer et al.[38] transplanted 10 patients with autologous mononuclear bone marrow stem cells via a balloon catheter placed into the infarct-related artery during balloon dilatation 5 to 9 days after acute myocardial infarction. After 3 months of follow-up, the infarct region had decreased significantly and showed significant improvement in stroke volume index, left ventricular end-systolic volume and contractility and myocardial perfusion of the infarct region.

Kang et al.[24] studied the evolution of 27 patients with reperfused STEMI who were randomly allocated to conventional therapy (7 patients), intracoronary transplantation of circulating blood-derived progenitor cells after bone marrow mobilization with G-CSF (10 patients) or mobilization alone (10 patients). Importantly, in this study patients allocated to conventional therapy underwent bare stent-based repair of the infarct-related artery 4 days after randomization. Similarly, patients treated with G-CSF alone or in combination with intracoronary infusion of bone marrow stem cells achieved stenting after having been treated with G-CSF during 4 days. At 6 months of follow-up, myocardial perfusion and left ventricular ejection fraction improved significantly in patients who received cell infusion. However, enrolment was stopped because of the observation that those patients randomized to G-CSF alone or in combination with intracoronary bone marrow stem cells transplantation before stenting had an unexpectedly high rate of in-stent restenosis. It must be pointed out that no increase in in-stent restenosis was noted in other coronary stem-cell infusion studies. All these trials did not use G-CSF. So it seems reasonable to conclude that G-CSF given before stenting can cause excessive in-stent restenosis and further clinical assessment of G-CSF mobilized stem cell therapy in the setting of recent coronary artery stenting is priority.

Fernandez-Aviles et al.[39] used bone marrow mononuclear cells from 20 patients with STEMI to assess both their myocardial regenerative capability *in vitro* and their effect on postinfarction left ventricular remodeling. The human bone marrow stem cells were grafted into cryoinjured mice heart slices and, after 1 week, acquired a cardiomyocyte phenotype and expressed cardiac proteins. In the clinical trial, an average of $78\pm41\times106$ bone marrow stem cells per patient was intracoronarally transplanted 13.5 ± 5.5 days after infarction, with no adverse effects on microvascular function or myocardial injury. No major cardiac events occurred up to 11 ± 5 months. At 6 months, magnetic resonance showed a decrease in the end-systolic volume, improvement of regional and global left ventricle function and increased thickness of the infarcted wall, while coronary restenosis was only 15%. Angiographic follow-up confirmed the aforementioned benefit on left ventricular outcome. Concordantly, PET and low dose dobutamine stress echocardiography showed recovery of viability in the infarcted wall. No changes were found in a non-randomized contemporary control group. Thus, these results indicate that intracoronary transplantation of autologous bone marrow stem cells after STEMI is feasible and safe in the short and mid-term follow-up, prevents left ventricular remodeling, leads to a significant recovery of cardiac function and seems to regenerate myocardial tissue.

Wollert et al.[40] included 60 patients who had had a myocardial infarction and underwent primary angioplasty. They randomly allocated patients to receive standard therapy (30 patients) versus intracoronary infusion of unselected bone marrow progenitor cells (30 patients). Bone marrow cells transplantation was made under a protocol similar to Strauer et al.[38] and all patients were evaluated by Magnetic Resonance Imaging, with a basal study 3.5 days after primary angioplasty and another at 6 months. There was a significant improvement in ejection fraction within the cell therapy group (6.7%, p= 0.0026), but not in the control group (0.7%). It is important to point out that this improvement occurred in all groups of patients, especially in those reperfused. As described in the safety endpoints, electrophysiological study was made for exhaustive arrhythmia analysis at 6 months. No malignant arrhythmias were induced.

Chen et al.[41] studied the evolution of 69 patients with reperfused STEMI who were randomly allocated to conventional therapy (35 patients), or intracoronary transplantation of bone marrow mesenchymal stem cells. They aspirated bone marrow 8 days after the percutaneous coronary intervention and cultured for 10 days. Six milliliters of the cell suspension or standard saline (control group) was injected through the coronary artery following the protocol described by Strauer et al.[38] All patients were evaluated by positron emission tomography (PET), cardiac catheterization and cardiac echocardiography on the day of the transplantation, and 3 and 6 months after transplantation. Left ventricular ejection fraction 3 months after transplantation in the stem cell group increased significantly compared with that before transplantation and with the control group 3 months after injection. Perfusion defects detected by PET decreased significantly in the stem cell group after 3 months compared with those in the control group. Left ventricular end-diastolic volume and end-systolic volume decreased significantly. All this improvement was maintained at 6 months after the procedure, but without additional benefit.

significantly. All this improvement was maintained at 6 months after the procedure, but without additional benefit.

4.   Intracoronary Bone Marrow Cell Transplantation Therapy for Acute Myocardial Infarction into Perspective

Much excitement has surrounded recent breakthroughs in the field of adult stem-cell research and their implications for cell therapy in patients with acute ischemic heart disease. However, further proof of the efficacy and the safety of this therapy in the treatment of acute myocardial infarction is necessary.

According to the available clinical data presented in this review, it seems to be clear that, in patients with recent STEMI, intracoronary transplantation of autologous bone marrow-derived stem cells is a feasible and safe procedure that seems to diminish significantly the extent of left ventricular remodeling and promote a significant recovery of both global and segmental cardiac function. Moreover, although the mechanism of this putative beneficial effect remains to be elucidated, data from animal studies and from our parallel clinical and *in vitro* experiments strongly suggest that bone marrow cell therapy for STEMI might regenerate contractile myocardial tissue. Therefore, altogether these results demonstrate a favorable risk-benefit ratio for early intracoronary administration of hematopoietic progenitors in patients with acute myocardial infarction, which opens the way to the development of randomized large-scale clinical trials in this area. These trials should be compatible with simultaneous mechanistic clinical and basic research aimed at addressing some crucial questions still unsettled: How do adult bone-marrow stem cells contribute to repair in the setting of acute myocardial infarction? At least six different mechanisms might be proposed; transdifferentiation, dedifferentiation, transdetermination, cell fusion, true pluripotent stem-cell behavior, and the production of trophic factors. It is likely that our current knowledge of cell markers is inadequate to define cell populations accurately, so it is possible that cells with true multipotency may have contaminated experiments previously reported as examples of transdifferentiation. What will be the ideal source of adult stem cells in patients with acute myocardial infarction? Bone marrow stem cells would seem simple, cheap, and apparently widely applicable. What is the best route of administration? So far only percutaneous intracoronary release and mobilization of stem cells with G-CSF have been tested. When should cell transplantation be performed? Experimental studies suggest that stem-cell transplantation is most successful after the inflammatory reaction is resolved but before scar expansion. How many times should cell transplantation be performed? Several clinical studies have demonstrated that stem cells can improve cardiac function in patients with old myocardial infarction, so compared with single autologous stem-cell transplantation in the acute phase, successive transplantations may improve the benefit of this therapy.

We are optimistic that stem-cell transplantation is likely to be of future benefit to all patients with acute myocardial infarction and that new tools, such as magnetic resonance, will help to refine patient selection and lead to a better assessment of results. Finally, lessons from the past suggest that in this field, a close collaboration between clinical and non-clinical scientists is of the utmost importance.

5.   Acknowledgments

Our work has been funded by unrestricted grants from the Spanish Ministry of Health and the Spanish Network for Cardiovascular Research RECAVA (National Health Institute "Carlos III"). The authors greatly appreciate the

198 F. Fernández-Avilés et al.

assistance of Pedro Guerra and Gonzalo Peña in preparing the figures of this chapter.

6. References

1. British Heart Foundation. Coronary heart disease statistics. www.bhf.org.uk. 2002; BHF Statistics Database.
2. Reddy KS, Global perspective on cardiovascular disease. In: Yusuf S, Cairns JA, Camm AJ, Fallen EL , Gersh BJ, eds, 2nd end (BMJ Books; London, 2003) 91–102.
3. Antman EM, Van de Werf F. Pharmacoinvasive therapy. The future of treatment for ST-elevation myocardial infarction. Circulation 2004; 109: 2480–2486.
4 Eagle KA, Goodman SG, Avezum A, Budaj A, Sullivan CM, Lopez-Sendon J; GRACE Investigators. Practice variation and missed opportunities for reperfusion in ST-segment-elevation myocardial infarction: findings from the Global Registry of Acute Coronary Events (GRACE). Lancet 2002;359:373–377.
5. Ryan TJ, Antman EM, Brooks NH, et al. 1999 update: ACC/AHA Guidelines for the Management of Patients With Acute Myocardial Infarction: Executive Summary and Recommendations: A report of the American College of Cardiology/American Heart Association Task Force on Practice Guidelines (Committee on Management of Acute Myocardial Infarction). Circulation 1999;100:1016–1030.
6. Pfeffer MA, Braunwald E. Ventricular remodeling after myocardial infarction: experimental observations and clinical implications. Circulation 1990; 81: 1161–1172.
7. Bolognese L, Carrabba N, Parodi G, Santori GM, Buonamici P, Cerisano G, et al. Impact of microvascular dysfunction on left ventricular remodeling and long-term clinical outcome after primary coronary angioplasty for acute myocardial infarction. Circulation 2004; 109: 1121–1126.
8. Tosh D, Slack JMW. How cells change their phenotype. Nat Rev Mol Cell Biol 2002; 3: 187–194.
9. Beltrami AP, Barlucchi L, Torella D, Baker M, Limana F, Chimenti S, et al. Adult cardiac stem cells are multipotent and support myocardial regeneration. Cell 2003; 114: 763–776.
10. Beltrami AP, Urbanek K, Kajstura J, Yan SM, Finato N, Bussani R, et al. Evidence that human cardiac myocytes divide after myocardial infarction. N Engl J Med 2001; 344: 1750–1757.
11. Anversa P, Nadal-Ginard B. Myocyte renewal and ventricular remodeling. Nature 2002; 415: 240–243.
12. Nadal-Ginard B, Kajstura J, Leri A, Anversa P. Myocyte death, growth, and regeneration in cardiac hypertrophy and failure. Circ Res 2003; 92: 139–150.
13. Quaini F, Urbanek K, Beltrami AP, Finato N, Beltrami CA, Nadal-Ginard B, et al. Chimerism of the transplanted heart. New Engl J Med 2002; 346: 5–15.
14. Thiele J, Varus E, Wickenhauser C, Kvasnicka HM, Metz KA, Beelen DW. Regeneration of heart muscle tissue: quantification of chimeric cardiomyocytes and endothelial cells following transplantation. Histol Histopathol 2004; 19: 201–209.

15. Deb A, Wang S, Skelding KA, Miller D, Simper D, Caplice NM. Bone marrow-derived cardiomyocytes are present in adult human heart: A study of gender-mismatched bone marrow transplantation patients. Circulation 2003;107:1247–9.
16. Orlic D, Kajstura J, Chimenti S, Jakoniuk I, Anderson SM, Li B, et al. Bone marrow cells regenerate infarcted myocardium. Nature 2001; 410: 701–705.
17. Orlic D, Kajstura J, Chimenti S, Limana F, Jakoniuk I, Quaini F, et al. Mobilized bone marrow cells repair the infarcted heart, improving function and survival. Proc Natl Acad Sci 2001; 98: 10344–10349.
18. Tomita S, Mickle DA, Weisel RD, Jia ZQ, Tumiati LC, Allidina Y, et al. Improved heart function with myogenesis and angiogenesis after autologous porcine bone marrow stromal cell transplantation. J Thorac Cardiovasc Surg 2002; 123: 1132–1140.
19. Mangi AA, Noiseux N, Kong K, He H, Rezvani N, Ingwall JS, et al. Mesenchymal stem cells modified with Akt prevent remodeling and restore performance of infracted hearts. Nat Med 2003; 9: 1195–1201.
20. Balsam LB, Wagers AJ, Christensen JL, Kofidis T, Weissman IL, Robbins RC. Haematopoietic stem cells adopt mature haematopoietic fates in ischaemic myocardium. Nature 2004; 428: 668–73.
21. Murry CE, Soonpaa MH, Reinecke H, Nakajima H, Nakajima HO, Rubart M, et al. Haematopoietic stem cells do not transdifferentiate into cardiac myocytes in myocardial Infarcts. Nature 2004; 428: 664–668.
22. Vulliet PR, Greeley M, Halloran M, MacDonald A, Kittelson MD. Intra-coronary arterial injection of mesenchymal stromal cells and microinfarction in dogs. Lancet 2004; 363: 783–84.
23. Silvestre JS, Gojova A, Brun V, Potteaux S, Esposito B, Duriez M, et al. Transplantation of bone marrow-derived mononuclear cells in ischemic apolipoprotein E-knockout mice accelerates atherosclerosis without altering plaque composition. Circulation 2003; 108: 2839–2842.
24. Kang HJ, Kim HS, Zhang SY, Park KW, Cho HJ, Koo BK, et al. Effects of intracoronary infusion of peripheral blood stem-cells mobilized with granulocyte-colony stimulating factor on left ventricular systolic function and restenosis after coronary stenting in myocardial infarction: the MAGIC cell randomized clinical trial. Lancet 2004; 363: 751–756.
25. Chien KR. Lost in translation. Nature 2004; 428: 607–608.
26. Matsubara H. Risk to the coronary arteries of intracoronary stem cell infusion and G-CSF cytokine therapy. Lancet 2004: 746–747.
27. Hamano K, Nishida M, Hirata K, Mikamo A, Li TS, Harada M, et al. Local implantation of autologous bone marrow for therapeutic angiogenesis in patients with ischemic heart disease: clinical trial and preliminary results. Jpn Circ J 2001;65:845–847.
28. Menasche P, Hagege AA, Vilquin JT, Desnos M, Abergel E, Pouzet B, Bel A, Sarateanu S, Scorsin M, Schwartz K, Bruneval P, Benbunan M, Marolleau JP, Duboc D. Autologous skeletal myoblast transplantation for severe postinfarction left ventricular dysfunction. J Am Coll Cardiol. 2003;41:1078–83.
29. Herreros J, Prosper F, Perez A, Gavira JJ, Garcia-Velloso MJ, Barba J, et al. Autologous intramyocardial injection of cultured skeletal muscle-derived stem cells in patients with non-acute myocardial infarction. Eur Heart J 2003;24: 2012–2020.

30. Pagani FD, DerSimonian H, Zawadzka A, Wetzel K, Edge AS, Jacoby DB, et al. Autologous skeletal myoblasts transplanted to ischemia-damaged myocardium in humans. Histological analysis of cell survival and differentiation. J Am Coll Cardiol 2003;41:879–888.
31. Galinanes M, Loubani M, Davies J, Chin D, Pasi J, Bell PR. Autotransplantation of unmanipulated bone marrow into scarred myocardium is safe and enhances cardiac function in humans. Cell Transplant 2004;13:7–13.
32. Smits PC, van Geuns RJ, Poldermans D, Bountioukos M, Onderwater EE, Lee CH, et al. Catheter-based intramyocardial injection of autologous skeletal myoblasts as a primary treatment of ischemic heart failure: clinical experience with six-month follow-up. J Am Coll Cardiol 2003;42:2063–2069.
33. Tse HF, Kwong YL, Chan JK, Lo G, Ho CL, Lau CP. Angiogenesis in ischaemic myocardium by intramyocardial autologous bone marrow mononuclear cell implantation. Lancet 2003;361:47–49.
34. Perin EC, Dohmann HF, Borojevic R, Silva SA, Sousa AL, Mesquita CT, et al. Transendocardial, auotologous bone marrow cell transplantation for severe, chronic ischemic heart failure Circulation. 2003;107:2294–2302.
35. Fuchs S, Satler LF, Kornowski R, Okubagzi P, Weisz G, Baffour R, et al. Catheter-based autologous bone marrow myocardial injection in no-option patients with advanced coronary artery disease. A feasibility study. J Am Coll Cardiol 2003;41:1721–1724.
36. Kuethe F, Figulla HR, Voth M, Richartz BM, Opfermann T, Sayer HG, et al. Mobilization of stem cells by granulocyte colony-stimulating factor for the regeneration of myocardial tissue after myocardial infarction. Dtsch Med Wochenschr 2004;129:424–428.
37. Assmus B, Schächinger V, Teupe C, Britten M, Lehmann R, Döbert N, et al. Transplantation of progenitor cells and regeneration enhancement in acute myocardial infarction (TOPCARE-AMI). Circulation 2002; 106: 3009–3017.
38. Strauer BE, Brehm M, Zeus T, Köstering M, Hernandez A, Sorg RV, et al. Repair of infarcted myocardium by autologous intracoronary mononuclear bone marrow cell transplantation in humans. Circulation 2002; 106: 1913–1918.
39. Fernandez-Aviles F, San Roman JA, Garcia-Frade J, Fernandez ME, Penarrubia MJ, de la Fuente L, et al. Experimental and clinical regenerative capability of human bone marrow cells after myocardial infarction. Circ Res. 2004;95:742–748.
40. Wollert KC, Meyer GP, Lotz J, Ringes-Lichtenberg S, Lippolt P, Breidenbach C, et al. Intracoronary autologous bone-marrow cell transfer after myocardial infarction: the BOOST randomised controlled clinical trial. Lancet 2004;364:141–148.
41. Chen SL, Fang WW, Ye F, Liu YH, Qian J, Shan SJ, Zhang JJ, Chunhua RZ, Liao LM, Lin S, Sun JP. Effect on left ventricular function of intracoronary transplantation of autologous bone marrow mesenchymal stem cell in patients with acute myocardial infarction. Am J Cardiol. 2004;94:92–5.
42. Sakakibara Y, Tambara K, Lu F, Nishina T, Nagaya N, Nishimura K et al. Cardiomyocyte transplantation does not reverse cardiac remodelling in rats with chronic myocardial infarction. Ann Thorac Surg 2002; 74: 25–30.
43. Li RK, Mickle DA, Weisel RD, Rao V, Jia ZQ.. Optimal time for cardiomyocyte transplantation to maximize myocardial function after left ventricular injury. Ann Thorac Surg 2001; 72: 1957–1963.

44. Cerqueira MD, Weissman NJ, Dilsizian V, Jacobs AK, Kaul S, Laskey WK, et al. Standardized myocardial segmentation and nomenclature for tomographic imaging of the heart. Circulation 2002; 105: 539–542.
45. Baer FM, Voth E, Scheneider CA, Theissen P, Schicha H, Sechtem U. Comparison of low-dose dobutamine-gradiente-echo magnetic resonance imaging and positron emission tomography with [18F] fluorodeoxyglucose in patients with chronic coronary artery disease. Circulation 1995; 91: 1006–1015.
45. Baer FM, Voth E, Scheneider CA, Theissen P, Schicha H, Sechtem U. Comparison of low-dose dobutamine-gradiente-echo magnetic resonance imaging and positron emission tomography with [18F] fluorodeoxyglucose in patients with chronic coronary artery disease. Circulation 1995; 91: 1006–1015.
46. Cwajg JM, Cwajg E, Nagueh SF, He ZX, Qureshi U, Olmos LI, et al. End-diastolic wall thickness as a predictor of recovery of function in myocardial hibernation: relation to rest-redistribution T1-201 tomography and dobutamine stress echocardiography. J Am Coll Cardiol 2000; 35: 1152–1161.
47. Barbato E, Aarnoudse W, Aengevaeren WR, Werner G, Klauss V, Bojara W, et al; Week 25 study group. Validation of coronary flow reserve measurements by thermodilution in clinical practice. Eur Heart J 2004; 25. 219–223.

13
Mobilizing Bone Marrow Stem Cells for Myocardial Repair After Acute Myocardial Infarction

STEPHEN G. ELLIS* AND OUSSAMA WAZNI

1. Introduction

Bone marrow cell mobilization was first used for allogenic bone marrow transplantation. Cytometric analysis of CD34+ cells was used to estimate the quantity of hematopoietic cells mobilized. Mobilization of the bone marrow was initially achieved using granulocyte colony stimulating factor G-CSF. Patients undergoing autologous bone marrow transplantation who received G-CSF had a surge in the number of CD34+ cells. More recently GCSF given to normal donors to collect cells for allogeneic transplantation had been shown to increase the number of circulating CD34+ cells.[1-6]

After an acute myocardial infarction (AMI) there is a very narrow window in which revascularization may result in myocardial salvage. Sheiban et al. showed that primary PTCA for patients with AMI is effective in improving LV function if performed within four hours from symptom onset by preventing LV enlargement and remodeling. However, beyond this window it is likely that revascularization may not prevent negative remodeling and meaningful myocardial salvage.[7] This has led to a steady effort to find a means by which myocardial recovery can be achieved. It is hoped that stem cell therapy, of which mobilization is only one dimension, could help in realizing the goal of myocardial regeneration.

Direct evidence of bone marrow mobilization was demonstrated by Quaini et al., who showed that undifferentiated cells, some of which were Y chromosome, had populated hearts from female donors in male recipients. This was thought to be due to translocation from the bone marrow of the male recipients to the female donor hearts.[8]

Myocardial ischemic insult results in cardiomyocyte hypertrophy, which leads to genetic changes resulting in apoptosis of cardiac myocytes, progressive collagen replacement, and heart failure. This has been termed cardiac

*Cleveland Clinic; Phone: 216-445-6712; e-mail: ellis@ccf.org.

remodeling. After large infarcts, lineage-negative, c-kit–positive CD34-positive and highly enriched hematopoietic stem cells (side population) of the bone marrow have been suggested to migrate to damaged areas and promote repair.[9]

These studies have produced interest in the mobilization of the bone marrow for induction of myocardial repair after acute myocardial infarction via pathways dependent on elements in the adult bone marrow.

There are several aspects to bone marrow mobilization utilized to improve myocardial repair. First, there are studies that have shown that as a result of ischemia or exogenously administered cytokines there is clearly mobilization of bone marrow cells that then take residence in recently injured myocardium.[9] A second set of studies address not only mobilization and homing into the myocardium but also demonstrate that bone marrow derived angioblasts differentiate into vascular structures in the injured myocardium, and that there is also actually transdifferentiation of myocardial-homed bone marrow hematopoietic stem cells into cardiac myocytes. Therefore there are several different avenues whereby mobilization of BM stem cells could promote myocardial healing and preservation of function after an acute insult.

In this chapter we will review some of the studies that address each of these aspects of this exciting topic.

2.   Mobilizing Stem Cells

Orlic et al. first reported in 2001 that injection of bone marrow stem cells into injured myocardium resulted in the apparent transdifferentiation of these cells into myocardial cells, and caused improvement in function.[10,11] Similarly, Jackson et al. showed that when bone marrow side population cells are injected into lethally irradiated mice with induced myocardial infarction these cells homed to the injured myocardium, then migrated into ischemic cardiac muscle and blood vessels, differentiated to cardiomyocytes and endothelial cells, and contributed to the formation of functional tissue.[12]

Kocher et al. demonstrated that CD34+ cell fraction was rich in endothelial cells and angioblasts. CD34+ cells (>98% purity, containing both hematopoietic and endothelial progenitors) resulted in infiltration of the infarct zone within 48 h of LAD ligation, but this did not occur in unaffected myocardium or myocardium of sham-operated rats. Histological examination revealed that the injection of CD34+ cells resulted in a significant increase in infarct zone microvascularity, cellularity and numbers of factor-VIII+ angioblasts and capillaries, and was also accompanied by reduction in matrix deposition and fibrosis in comparison to controls. This translated into improved myocardial function compared to controls.[13]

Similarly, Schuster et al. elegantly demonstrated that human CD34+ cells mobilized by GCSF in healthy human donors when injected into mice with LAD ligation homed predominantly to damaged myocardium. They were also able to demonstrate induction of neovascularization measured by increased number of vessels. Mice that received the CD34+ cells also had less apoptosis and enhanced cardiomyocyte survival and regeneration resulting in reduced fibrosis and improvement in cardiac function.[14]

Exogenous administration of cytokines such as GCSF, GMCSF or VEGF can lead to more mobilization and better homing of these cells. More recently the exogenous administration of various cytokines has been demonstrated to have positive effects on the mobilization of progenitor cells. Kalka et al. studied the effect of vascular endothelial growth factor (VEGF) on the endothelial progenitor cells (EPC) population in patients with critical limb ischemia undergoing intramuscular phVEFG165 gene transfer and in patients with critical limb ischemia who received intramuscular saline only. They found that the patients who received the VEGF had much higher counts of circulating EPC's compared to the patients who received saline. This effect was seen up to 4 weeks after initial injection. Similarly Kalka et al. in another study showed that increased circulating EPC's in patients receiving intramyocardial VEGF165 compared to patients who did not.[15-18]

Seiler et al. reported the effects of intracoronary and systemic administration of granulocyte-macrophage colony stimulating factor (GM-CSF) in patients with coronary artery disease. Twenty-one patients who were not amenable to or refused coronary bypass surgery participated in this randomized, double blind, placebo-controlled study. Ten individuals received GM-CSF via intracoronary infusion into the vessel believed to supply ischemic myocardium, followed by systemic administration of GM-CSF daily for two weeks. Analysis of mobilization of bone marrow stem cells was not performed in this study, but because the leukocyte counts were only twice the baseline values, it was suggested that only modest BMSC mobilization was achieved.

The type of bone marrow cells responsible for myocardial regeneration is under contention. Kawada et al., in an experiment in which irradiated mice were transplanted with either whole bone marrow cells or hematopoietic stem cells after ligation of the left anterior descending artery and treatment with GCSF, were able to demonstrate that is was in fact bone marrow derived mesenchymal stem cells that trans-differentiated into myocardial cells and not hematopoietic stem cells.[19]

Orlic et al. studied the response to GCSF and stem cell factor on infarcted myocardium. Splenectomized mice were injected with subcutaneous stem cell factor (SCF) and GCSF prior to and after ligation of the LAD. Controls were splenectomized infarcted and sham operated (SO) mice injected with saline. In this study, BMC mobilization by SCF and G-CSF resulted in a dramatic increase in survival of infarcted mice; with cytokine treatment, 73% of mice (11 of 15) survived 27 days, whereas mortality was very high in untreated infarcted mice. A band of newly formed myocardium occupying most of the damaged area characterized cardiac repair. The developing tissue extended from the border zone to the inside of the injured region and from the endocardium to the epicardium of the left ventricular free wall. In the absence of cytokines, myocardial replacement was never observed, and healing with scar formation was apparent. In addition, connexin43, a marker of viable and functioning myocardial cells, was clearly detectable in the newly formed myocardial cells derived from BMC at 9 days after implantation and it acquired a more mature pattern of distribution at 27 days. Consistent with the identification of contractile activity in the repairing myocardium, the expression of connexin43 suggests that operative gap junctions were developed between myocardial cells.[20]

Adachi et al. demonstrated that GCSF is able to mobilize and home side population bone marrow cells. Hearts of mice that had undergone coronary occlusion were isolated and digested with collagenase. Infiltrating cells in the heart were collected using Percoll density gradients. The infiltrating cells were sorted for side population a unique bone marrow cell fraction, which is rich in hematopoietic stem cells with staining by a Hoechst dye.

One to 14 days after myocardial infarction, hundreds of infiltrating SP cells were found in the infarcted zone. There were only a few SP cells in hearts without infarction. Infiltrating SP cells were increased in the 4-day G-CSF treated group compared with the placebo group. SP cells in the infarcted hearts of mice were positive for b-galactosidase indicating the bone marrow origin of these cells in these mice which had been transplanted with bone marrow from ROSA 26 (b-galactosidase transgenic) mice.[21]

Takahashi et al. demonstrated that circulating EPC's are mobilized endogenously in response to tissue ischemia or exogenously by cytokine therapy and thereby augment neovascularization of ischemic tissues.

The development of regional ischemia in both mice and rabbits increased the frequency of circulating EPC's. In this study the effect of ischemia-induced EPC mobilization in mice was demonstrated by enhanced ocular neovascularization after cornea micropocket surgery in mice with hind limb ischemia compared with that in non-ischemic control mice. In rabbits with hind limb ischemia, circulating EPC's were further augmented after pretreatment with GM-CSF, with a corresponding improvement in hind limb neovascularization. Transgenic tagged donor EPC's expressing galactosidase were used to prove that the cells contributing to corneal neovascularization were specifically mobilized from the bone marrow in response to ischemia and GM-CSF.[9]

Another potential factor that can play a role in the mobilization of bone marrow cells is stromal derived factor 1SDF-1. SDF-1 is a chemokine of the CXC family. CXCR4 is the only known receptor of SDF-1.[22-24] Yamagushi et al. demonstrated that SDF-1 up-regulates VEGF expression in an ischemic model. They also found that SDF-1 recruited transplanted EPC's from the systemic circulation.[22]

Recent reports indicate that SDF-1 is a strong chemo attractant for CD34+ cells, which express CXCR4, the receptor for SDF-1. It plays an important role in hematopoietic stem cell trafficking between the peripheral circulation, bone marrow and ischemic tissue, and exerts a strong chemoattractant effect on circulating EPC's augmenting the effect of endogenous angiogenic/chemoattractant factors.[22-24]

All of the previous studies involved the induction of the BM cells around the time period of the acute induction of ischemia. Not many studies have addressed the issue and feasibility of BM mobilization for the treatment of remotely infarcted hearts. Recently Askari et demonstrated that stem-cell mobilization alone did not lead to significant engraftment of circulating cells in ischemic cardiomyopathy at a time remote from the myocardial infarction. However when cells that express SDF-1 were injected into the myocardium there was significant homing of bone marrow derived cells. However their group did not observe regeneration of cardiac cells raising the possibility that those signaling molecules that direct stem-cell transdifferentiation towards a cardiac myocyte phenotype are only transiently expressed[24] and possibly only during the acute insult.

3.   Initial Human Experience

Initial experience with stem cell mobilization in humans seems promising. Two strategies with respect to the use of mobilizing techniques have been implemented. In one strategy only GCSF administration is performed. In a more extensive strategy peripheral blood cells mobilized by GCF are collected and then injected into the coronaries of patients after a myocardial infarction.

In the TOPCARE-AMI trial the transplantation of progenitor cells was associated with better left-ventricular function. LV function after progenitor cell therapy. The LV EF increased by up to 8.7% four months following intracoronary progenitor cell infusion. Also, analysis of LV function by MRI one year after progenitor cell infusion documented a sustained improvement in global EF, and revealed the lack of infarct expansion as evidenced by reduced end-systolic volumes and unchanged end-diastolic volumes as well as absent reactive hypertrophy of non-infarcted segments as evidenced by a preserved significant reduction of LV mass between month 4 and month 12 compared to the acute phase post-MI.[25]

The MAGIC trial compared the use of GCSF only to the intracoronary infusion of cells collected after mobilization with GCSF. In this trial administration of GCF alone resulted in no discernible improvements in left ventricular function at six months. In the cell infusion group, however, there were statistically significant improvements in left ventricular function and dimensions.[26]

4.   Potential Risks

There have been recent concerns with the use of GCSF. There was an increased risk of restenosis in patients receiving GCSF in the Magic Trial.[26] There have also been concerns that the mobilization of inflammatory cells may lead to higher risk of myocardial rupture after myocardial infarction. GCSF use has also been associated with spleen rupture in a peripheral blood progenitor cell donor.[27]

5.   Controversies

Two recent studies in *Nature* cast doubts as to the ability of stem cells to home to damaged myocardium, let alone transdifferentiate into myocardial cells. Murry et al. and Balsam et al. showed that genetically tagged cells injected into myocardium demonstrated no transdifferentiation when injected into freshly damaged myocardium.[28,29] The methods used to identify and track the cells were different than those in Orlic's original early reports. In the original work by Orlic et al., antibody tagging that is less specific was used to track BM cells. These antibodies could have tagged endogenous myocardial elements. It is accepted today that genetic tagging is much more reliable. Murray et al. used stem cells that were tagged with the LacZ gene which is expressed only when these cells are located in heart tissue. When these cells were directly injected into infarcted myocardium hardly any LacZ was expressed. Balsam et al. using a different tag, the green fluorescent protein, showed that stem cells with this tag did not trans-differentiate into cardiac cells. Also Balsam et al. showed that GFP tagged cells that were continuously infused into mice with infarcted hearts did not home into the myocardium or become cardiac cells.[29]

Given these contradictory reports there have been recent calls to make research in this field more uniform and standardized. However, this should not hinder further investigation into this very exciting field.[30]

6.   References

1. Bolwell BJ, Fishleder A, Andresen SW, Lichtin AE, Koo A, Yanssens T, Burwell R, Baucco P, Green R. G-CSF primed peripheral blood progenitor cells in autologous bone marrow transplantation: parameters affecting bone marrow engraftment. *Bone Marrow Transplant.* 1993;12:609–14.
2. Bishop MR, Tarantolo SR, Jackson JD, Anderson JR, Schmit-Pokorny K, Zacharias D, Pavletic ZS, Pirruccello SJ, Vose JM, Bierman PJ, Warkentin PI, Armitage JO, Kessinger A. Allogeneic-blood stem-cell collection following mobilization with low-dose granulocyte colony-stimulating factor. *J Clin Oncol.* 1997;15:1601–7.

3. Russell JA, Luider J, Weaver M, Brown C, Selinger S, Railton C, Karlsson L, Klassen J. Collection of progenitor cells for allogeneic transplantation from peripheral blood of normal donors. *Bone Marrow Transplant.* 1995;15:111–5.
4. Grigg AP, Roberts AW, Raunow H, Houghton S, Layton JE, Boyd AW, McGrath KM, Maher D. Optimizing dose and scheduling of filgrastim (granulocyte colony-stimulating factor) for mobilization and collection of peripheral blood progenitor cells in normal volunteers. *Blood.* 1995;86:4437–45.
5. Bolwell BJ, Goormastic M, Yanssens T, Dannley R, Baucco P, Fishleder A. Comparison of G-CSF with GM-CSF for mobilizing peripheral blood progenitor cells and for enhancing marrow recovery after autologous bone marrow transplant. *Bone Marrow Transplant.* 1994;14:913–8.
6. Chao NJ, Schriber JR, Grimes K, Long GD, Negrin RS, Raimondi CM, Horning SJ, Brown SL, Miller L, Blume KG. Granulocyte colony-stimulating factor "mobilized" peripheral blood progenitor cells accelerate granulocyte and platelet recovery after high-dose chemotherapy. *Blood.* 1993;81:2031–5.
7. Sheiban I, Fragasso G, Lu C, Tonni S, Trevi GP, Chierchia SL. Influence of treatment delay on long-term left ventricular function in patients with acute myocardial infarction successfully treated with primary angioplasty. *Am Heart J.* 2001;141:603–9.
8. Quaini F, Urbanek K, Beltrami AP, Finato N, Beltrami CA, Nadal-Ginard B, Kajstura J, Leri A, Anversa P. Chimerism of the transplanted heart. *N Engl J Med.* 2002;346:5–15.
9. Takahashi T, Kalka C, Masuda H, Chen D, Silver M, Kearney M, Magner M, Isner JM, Asahara T. Ischemia- and cytokine-induced mobilization of bone marrow-derived endothelial progenitor cells for neovascularization. *Nat Med.* 1999;5:434–8.
10. Orlic D, Kajstura J, Chimenti S, Bodine DM, Leri A, Anversa P. Transplanted adult bone marrow cells repair myocardial infarcts in mice. *Ann N Y Acad Sci.* 2001;938:221–9; discussion 229–30.
11. Orlic D, Kajstura J, Chimenti S, Limana F, Jakoniuk I, Quaini F, Nadal-Ginard B, Bodine DM, Leri A, Anversa P. Mobilized bone marrow cells repair the infarcted heart, improving function and survival. *Proc Natl Acad Sci U S A.* 2001;98:10344–9.
12. Jackson KA, Majka SM, Wang H, Pocius J, Hartley CJ, Majesky MW, Entman ML, Michael LH, Hirschi KK, Goodell MA. Regeneration of ischemic cardiac muscle and vascular endothelium by adult stem cells. *J Clin Invest.* 2001;107:1395–402.
13. Kocher AA, Schuster MD, Szabolcs MJ, Takuma S, Burkhoff D, Wang J, Homma S, Edwards NM, Itescu S. Neovascularization of ischemic myocardium by human bone-marrow-derived angioblasts prevents cardiomyocyte apoptosis, reduces remodeling and improves cardiac function. *Nat Med.* 2001;7:430–6.
14. Schuster MD, Kocher AA, Seki T, Martens TP, Xiang G, Homma S, Itescu S. Myocardial neovascularization by bone marrow angioblasts results in cardiomyocyte regeneration. *Am J Physiol Heart Circ Physiol.* 2004;287:H525–32.
15. Kalka C, Asahara T, Krone W, Isner JM. [Angiogenesis and vasculogenesis. Therapeutic strategies for stimulation of postnatal neovascularization]. *Herz.* 2000;25:611–22.
16. Kalka C, Masuda H, Takahashi T, Gordon R, Tepper O, Gravereaux E, Pieczek A, Iwaguro H, Hayashi SI, Isner JM, Asahara T. Vascular endothelial growth

factor(165) gene transfer augments circulating endothelial progenitor cells in human subjects. *Circ Res*. 2000;86:1198–202.

17. Kalka C, Masuda H, Takahashi T, Kalka-Moll WM, Silver M, Kearney M, Li T, Isner JM, Asahara T. Transplantation of ex vivo expanded endothelial progenitor cells for therapeutic neovascularization. *Proc Natl Acad Sci U S A*. 2000;97:3422–7.

18. Kalka C, Tehrani H, Laudenberg B, Vale PR, Isner JM, Asahara T, Symes JF. VEGF gene transfer mobilizes endothelial progenitor cells in patients with inoperable coronary disease. *Ann Thorac Surg*. 2000;70:829–34.

19. Kawada H, Fujita J, Kinjo K, Matsuzaki Y, Tsuma M, Miyatake H, Muguruma Y, Tsuboi K, Itabashi Y, Ikeda Y, Ogawa S, Okano H, Hotta T, Ando K, Fukuda K. Non-hematopoietic mesenchymal stem cells can be mobilized and differentiate into cardiomyocytes after myocardial infarction. *Blood*. 2004.

20. Orlic D. Stem cell repair in ischemic heart disease: an experimental model. *Int J Hematol*. 2002;76 Suppl 1:144–5.

21. Adachi Y, Imagawa J, Suzuki Y, Yogo K, Fukazawa M, Kuromaru O, Saito Y. G-CSF treatment increases side population cell infiltration after myocardial infarction in mice. *J Mol Cell Cardiol*. 2004;36:707–10.

22. Yamaguchi J, Kusano KF, Masuo O, Kawamoto A, Silver M, Murasawa S, Bosch-Marce M, Masuda H, Losordo DW, Isner JM, Asahara T. Stromal cell-derived factor-1 effects on ex vivo expanded endothelial progenitor cell recruitment for ischemic neovascularization. *Circulation*. 2003;107:1322–8.

23. Penn MS, Zhang M, Deglurkar I, Topol EJ. Role of stem cell homing in myocardial regeneration. *Int J Cardiol*. 2004;95 Suppl 1:S23–5.

24. Askari AT, Unzek S, Popovic ZB, Goldman CK, Forudi F, Kiedrowski M, Rovner A, Ellis SG, Thomas JD, DiCorleto PE, Topol EJ, Penn MS. Effect of stromal-cell-derived factor 1 on stem-cell homing and tissue regeneration in ischaemic cardiomyopathy. *Lancet*. 2003;362:697–703.

25. Schachinger V, Assmus B, Britten MB, Honold J, Lehmann R, Teupe C, Abolmaali ND, Vogl TJ, Hofmann WK, Martin H, Dimmeler S, Zeiher AM. Transplantation of progenitor cells and regeneration enhancement in acute myocardial infarction: final one-year results of the TOPCARE-AMI Trial. *J Am Coll Cardiol*. 2004;44:1690–9.

26. Kang HJ, Kim HS, Zhang SY, Park KW, Cho HJ, Koo BK, Kim YJ, Soo Lee D, Sohn DW, Han KS, Oh BH, Lee MM, Park YB. Effects of intracoronary infusion of peripheral blood stem-cells mobilised with granulocyte-colony stimulating factor on left ventricular systolic function and restenosis after coronary stenting in myocardial infarction: the MAGIC cell randomised clinical trial. *Lancet*. 2004;363:751–6.

27. Balaguer H, Galmes A, Ventayol G, Bargay J, Besalduch J. Splenic rupture after granulocyte-colony-stimulating factor mobilization in a peripheral blood progenitor cell donor. *Transfusion*. 2004;44:1260–1.

28. Murry CE, Soonpaa MH, Reinecke H, Nakajima H, Nakajima HO, Rubart M, Pasumarthi KB, Virag JI, Bartelmez SH, Poppa V, Bradford G, Dowell JD, Williams DA, Field LJ. Haematopoietic stem cells do not transdifferentiate into cardiac myocytes in myocardial infarcts. *Nature*. 2004;428:664–8.

29. Balsam LB, Wagers AJ, Christensen JL, Kofidis T, Weissman IL, Robbins RC. Haematopoietic stem cells adopt mature haematopoietic fates in ischaemic myocardium. *Nature*. 2004;428:668–73.

30. Chien KR. Stem cells: lost in translation. *Nature*. 2004;428:607–8.

Percutaneous Stem Cell
Transplantation

14
Percutaneous Myoblast Transplantation: Steps In Translational Research

Nabil Dib[*]

1. Introduction

Epicardial local delivery might be one easy and reliable method of delivery. It has been used for gene[1] and cell therapy.[2-4] Endocardial local delivery have been used for gene therapy. In a phase one clinical trial to assess the safety and feasibility of catheter-based myocardial gene transfer for therapeutic angiogenesis. The procedure has been shown to be feasible and safe.[5,6] Cell therapy involving bone marrow transplantation for ischemic cardiomyopathy has been used successfully with trend toward efficacy.[7] Percutaneous myoblast transplantation has been done successfully in Europe under both three dimensional and two dimensional guidance for myocardial regeneration.[8,9] We have been working over the last four years on developing the methods for catheter base cell therapy for myocardial regeneration with the goal of treating patients suffering of myocardial infarction or heart failure secondary to myocardial infarction. We developed percutaneously a swine model of myocardial infarction to simulate myocardial infarction in human and the intention was to use catheter that will be used in human for cell transplantation. The procedure described in detail in the chapter "A Porcine Model of Myocardial Infarction for Evaluation of Cell Transplantation."

As discussed in previous chapters, myocardial infarction results in the death of cardiomyocytes. Cell transplantation has been suggested as a method of regenerating the scarred myocardium, and a variety of cells types, including embryonic stem cells, cardiomyocytes, mesenchymal stem cells, hematopoetic stem cells, and autologous myoblasts, have been proposed for replacing nonfunctioning tissue. Although epicardial transplantation has been the most common route of delivery for cell transplant, an endoventricular approach has several theoretical advantages, including that the procedure can be: (1) used in high-risk patients, (2) repeated with minimal risk to

---

*Nabil Dib, Arizona Heart Institute and Heart Hospital, Phoenix, AZ, 85006

the patient, (3) associated with a lower morbidity rate than surgery, and (4) used to treat areas normally inaccessible by surgery (such as the septum). At present, several endoventricular devices are under evaluation (Figure 1). They can be divided into two categories: the three-dimensional (3-D) guidance catheter delivery system manufactured by Cordis Corp. (Miami Lakes, FL), and the two-dimensional (2-D) fluoroscopy guidance systems manufactured by Bioheart, Inc. (Santa Rosa, CA), TransVascular, Inc. (Menlo Park, CA), Biocardia, Inc., (South San Francisco, CA) and Boston-Scientific/Scimed, Inc. (Natick, MA).

Endoventricular delivery is more challenging than surgical injection. Safe, accurate and reproducible, endoventricular delivery of cells ideally incorporates knowledge of the internal architecture of the ventricle, the position and

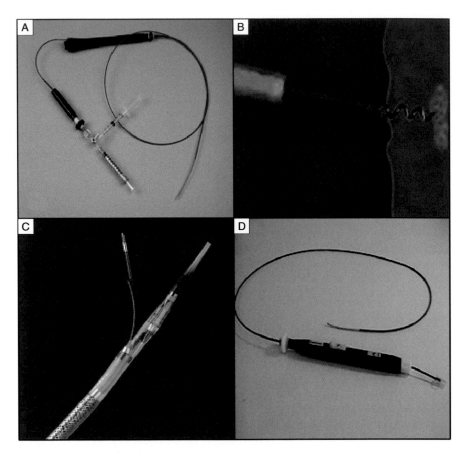

FIGURE 1. The four catheter types available for intromyocardial delivery are pictured as follows: (A) Myostar™ [Cordis Corp.], (B) Helical Injection Character™ [Biocardia, Inc.], (C) TransAccess® MicroLume™ [Transvascular, Inc.], (D) MyoCath™ [Bioheart, Inc.]

orientation of the catheter tip in space, catheter maneuverability, and the ability to penetrate and inject into the thin, scarred myocardium.

In this chapter, we will review our work of benchmark testing and preclinical evaluations that include catheter–cell biocompatibility, feasibility of percutaneous cell delivery, bioretention and distribution, and safety and efficacy. We hope these steps will serve as a platform for the researchers who are interested in translational research on stem cell therapy that leads to clinical application.

2. Equipment

Endocardial methods of delivery could be devided to 3-D delivery (NOGAS-TAR® Mapping Catheter and MyoStar™ Injection Catheter, Cordis) and 2-D giudance.

As it is demonstrated in this chapter using 3-D guidance cordis catheter one can reconstruct the left ventricle and identify myocardial infarction and distribute the transplant sites. That might potentially have two advantages first avoid local toxicity (figure 2) by avoiding multiple injections at the same

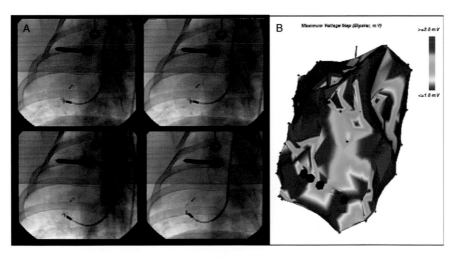

FIGURE 2. Visualization of 2-dimensional fluoroscopy and 3-dimensional NOGA MyoStar™ visualization of catheter dye injections performed near the apex of a porcine heart that had undergone coil-induced occlusion of the left anterior descending artery 30 days before. (A) Using fluoroscopic imaging, it appears that the four different injections of contrast dye into infarcted tissue are overlapping. (B) Using the 3-dimensional NOGA system, the spacial distribution of each injection is apparent. A user-defined color gradient (vertical bar on right) shows the voltage potential of the heart. Red=infarcted tissue; Blue, purple, and green=healthy tissue; Yellow=border zone

sites and second the distribution of the transplant sites might play role in the final outcome on efficacy. Our review focuses on the Cordis 3-D system.

The Cordis system and accompanying computer software (Figures 3 and 4) includes a locator pad (fixed beneath the patient table) with three coils that emit a low energy magnetic field (1, 2, 3 kHz) and also incorporates a stationary reference catheter with a magnetic field sensor, a mapping catheter, and a needle injection catheter with a magnetic field sensor and a Silicon Graphics (Mountain View, CA) processor. The emitted fields possess well-known temporal and spatial distinguishing characteristics that "code" the mapping space around the patient's chest. Sensing of the magnetic field by the location sensor enables determination of the location and orientation of the catheter in 6° of freedom. The system uses a triangulation algorithm to determine the position of the catheter tip in 3-D space (Figure 3).

When the catheter is in contact with endocardium, two electrodes on the distal tip permit measurement of a voltage potential across a short segment of endocardium. Data taken during these measurements are processed to generate a 3-D, color-coded, voltage map representation of the left ventricle (LV) that clearly demarcates the area of myocardial infarction. When the LV map is complete, the mapping catheter is exchanged for a modified catheter that allows endocardial injection through a needle on the distal tip (Figure 5). The catheter tip can be bent (to angles > 90°) by using the knob on the handle

Catheter Tip Location

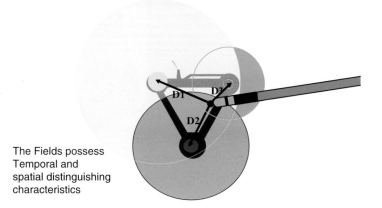

The Fields possess Temporal and spatial distinguishing characteristics

FIGURE 3. The location pad is fixed beneath the patient table, and the emitted fields possess well known temporal and spatial distinguishing characteristics that "code" the mapping space around the patient's chest. When the catheter is in contact with endocardium, two electrodes on the distal tip permit measurement of a voltage potential across a short segment of endocardium. The system uses a triangulation algorithm to determine the position of the catheter tip in 3-D space.

Biosense NOGA Mapping System

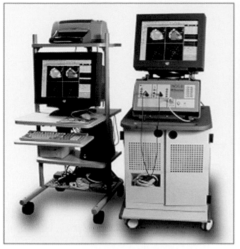

**Workstation able to reconstruct
the LV in 3-D image**

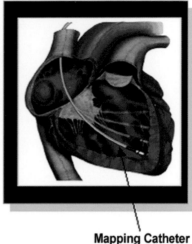

Mapping Catheter

FIGURE 4. The Cordis system is pictured at left, and a diagram showing the position of the mapping catheter in the left ventricle is shown at right.

of the catheter to orient the catheter tip during the advancement into the left ventricle (Figure 6). This hollow, steerable catheter has a 27-gauge nitinol needle on the distal tip, and a luer lock syringe can be attached to the proximal end so that a 1-cc syringe can be fitted to load a cell or gene sample into the lumen of the needle (Figure 5). There is a separate handle for needle injection with a knob that can advance and retrieve the needle (Figure 7). The needle length can be adjusted 2-10 mm by rotating the knob clockwise or counterclockwise (Figure 8). The recommended needle length is 60% of the myocardial wall thickness.

3.   Experiments

3.1.   Catheter-Cell Biocompatibility

Passage of cells or other biological agents through an injection catheter exposes them to shearing forces, pressure, and to the surface material of the catheter inner lumen. Surprisingly, there is little published data regarding the recovery, survival, and biological activity of agents delivered in this manner. It is a requirement by the regulatory authority that catheter and cells are intended to be used in human should be tested by asseesing the effects of physical forces on cell survival.

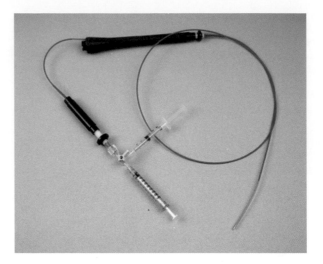

FIGURE 5. The needle injection catheter with luer lock syringe is shown ready for cell or gene injection.

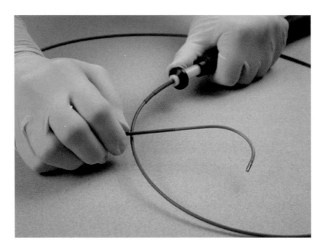

FIGURE 6. The needle injection catheter has a knob on the handle that can bend the catheter at angles > 90°.

We suggest that survival parameters of each cell type be carefully assessed prior to *in vivo* injections. In our experience, the main factors that affect cell survival include the speed of injection, the composition of solution they are suspended in, and the cell type. Adjusting the amount of solution injected over time (flow rate) may be necessary depending on the cell type and the viscosity of the solution. We have found that injecting 0.25 ml (10-100 million cells/ml) over 15-20 seconds preserves myoblast viability.

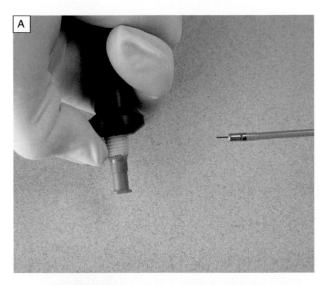

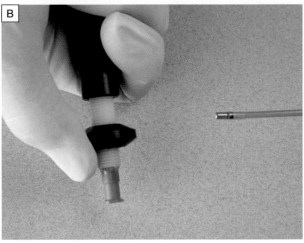

FIGURE 7. A special knob on the handle of the needle injection is used to A) advance an B) retrieve the needle.

3.2.   Animal Model

For catheter-based cell transplantation studies, a large animal model is required to simulate conditions in the human. We have used a swine model of myocardial infarction produced by coil placement in the left anterior descending (LAD) artery. We prefer a coil model to surgical ligation because our mortality rate has been much lower with coils (9% versus 50%). By placing coils distal to the diagonal, one can produce ejection fractions of 44% at one month and 41% at three months following myocardial infarction (Figure 9).

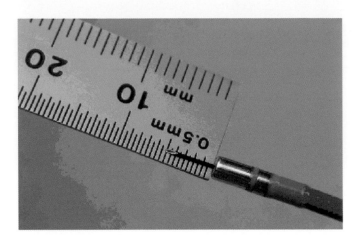

FIGURE 8. Needle length can be adjusted 2-10 mm by rotating the knob clockwise or counterclockwise and may be measured using a ruler. The appropriate needle length is based on the wall thickness.

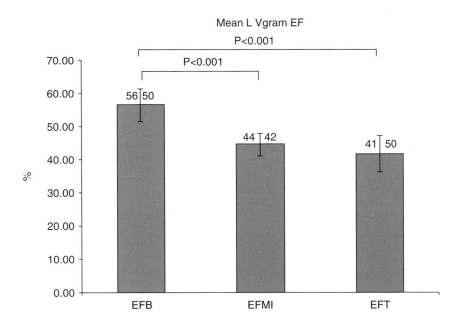

FIGURE 9. Ejection fraction in a swine model of myocardial infarction.

The full details of this model are described in the chapter text "A Porcine Model of Myocardial Infarction for Evaluation of Cell Transplantation" to help those interested in evaluating cell therapy or catheter technology reproduce the results. The FDA has accepted the described model for evaluation of cell therapy for regeneration of myocardial infarction.

3.3.   Feasibility of Catheter-Based Cell Delivery

Numerous tracer substances have been delivered to normal or damaged myocardial tissue using the MyoStar™ system (Figures 10), including dyes, recombinant viral vectors, contrast agents, The detection of these relatively inert substances by gross pathology and/or MRI has encouraged the evaluation of cell transplantation into infarcted tissue. We have used our model of myocardial infarction to demonstrate the feasibility of endoventricular delivery of porcine myoblasts to infarcted regions of the swine heart (Figure 11, 12).[10] At 10 days post-cell transplantation, multinucleated myotubes were observed. Catheter-based, autologous, bone-marrow cell delivery has also proven to be safe and possibly effective in humans with end-stage ischemic heart disease,[11,7] demonstrating increased perfusion.

3.4.   Bioretention and Biodistribution

Endoventricular injection carries the risk of pericardial effusion or cell leakage back into the circulatory system. Leakage may result only in cell loss, or it may have more detrimental effects, such as distal embolization. In our preliminary studies using the Cordis Myostar™ injection system in the swine infarction model, we tracked iridium-labeled myoblasts and found 4.1% in

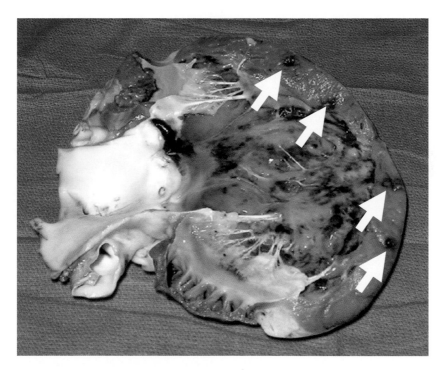

FIGURE 10. Methylene blue dye as injected using the MyoStar™ injection catheter.

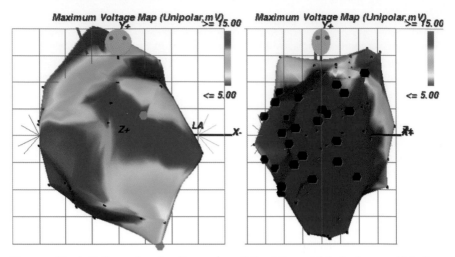

FIGURE 11. A 3-dimensional voltage map of the left ventricle is shown: A) before myocardial infarction, and B) after myocardial infarction. (Blue and Green = normal voltage, Red = low voltage, representing myocardial infarction, Black markers represent the site of cell transplants).

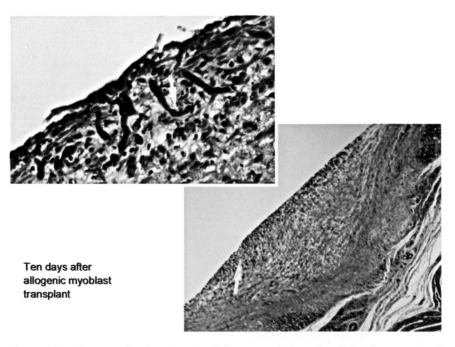

FIGURE 12. Photographs showing: (top left, at arrow) myotubes formed as a result of myoblast fusion, and (lower right, at arrow) an area of myocardial infarction and cell transplant.

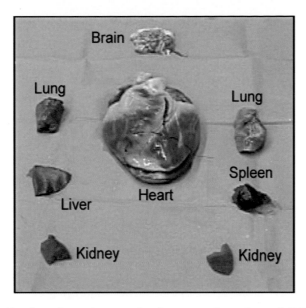

FIGURE 13. Porcine tissue harvested after transplantation of Iridium-labeled myoblasts to measure retention and detect distribution to other tissues.

the infarct region, none in remote regions of the heart, 5% in the lungs, <1% in the spleen, and none in the brain, liver, or kidneys (Figure 13). This suggests endoventricular cell transplantation into scar tissue is feasible and poses minimal risk for systemic embolization.. Overall, it appears that bioretention and distribution are affected by cell dose and volume; determining optimal protocols for these factors is likely to impact safety and efficacy of cell transplantation.

It is generally assumed that cell survival will be vital for transplant success, yet it is clear that in current clinical protocols only a minority of transplanted cells engraft and survive.[12] Survival may be affected by several parameters, including the overall health of tissue receiving the transplant, initial cell viability, catheter-cell biocompatibility, secretion of growth or apoptotic factors, and the degree of inflammatory response.

3.5.   Safety and Efficacy

Endoventricular injection catheters have an exemplary safety record, with few reports of myocardial rupture leading to cardiac tamponade from overly aggressive catheter manipulation or from injection. In our recent preclinical testing, cell transplantation was performed on 32 swine that were models of myocardial infarction, and there were no perforations or significant complications.

Delivering cells to scar tissue is more challenging than injection into ischemic or normal myocardium because the scarred myocardium is thin (Figure 14) yet hard to penetrate. Needle length should be adjusted to a depth ~60% of the wall thickness to avoid penetration of the wall and cell leakage to the systemic circulation.

In some cases, the catheter is pushed backward during needle advancement (Figure 15). Injecting into the apex should be avoided even in the normal

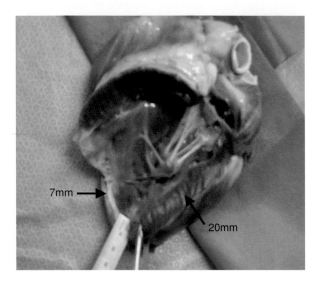

FIGURE 14. Photograph showing a normal wall thickness (20 mm) and an area of myocardial infarction (7 mm).

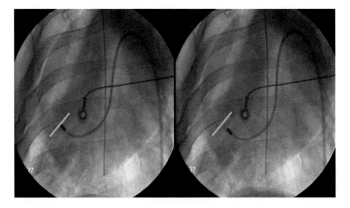

FIGURE 15. Flouroscopy demonstrating needle advancement causing backward motion of the catheter instead of needle penetration.

swine heart because the wall is very thin in this location (~2 mm) (Figure 16). The area of the mitral valve should also be avoided to eliminate the possibility of damaging the valve structure. Instances of sustained ventricular tachycardia (SVT) or premature ventricular contractions (PVCs) do sometimes occur, but are primarily related to the presence of the catheter itself, or to the injection process—they usually resolve quickly without the need for cardiac defibrillation if the catheter is repositioned.[10] Despite the difficulty of injecting infarcted tissue, we have found PVCs caused by needle injection are much less common in the infarct model than in the normal swine myocardium (30% versus 90%; Figure 17).

In our infarction model, transplantation of myoblasts using up to 600 million cells yielded no ventricular arrhythmias, as judged by monitoring with an implanted loop recorder, during the two months following the procedure (Figure 18).

Our evaluation showed improvements in the viability of the scar in the locations where myoblasts were transplanted; the average voltage in the area of the myocardial infarction improved (7.2 millivolts in the control group vs. 9.5 millivolts in the treated arm) two months after myoblast transplantation as assessed by NOGASTAR® mapping (Figures 19, 20). In addition, there

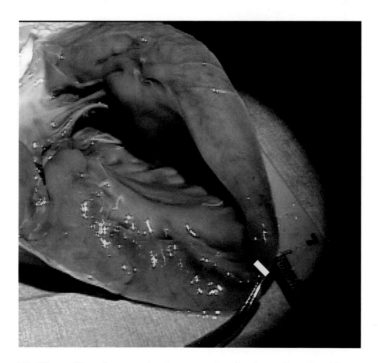

FIGURE 16. The wall at the apex in the normal swine heart is quite thin, measuring ~2 mm.

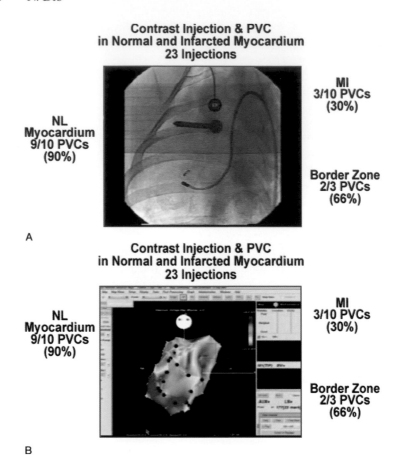

FIGURE 17. A) Fluoroscopic image shows the MyoStar™ catheter inside the left ventricle and a contrast injection, B) NOGASTAR® mapping shows the location of the injection (Red=scar, Green=normal tissue and border).

were trends indicating improvements in heart function as evaluated by measuring the cardiac index (0.65 in the control group vs. 0.83 in the treatment group) and ejection fraction (43.5% in controls vs. 52.5% in treated swine) (Figure 21).

The first patient in the United States to undergo myoblast transplantation via catheter using the NOGA 3-D imaging system took place on November 30, 2004 at the Arizona Heart Hospital. The 51-year old male had a heart attack on January 24, 2004 and had an ejection fraction of 27%. The patient was transplanted with 30 million cells and the procedure was uneventful.

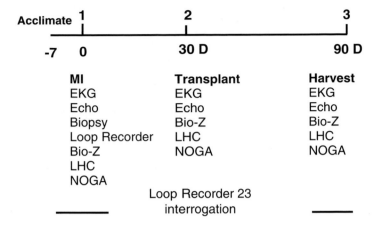

FIGURE 18. Flow chart for myoblast transplantation using the Myostar™ catheter injection catheter in the swine myocardial infarction model. The nuber 1,2 and 3 reflect the number of procedure. D= day. Bioz; a non-invasive assessment of cardiac output and index.

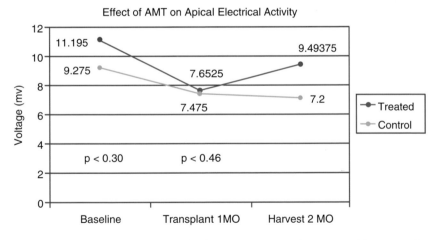

FIGURE 19. Comparison of voltage in the treatment [autologous myoblast transplant (AMT)] and control arms.

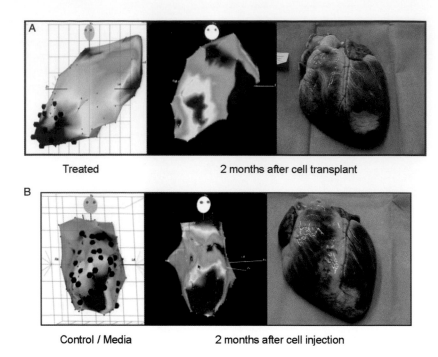

Treated   2 months after cell transplant

Control / Media   2 months after cell injection

FIGURE 20. Diagram showing improvement in viability as reflected by comparing the voltage map in the A) treatment and B) control arms. Red color represnet the size of myocardial infarction. Blue and Green represent normal myocardium.

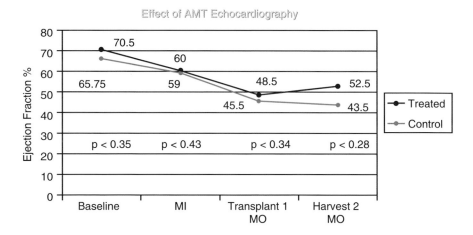

FIGURE 21. Graph showing a trend toward improvement in ejection fraction in the treatment arm as compared to the control arm.

4.   Conclusions

Early results of endoventricular cell transplantation demonstrate that this approach is feasible and safe in the models tested. The procedure is likely to have application in a majority of patients with previous myocardial infarction and congestive heart failure as the risks associated with a minimally invasive endoventricular injection are potentially lower than those linked with direct epicardial injection. The use of 3-D guidance appears to be key in accurately targeting areas that need to be treated, and catheters and cell preparations to be used in humans should be pretested for biocompatibility and safety. While catheter injection of cells is a relatively new innovation, the ability to access the heart without having to perform a median sternotomy will certainly encourage further evaluation of its potential for delivering many therapeutic biologic agents.

5.   References

1. Fortuin FD, Vale P, Losordo DW et al. One-year follow-up of direct myocardial gene transfer of vascular endothelial growth factor-2 using naked plasmid deoxyribonucleic acid by way of thoracotmy in no-opion patients, *J. Am. Coll. Cardiol.* 92, 436–9 (2003).
2. Menasche P, Hagege AA, Vilquin JT, et al. Autologous skeletal myoblast transplantation for severe postinfarction left ventricular dysfunction. *J. Am. Coll. Cardiol.* April 2, 1078–83 (2003).
3. Dib N, McCarthy P, Campbell A, et al. Feasiblility and Safety of Autologous Myoblast Transplantation in Patients with Ischemic Cardiomyopathy, *Cell Transplantation.* 14, (2003).
4. Dib N, McCarthy P, Dinsmore J, et al. Safety and Feasibility of autologous Myoblast Transplantation in Patients with Ischemic Cardiomyopathy: Interim results from the United States Experience, *Circulation.* 106, II-463 (2002).
5. Vale PR, Losordo DW, Milliken CD, et al. Randomized, single-blind, placebo-controlled pilot study of catheter-based myocardial gene transfer for therapeutic angiogenesis using left ventricular electromechanical mapping in patiens with chronic myocardial ischemia, *Circulation.* 103, 2138–43 (2001).
6. Fuchs S, Dib N, Cohen B, et al. A Randomized Double Blind Placebo Controlled multicenter Pilot Study of the Safety and Feasiblity of $Ad_{GV}VEGF121.10$ via an Intramyocardial Injection Catheter in Patients With Advanced Coronary Artery Disease, *J. Am. Coll. Cardiol.* 41, 21A (2003)
7. Fuchs S, Satler LF, Kornowski R, et al. Catheter-based autologous bone marrow myocardial injection in no-option patients with advanced coronary artery disease: a feasibility study, *J. Am. Coll. Cardiol.* 41, 1721–4 (2003).
8. Smits PC, van Geuns RJ, Poldermans D, et al. Catheter-based intramyocardial injection of autologous skeletal myoblasts as a primary treatment of ischemic heart failure: clinical experience with six-month follow-up, *J. Am. Coll. Cardiol.* 42,2063–9 (2003)

9. Ince H, Petzsch M, Rehders TC, et al. Transcatheter transplantation of autologous skeletal myoblasts in postinfarction patients with severe left ventricular dysfunction, *J. Endovasc. Ther.* 6, 695–704 (2004).
10. Dib N, Diethrich EB, Campbell A, et al. Endoventricular transplantation of allogenic skeletal myoblasts in a porcine model of myocardial infarction, *J. Endovasc. Ther.* 9, 313–9 (2002).
11. Perin EC, Dohmann HF, Borojevic R, et al. Transendocardial, autologous bone marrow cell transplantation for severe, chronic ischemic heart failure, *Circulation.* 107, 2294–302 (2003).
12. Pagani FD, DerSimonian H, Zawadzka A, et al. Autologous skeletal myoblasts transplanted to ischemia-damaged myocardium in humans. Histological analysis of cell survival and differentiation, *J. Am. Coll. Cardiol.* 41, 879–88 (2003).

15
A Porcine Model of Myocardial Infarction for Evaluation of Cell Transplantation

NABIL DIB, EDWARD B. DIETHRICH, ANN CAMPBELL, NOREEN GOODWIN, BARB ROBINSON, JAMES GILBERT, DAN W. HOBOHM, AND DORIS A. TAYLOR

1. Introduction

Myoblast transplantation is a promising new treatment for patients with congestive heart failure or myocardial infarction. Successful autologous myoblast transplantation to the myocardium has been demonstrated in a variety of animal models,[1-4] where survival and engraftment of the injected myoblasts was verified by the presence of labeled skeletal cells[4] and multinucleated myotubules characteristic of skeletal muscle in myocardial tissue.[3]

After injection into a damaged myocardium, skeletal myoblasts can differentiate and develop into striated cells, becoming integrated into the scar.[2] More importantly, transplantation of myoblasts is correlated with improved myocardial performance.[2] Taylor and colleagues[2] demonstrated improved cardiac performance after transplanting autologous myoblasts into 12 cryoinjured rabbit hearts.

More recently, autologous myoblast transplantation has been applied as an adjunct to coronary artery bypass grafting in humans with severe ischemic heart failure. In their early report, Menasché et al.[5] reported successful autologous myoblast transplantation associated with concurrent improvement in myocardial function. In this study, myoblasts were delivered by direct injection into the epicardial surface of the infarcted myocardium during a thoracotomy for bypass surgery. While surgical transplantation of myoblasts into injured myocardium appears promising, a less invasive means of delivering the myoblasts would be preferable.

In this preliminary report, we evaluated the feasibility of injecting skeletal myoblasts into infarcted porcine heart via a percutaneous endocardial delivery approach. Our objectives were to histologically confirm endoventricular delivery and engraftment of myoblasts into the damaged myocardium >1 week after injection.

231

2.   Methods

2.1.   Animal Preparation

A swine model was studied using guidelines published in the Guide for the Care and Use of Laboratory Animals (DHHS publication number NIH 85-23, revised 1985) and Subchapter A of the Federal Animal Welfare Act written by the United States Department of Agriculture. The study protocol was approved by our institution's Animal Care and Use Committee.

One 7-month-old male swine weighing 43.5 kg underwent baseline cardiovascular evaluation and served as the recipient animal for myoblast transplantation. A 12-lead electrocardiogram (ECG) was obtained (Figure 1), and 2-dimensional transthoracic echocardiography was performed to assess wall motion and ejection fraction. An 8-F arterial sheath was inserted into the right femoral artery using a cutdown technique, and selective left and right coronary angiography (Figure 2) and left ventriculography were performed using the right anterior oblique and left anterior oblique projections.

NOGA Biosense Navigational System (Biosense Webster, Diamond Bar, CA, USA) via a 7-F NOGA B-curve catheter advanced through the 8-F sheath into the left ventricle. The electromechanical activity of the

Pre-infarction	Immediately following infarction
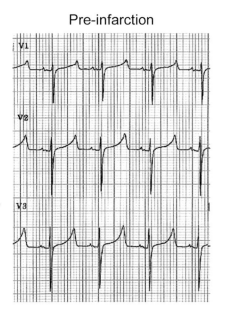	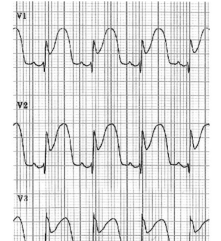

FIGURE 1. Comparison of the electrocardiograms before and after infarction via LAD coil placement.

myocardium was determined (Figure 3) based on the maps constructed from 35 acquired points, as described previously.[6]

Concurrent with the femoral cutdown, a 6-cm incision was made longitudinally along the right hind leg. Under sterile conditions, a 5-g segment of the thigh muscle was removed with a sharp dissection technique. The incision was closed in layers. The muscle segment was placed immediately in a cell transportation medium on ice and sent to a cell culturing facility for myoblast expansion.

2.2. Infarction Model

An anterior infarct was induced in the host swine via coil embolization using individual 3- and 4-mm Vortx coils (Boston Scientific/Target, Natick, MA, USA) delivered to the middle left anterior descending (LAD) artery. Coronary occlusion occurred 2 minutes after coil placement, as demonstrated by coronary angiography. A postinfarction left ventriculogram, echocardiogram, and ECG were performed within 5 minutes of infarction. Significant ventricular arrhythmias were treated with a 2% intravenous lidocaine bolus and electrical cardioversion. The femoral artery was sutured, the incision was closed, and the animal was recovered per standard operating procedures. Postprocedural discomfort was treated with intramuscular butorphanol tartrate (Dolorex, 1.0 mL).

Baseline   Post Infarct

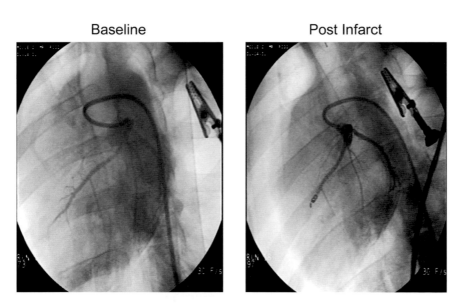

FIGURE 2. Coronary angiograms in the left anterior oblique view at baseline and after infarction.

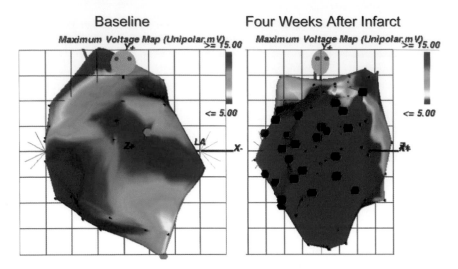

FIGURE 3. Baseline 3D electromechanical mapping of left ventricle and 4 weeks after infarction, showing the cell injection sites (black markers).

2.3. Myoblast Isolation

Although autologous myoblasts were isolated from the host animal, an unexpected bacterial contamination of the cell preparation required a second biopsy from another pig of similar age and weight to the recipient. The allogenic skeletal muscle myoblasts were isolated through a series of steps described previously,[3] involving mechanical dissection, washing, and resuspension. The cells were plated in a growth medium composed of Dulbecco's Modified Eagle Medium (Gibco, Grand Island, NY, USA) with 10% (vol/vol) fetal bovine serum (Hyclone, Logan, UT, USA) and 0.5% (vol/vol) gentamicin (Gibco). The cells were maintained at <70% density and allowed to expand over a 4-week period, replacing one half of the growth medium with fresh medium every other day. Cells were visually examined daily and growth curves were obtained.

In preparation for cell injection, the myoblasts were harvested using 0.05% trypsin/ethylenediaminetetraacetic acid (Gibco); trypsin was inactivated by the addition of growth medium containing fetal bovine serum. The cells were centrifuged and washed twice. The resulting cell pellet was resuspended in 2.5 mL of serum-free Dulbecco's Modified Eagle Medium.[3]

2.4. Allogenic Myoblast Transplantation

Four weeks after creating the infarction, the animal was anesthetized with intramuscular Telozol (tiletamine hydrochloride and zolazepam hydrochloride; 500 mg), intubated, and mechanically ventilated with 2% isoflurane and 3-L/min oxygen. An 8-F arterial sheath was inserted into the left femoral artery using a cutdown technique and cardiovascular assessments were repeated (ECG, echocardiography, left ventriculography, and coronary angiography). Electromechanical mapping identified the infarcted area.

Using a B-curve needle injection catheter (Biosense Webster) calibrated to extend 4 to 5 mm into the endocardium, approximately 200 million cells in the 2.5-mL suspension were injected into 25 arbitrarily selected sites (0.1 mL each) at the center and periphery of the infarcted myocardium. Penetration of the endocardium was verified by ST elevations and premature ventricular contractions during needle advancement. The injection sites were delineated on the electromechanical map (Figure 3). After the injections were completed, the sheath was removed, the femoral artery was sutured, and the animal was allowed to recover.

Ten days later, the animal was anesthetized as described previously and euthanized. The heart was harvested, rinsed in saline, and preserved in 10% formalin prior to section in 5-mm increments from apex to base. Thin sections (8 μm) from the infarct region were stained either with hematoxylin and eosin (H&E) or Masson's trichrome.

3.   Results

At the baseline cardiovascular examination, the animal demonstrated normal sinus rhythm (Figure 1), wall motion, and ejection fraction (55%–60%). Angiography (Figure 2) indicated patent coronary arteries but with mild apical hypokinesis. Electromechanical mapping (Figure 3) was consistent with these findings and showed voltage with mildly abnormal local shortening at the apex.

Immediately after infarction, echocardiography indicated akinesis of the anteroseptal segment with an ejection fraction of 45%. Severe left ventricular apical and anteroapical hypokinesis was seen. ST elevations and anterior Q-wave disturbances were also apparent (Figure 1). Four weeks later, left ventricular deterioration was still present. Electromechanical mapping was consistent with myocardial infarction (Figure 3). Voltages in the averaged apical and combined septal regions had decreased from 9.3 mV to 4.3 mV and from 11.0 mV to 5.4 mV, respectively. There was also a concomitant decrease in the local shortening of the septal regions (10.5% to −1.4%).

With the exception of a premature ventricular systolic beat and occasional intermittent ventricular tachycardia, no sustained ventricular arrhythmias occurred during endoventricular injection. No obvious changes in voltage were noted during or after the injection period. Ten days after allogenic cell transfer, macroscopic assessment revealed an anterior apical scar encompassing approximately 20% of the myocardium. Histologically, this was reflected by a dense matrix interspersed with areas containing what appeared to be muscle-derived cells (Figure 4). High-power micrographs of the endocardium showed eosinophilic cells with central nuclei that appeared to be myoblasts. In some cases, these myoblasts were forming multinucleated myotubes. An extensive cellular inflammatory reaction was also seen, indicative of the rejection of donor allogenic cells.

4.   Discussion

Ischemic cardiomyopathy and congestive heart failure are leading causes of cardiovascular morbidity and mortality. Several models for myocardial injury have been used in previous transplantation studies, including cryolesion and coronary artery ligation techniques.[2,7] While these models have been useful in evaluating myoblast transplantation, the occlusion coil technique we employed may be the safest and most representative of clinical ischemic

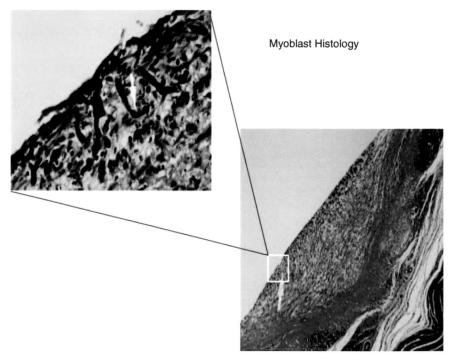

Myoblast Histology

FIGURE 4. Low-power view (right) of infarcted myocardium (Masson's trichrome) after myoblast injection. The area in the lower right hand corner is normal myocardial tissue that stains red. The blue stained area is indicative of the fibrotic cells found in the scarred infarcted area. The red stippled area on the endocardial surface (arrow) contains proliferating myoblasts that are better appreciated in the high-power view (upper left; H&E ×200). The myoblasts are forming multinucleated myotubes (arrow). A cellular reaction confirms engraftment and rejection by the allogenic host.

injury. It provides a less invasive, endovascular approach to total LAD occlusion that closely approximates the pathology of a myocardial infarct, especially when compared to the epicardial injury produced by the cryolesion technique. Gross and histological examinations of the myocardium in our animal showed fibrotic scarring at the apex of both ventricles and in the left ventricular anterolateral wall. Further elucidation of this infarction model is underway.

Regeneration of myocardial muscle after autologous myoblast transplantation has the potential to improve both morbidity and mortality in patients with myocardial infarction, cardiomyopathy, and congestive heart failure. Experimentally, myoblasts have been delivered into the injured heart using a number of methods, including intravascular infusion into the coronary circulation[4]; however, direct injection of myoblasts into injured myocardium results in a higher proportion of engrafted cells.[4]

In the past, direct myoblast transfer has been successfully accomplished primarily during open-heart surgery, where the cells were injected into the epicardial surface. More recently, catheter-based endoventricular delivery of myoblasts into normal pig myocardium has been reported, with recovery of viable cells after 48 hours.[8] Strauer et al.[9] performed catheter-based endoventricular transplantation of bone marrow cells into the infarcted myocardium, which suggested that catheter-based delivery is possible. However, the much smaller bone marrow–derived cells they used did not address the potential problems associated with injection of skeletal myoblasts into a scar.

In our study, we demonstrated that catheter-based endoventricular cell delivery into the scarred myocardium is technically feasible via a needle-containing catheter inserted through the femoral artery. To accomplish this, we first had to map the infarcted area. Using the NOGA system, we were then able to monitor and record the injections into the endocardium, which was verified by a premature ventricular contraction at the time of needle extension into the wall. Myoblasts were then injected perpendicular to the endocardial surface.

Although cell delivery was presumed at the time of injection, no direct confirmation of injection was possible *in vivo*. However, histological examination of the heart 10 days after transplantation documented survival and engraftment of the transplanted myoblasts, which agrees with previous studies in which autologous myoblasts were directly transplanted into the injured myocardium during open-heart surgery in a rabbit model.[2-4] The presence of multinucleated myotubes in the injected myocardium provided evidence of the skeletal origin of the cells[2] and suggests that transplanted myoblasts survived and were able to fuse and engraft despite the anticipated active rejection of the allogenic donor cells.[4]

This study was a preliminary report in one animal to document the feasibility of delivering myoblasts into scarred heart using a less invasive catheter delivery system. Originally, this study called for transplantation of autologous myoblasts; however, contamination of the cell preparation prevented their use. In future studies, autologous myoblasts will be used for transplantation to avoid the concerns and complications of rejection.

In summary, our preliminary results indicate that delivery of skeletal myoblasts via a percutaneous endoventricular technique is technically feasible in a coil occlusion infarction model. This transluminal method of myoblast delivery may one day prove to be particularly advantageous in high-risk patients with cardiomyopathy and congestive heart failure.

5.   References

1. Yoon PD, Kao RL, Magovern GJ. Myocardial regeneration. Transplanting satellite cells into damaged myocardium. *Tex Heart Inst J.* 1995;22:119–125.
2. Taylor DA, Atkins BZ, Hungspreugs P, et al. Regenerating functional myocardium: improved performance after skeletal myoblast transplantation. *Nat Med.* 1998;4:929–933.
3. Atkins BZ, Lewis CW, Kraus WE, et al. Intracardiac transplantation of skeletal myoblasts yields two populations of striated cells in situ. *Ann Thorac Surg.* 1999;67:124–129.
4. Taylor DA, Silvestry SC, Bishop SP, et al. Delivery of primary autologous skeletal myoblasts into rabbit heart by coronary infusion: a potential approach to myocardial repair. *Proc Assoc Am Physicians.* 1997;109:245–253.
5. Menasché P, Hagege AA, Scorsin M, et al. Myoblast transplantation for heart failure. *Lancet.* 2001;357:279–280.
6. Kornowski R, Hong MK, Gepstein L, et al. Preliminary animal and clinical experiences using an electromechanical endocardial mapping procedure to distinguish infarcted from healthy myocardium. *Circulation.* 1998;98:1116–1124.
7. Jain M, DerSimonian H, Brenner DA, et al. Cell therapy attenuates deleterious ventricular remodeling and improves cardiac performance after myocardial infarction. *Circulation.* 2001;103:1920–1927.
8. Deutsch E, Tarazona N, Du B, et al. Autologous skeletal muscle transplantation in the swine heart: feasibility and viability via endocardial delivery [Abstract]. *Circulation.* 1999;100;I–164.
9. Strauer BE, Brehm M, Zeus T, et al. Intracoronary, human autologous stem cell transplantation for myocardial regeneration following myocardial infarction (in German). *Dtsch Med Wochenschr.* 2001 Aug 24;126:932–938.

Tissue Engineering

16
Tissue Engineering for Myocardial Regeneration

RAVI K. BIRLA[*]

1.   Introduction

Congestive heart failure (CHF) is a major medical challenge in developed countries. There are currently 4.8 million patients in the U.S. living with CHF with an estimated economic cost of $23.2 billion annually.[1] Current therapeutic strategies to treat CHF are limited to surgical transplantation,[2] pharmacological intervention[3] and mechanical cardiac support.[4] Although these treatment options have significantly improved the quality of patient care, there are limitations to each approach.

Heart transplantation has been the most successful treatment option to treat severe CHF. As of March 2000, over 55,000 heart transplantations had been performed.[2] Although the short-term survival rate stands at 81%, widespread applicability of heart transplantation is often limited by a chronic shortage of donor organs.[5] Pharmacological interventions with diuretics, inotropes, vasolidators, ACE inhibitors, β-blockers, and antiarrhythmic drugs have demonstrated reduced mortality of CHF patients, but there has been little improvement in the quality of life and little improvement in the functional performance of the failing myocardium.[3] A significant percentage of patients receiving pharmacological treatment develop progressive congestive failure and may become candidates for more invasive treatments. Mechanical circulatory support devices are currently used as a bridge to cardiac transplantation. An estimated 300-400 patients use this technology annually in the U.S. as a bridge to cardiac surgery and an additional 6,000 patients annually use the support devices after cardiac surgery.[4] Current limitations of mechanical support devices include thromobogenicity, infections, device size and weight, and power transmission.

Cardiac tissue engineering may provide a potential solution to the donor heart crisis in the future. Research in the area of cardiac tissue engineering is

---
[*] Section of Cardiac Surgery, Department of Surgery, University of Michigan, Ann Arbor, MI 48109-2007

241

focused on the development of functional 3-dimensional cardiac muscle constructs. These constructs can be used clinically to patch areas of local infarcted. As technological advancements occur in the field, one can imagine the potential to generate complete ventricles in the laboratory and even bio-engineered hearts. Before that goal is attained there are many immediate benefits of tissue engineering models. One potential application of engineered cardiac muscle is in basic *in vitro* cardiology research. The most common *in vitro* model for cardiac research has been 2-D monolayer culture. However, monolayer cultures confine cells to a substrate surface and do not resemble the normal physiological organization of native cardiac tissue. Current 3-D models have many components of native cardiac tissue and represent a more physiological organization of cells in a complex 3-D lattice. Other potential applications of tissue engineered constructs include drug testing and as a drug delivery vehicle. Tissue engineering models also allow the detailed study of critical events in organogenesis such as the establishment of cell-cell communication, construction and modification of the extracellular matrix, and angiogenesis.

2.   Strategies for Cardiac Tissue Engineering

The field of cardiac tissue engineering is relatively new and the first published journal article appeared in 1997.[6] Since that time there have been about 40 journal articles and a few good reviews published in the field.[7-12] There have been several strategies for engineering 3-D cardiac tissue *in vitro* that are described in the current literature. These can be categorized as (1) utilizing polymeric scaffolding material as a support matrix, (2) incorporating cardiac myocytes within biodegradable gels, or (3) utilizing polymeric temperature sensitive surfaces.

Carrier and colleagues utilized fibrous meshes made from polyglycolic acid (PGA) as a scaffolding material for culturing neonatal cardiac myocytes.[13] PGA was processed into fibrous meshes to form disk-shaped constructs with a very high degree of porosity. The high porosity provided a site for cell attachment and adequate nutrient exchange during cell culture. These constructs were seeded with primary cardiac myocytes and several physiological metrics utilized to evaluate functionality. These tissue constructs were shown to express cardiac specific biochemical markers like connexin-43 and exhibited electro-physical characteristics comparable to neonatal heart tissue.[14,15] A perfusion apparatus was later shown to improve viability of the cardiac tissue construct.[16,17] In the presence of perfusion, the engineered constructs were able to maintain cell viability for a depth of up to 1 mm.[16] These studies were the first to demonstrate the formation of functional cardiac muscle utilizing scaffolding based strategies and represent a significant milestone in the field of cardiac tissue engineering.

Eschenhagen developed a 3-D model of tissue engineered heart muscle by culturing chick cardiac myocytes in a collagen matrix.[6] The resulting tissue constructs were shown to generate an active force of around 200 μN upon electrical stimulation. In addition, these constructs were responsiveness to external calcium, exhibited length-force characteristics and were responsive to cardio-active drugs. The initial model was refined to generate engineered heart tissue (EHT) by casting a mixture of neonatal cardiac myocytes and collagen into plastic molds.[18] The EHTs were capable of generating an active force of up to 500 μN[18] and exhibited several physiologically metrics of heart function. These included responsiveness to calcium, force-frequency relationship and length-force relationship. Detailed histological characterization of the EHTs demonstrated the presence of highly organized sarcomeres and a high degree of intercellular connectivity.[19] EHTs were later implanted in the peritoneum cavity and wrapped around the circumference of hearts from syngeneic rats and survival was shown for up to 14 and 28 days respectively.[20,21] The EHTs were also subjected to unidirectional stretch at 1.5 Hz and 20% stretch for 6 days which resulted in an peak force of 700 uN.[22] Eschenhagens model was the first 3-D model of cardiac muscle *in vitro* and represented seminal work in the field of cardiac tissue engineering.[6]

Okano utilized temperature sensitive polymer surfaces (TSS) to engineer 3-D cardiac tissue.[23,24] TSS are hydrophobic at 37°C, allowing the culture of a confluent monolayer of cardiac myocytes.[25] Reducing the temperature to 32°C promotes the transition of the hydrophobic surface to a hydrophilic surface. The hydrophilic surface does not promote cell attachment and causes the detachment of the 2-D monolayer of cardiac myocytes.[25] Two-dimensional sheets can be stacked together to form 3-D cardiac muscle constructs.[26] The sheets are physically layered on top of each other to form 3-D cardiac muscle. Cardiac muscle engineered using TSS was shown to form intercellular connections between underlying cell layers. These 3-D layered constructs were later implanted into nude rats and shown to generate 1200 μN of passive force after 21 days of implantation.[27] In addition, large amounts of neovascularization were demonstrated throughout the explanted constructs.[27] The most attractive feature of this model is the utilization of the TSS which eliminates the need for synthetic scaffolding materials in the contractile region of the tissue engineering cardiac muscle.

Akins utilized a rotating bioreactor system to promote the organization of isolated cardiac cells on the surface of microcarrier beads.[28] The resulting tissue constructs exhibited a high degree of spontaneous contractility and were responsive to cardio-active drugs. Histological evaluation showed the presence of well organized contractile proteins and the presence of intercellular connectivity. The model utilized by Akins is successful application of the self-organization of cells to form functional cardiac muscle.

Li utilized a gelatin mesh as the scaffolding material for engineering cardiac tissue and demonstrated improved ventricular function in a cryo-injury model with these constructs.[29-33] In addition, a 20% stretch at 1.3 Hz for 14 days resulted in a two-fold increase in the tensile strength of the construct.[34] Leor utilized alginate sponges for culturing primary cardiac cells[35,36] and demonstrated the feasibility of utilizing the engineered construct as a potential therapy for the treatment of infarcted myocardium.[35] These models again demonstrate the feasibility for the utilization of biodegradable matrices for the culture of cardiac myocytes resulting in the formation of functional 3-D cardiac muscle.

There have been several different strategies described in the literature to engineer functional 3-D cardiac muscle. However, there appears to be a common theme among researchers in this field. The first step has been to define conditions that promote the formation of 3-D cardiac muscle. The most common strategies have utilized biodegradable polymeric scaffolds, biodegradable gels or self-organization methods for the formation of 3-D tissue. Once a functional cardiac tissue construct is developed, protocols are implemented that promote the long term viability of the constructs. Chemical, electrical and mechanical signals from the external environment are often necessary to maintain long term viability of the engineered constructs. Finally, strategies are implemented to induce angiogenesis throughout the cross-section of the constructs and subsequent perfusion of the vascularized constructs. This defines a systematic approach towards the generation of functional 3-D cardiac muscle.

3.   Methodology for Cardioid Formation

The methodology for cardioid formation has been described in detail.[37] Cardioids are formed from the spontaneous delamination of a confluent monolayer of neonatal cardiac myocytes, Figure 1. A tissue culture surface is first coated with polydimethylsiloxane (PDMS) and then with natural mouse laminin to control the cell adhesion properties. Anchor points are prepared by soaking 6 mm long segments of size 0 braided silk sutures soaked in a high laminin concentration. The sutures are pinned 12 mm apart in the center of the culture surface. Cardiac cells are isolated from 2-3 day old neonatal rat hearts and plated at confluence on the culture surface. A cohesive cell monolayer forms within 2-3 days after cell plating. A continuous cell monolayer forms due to the high plating density. The cell monolayer initiates spontaneous contractions and the entire cell monolayer beats as a continuum during the entire culture period.

The contractility of the cell monolayer generates sufficient force to promote delamination of the monolayer from the underlying culture surface. Delamination initiates within two weeks days after initial cell plating. The delamination process begins at the periphery of the culture surface and progresses towards the center of the plate. At the center of the plate, the cohesive cell monolayer attaches to the anchor points on the culture surface. Subsequent remodeling results in cardioid formation. Cardioid formation is complete within three weeks after initial plating. Cardioids exhibit a very regular spontaneous contractility during culture and the frequency of

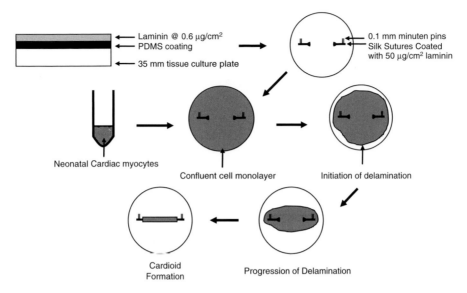

FIGURE 1. Methodology for cardioid formation.

contractions is typically 1-2 Hz. The length of cardioids is 12 mm and the diameter is typically about 200-300 μm. The cardioid model has several unique characteristics that make it an attractive model for cardiac muscle. Firstly, cardioid formation is dependent on the self-organization of individual cardiac cells into a 3-dimensional tissue construct. This process eliminates the need for synthetic scaffolding material in the contractile region of the tissue construct. This allows for cardioids to exhibit uninhibited repetitive contractions. Secondly, during cardioid formation, extracellular matrix (ECM) components are generated by the cardiac fibroblasts that are plated with the cardiac myocytes. This ECM is considered to be a suitable substrate for the generation of cardiac muscle and results in physiological functionality of the engineered construct. Thirdly, the entire process is spontaneous and allows for the individual cells to dictate the new 3-D environment. The 3-D organization of cardioids is not dictated by the geometry of pre-fabricated polymeric scaffolds.

The method for self-organization of 3-D tissue constructs was initially developed for skeletal myocytes.[38-41] The resulting tissue constructs were termed myooids. Myooids were engineered utilizing satellite cells isolated from adult soleus muscle and expanded in culture over a period of two weeks. The media was then changed to promote the fusion of individual myocytes. This resulted in myotube formation. Within two weeks of media transition, the entire culture surface became covered with contracting myotubes. The confluent monolayer of contracting myotubes promoted the delamination of the cell monolayer from the culture surface. The delaminating cell monolayer attached to anchor points at the center of the culture surface and subsequent remodeling resulted in myooid formation.

4.   The Delamination Process

The delamination process is central to cardioid formation. Several stages of the delamination process are shown in Figure 2. There are two variables that control the delamination process: formation of a cohesive cell monolayer and the properties of the adhesion protein used to coat the culture surface.

The formation of a cohesive cell monolayer is critical to cardioid formation. In the absence of a continuous cell monolayer, isolated cardiac myocytes are maintained in 2-D culture and do not delaminate to form cardioids. Initially, isolated cardiac cells are plated at a high density on a culture surface that has been coated with an adhesion protein. The high plating density promotes the formation of a cohesive cell monolayer and is necessary to compensate for the post-mitotic stage of the neonatal cardiac myocytes utilized for cardioid formation.

The cohesive cell monolayer exhibits spontaneous contractility in culture. The entire cell monolayer beats in continuum and exhibits a very regular frequency of 1-2 Hz. The spontaneous contractility of the cohesive cell monolayer results in delamination of the monolayer from the culture surface. Physical detachment of the cell monolayer from the underlying surface has been observed and the cell monolayer literally "tears" itself away from the culture surface. Initial detachment occurs at the periphery of the culture surface, Figure 2A. With each successive spontaneous contraction, the cell monolayer physically moves towards the center of the culture surface. The distance the cell monolayer travels with a single spontaneous contraction can be as much as 50 μN. After the initiation of delamination, the cohesive cell monolayer continues to move towards the center of the plate, Figure 2B. At the center of the plate, the cell monolayer delaminates around anchor points

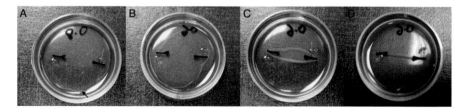

FIGURE 2. The delamination process. A. Delamination is initiated at the periphery of the culture surface. The cell monolayer can be seen to have detached from the surface (single arrow). B. The delaminating cell monolayer continues to move radially inwards, towards the center of the plate. C. Progression of the delaminating monolayer is guided by anchor points. D. At the center of the plate, the cell monolayer attaches to anchor points and remodels to form a 3-dimensional tissue construct, cardioid.

that were placed on the culture surface prior to cell plating, Figure 2C. The anchor points guide the delaminating cell monolayer and promote the formation of a three dimensional tissue construct, Figure 2D. In the absence of the anchor points, delaminating progresses in an uncontrolled manner and results in the formation of a mass of randomly organized tissue situated at any point on the culture surface.

Delamination of the cell monolayer is controlled by the properties of the adhesion protein utilized to coat the culture surface. The adhesion protein serves a two-fold purpose. Firstly, during the initial stages of culture, the adhesion protein promotes the adhesion of isolated cells to the culture surface and promotes the formation of a cohesive cell monolayer. Secondly, the surface adhesion protein controls the time for the initiation of monolayer delamination. The onset of delamination is dependant on the degradation of the adhesion protein. As the surface protein degrades, the cohesive cell monolayer is exposed to the hydrophobic PDMS surface. The PDMS surface does not promote cell adhesion, resulting in the delamination of the cell monolayer. During cardioid formation, natural mouse laminin is utilized at a surface concentration of 0.2-2.0 µg/cm^2 to promote the formation of a cohesive cell monolayer. This time period required for delamination to occur correlates with the surface laminin concentration. At a surface concentration of 0.2 µg/cm^2 delamination requires 10 days while at a concentration of 2.0 µg/cm^2 delamination requires 21 days.

5.   Histological Characterization of Cardioids

Cardioids show a very high density of cellular material and staining with hematoxylin & eosin verify the high degree of cellularity, Figure 3. We also evaluated the ultrastructure of cardioids by using transmission electron micrographs, Figure 4. We were able to show a single cardiac fibroblast surrounded by vast amounts of collagen, Figure 4A. The cardiac fibroblasts are a critical component of cardioids. The fibroblasts produce collagen, which provides mechanical stability to the cohesive cell monolayer during the

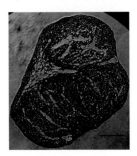

FIGURE 3. Histological evaluation of cardioids. Staining with hematoxylin and eosin. Scale bar represents 100 µm.

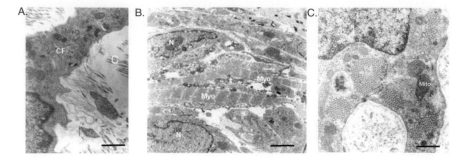

FIGURE 4. Electron micrographs of cardioids. A. Single cardiac fibroblast (CF) produces collagen (C). B. Longitudinal section showing the presence of multiple nuclei (N) and myofilaments (Myo). C. Cross section showing large amounts of contractile proteins (Myo) with associated mitochondria (Mito). Scale bars represent 1 μm for A, 2 μm for B and 400 nm for C.

delamination process. Cardioids also contain longitudinally aligned myofilaments with equally spaced z-lines, Figure 4B. Also evident are large amounts of myosin heads with surrounding actin molecules, organized as a hexagonal lattice, Figure 4C.

6.   Contractility Metrics of Cardioids

The contractility metrics of the cardioids that we evaluated include the active force, specific force (active force normalized to total cross-sectional area), time to peak tension (TPT) and half relaxation time ½ RT. We utilized a custom made testing system to evaluate the contractility metrics of cardioids. The system has been described in detail.[42] The cardioids are tested in the 35 mm culture dishes that were utilized during cardioid formation. One end

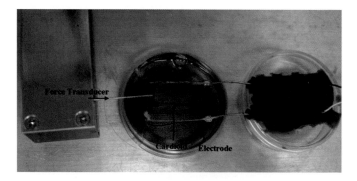

FIGURE 5. Contractility evaluation of cardioids. Cardioids are stimulated between parallel platinum electrodes and an optical force transducer is used to measure the active force generated.

of the cardioid is attached to a force transducer arm while the other end remains pinned to the culture surface. The cardioids are stimulated using parallel platinum electrodes. Twitch force is evaluated by using a stimulating using a single 5 V electrical impulse with a frequency of 1 Hz and a pulse width of 10 ms. Individual force tracings are digitally recorded using LabVIEW and can be processed to determine the peak active force, TPT and ½ RT.

The twitch force generated by cardioids was found to be in the range 75-125 µN, Figure 6A and a specific force of 2.4-4.0 kN/m². The average TPT was calculated to be 230 ms while the average ½ RT was calculated to be 212 ms. An adult rat papillary muscle generates a peak active of approximately 8130 µN[43] and a specific force of about 44.4 kN/m².[43] Thus, the force generating capability of the cardioids is an order of magnitude less than that for normal cardiac tissue. This could be due to the early developmental stage of the neonatal cardiac myocytes utilized in our model. Developmentally immature cardiomyocytes are known to contain significantly smaller amounts of contractile proteins per unit cross-section of cardiac tissue.[44] The average TPT and ½ RT of an adult papillary muscle are 185 ms and 118 ms respectively.[43] The rate of contraction and relaxation of cardioids is comparable to that of normal adult tissue.

To further characterize the cardiac specific phenotype of cardioids, we electrically paced the cardioids at physiological frequencies of 1-7 Hz, Figure 6B. At a frequency of 1 Hz, the number of active contractions was proportional to the number of stimulation impulses. In addition, we did not observe any signs of muscle fatigue during electrical pacing at any of the stimulation frequencies tested. The ability to electrically pace the cardioids did provide some evidence of cardiac specific phenotype and does suggest the functional arrangement of cardiac cells within 3-D cardioids.

7.   Physiological Metrics of Cardioid Function

In order to evaluate the physiological response of cardioids, we evaluated the responsiveness to calcium, the length-force relationship and

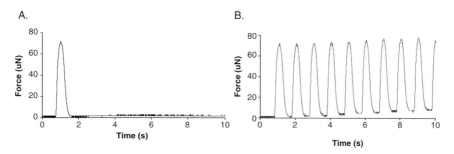

FIGURE 6. Contractility of cardioids. (A) Cardioids can be electrically stimulated using a 5V, 1Hz, 5ms impulse to generate an active force of 75µN. (B) Cardioids can be electrically paced at a frequency of 1Hz.

the responsiveness to epinephrine. The calcium sensitivity of cardioids was found be similar to that of normal cardiac tissue. In the absence of calcium, cardioids were not able to generate any measurable force upon electrical stimulation, Figure 7. Increasing the calcium concentration resulted in a proportional increase in active force production. At saturating levels of calcium, increasing the calcium concentration had no effect on the active force of cardioids. This gave rise to a sigmoidal calcium sensitivity curve, typical of normal cardiac muscle and is indicative of a functional calcium signaling cascade.

We also determined the length-force characteristics of cardioids, Figure 8. As the length of cardioids was increased, there was a proportional rise in active force production. This gave rise to the ascending limb of the curve. Increasing the length any further did not result in an increase in force

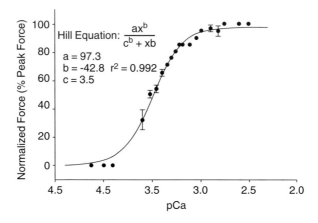

FIGURE 7. Calcium sensitivity curve for cardioids.

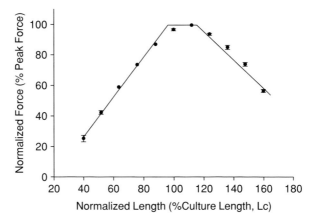

FIGURE 8. Length force relationship for cardioids.

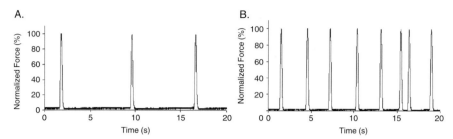

FIGURE 9. Responsiveness of cardioids to epinephrine. (A) Spontaneous contractility of cardioids. In the absence of any electrical stimulation, cardioids spontaneously contracted at a frequency of about 0.15Hz. (B) Responsiveness to Epinephrine. Addition of 0.6 μg/ml of epinephrine resulted in an increase in the spontaneous contractility of cardioids to a frequency of about 0.4Hz.

production giving rise to a plateau region. Any additional increase in length resulted in a decrease in force production, giving rise to the descending limb of the curve. The length-force curve that we obtained for cardioids is characteristic of muscle tissue and indicates the presence of functional sarcomeres.

We evaluated the responsiveness of cardioids to epinephrine, Figure 9. The bath epinephrine concentration was gradually increased to 0.6 μg/ml and the spontaneous contractility of the cardioids was evaluated. The spontaneous contractility of the cardioids increased from a baseline value of about 0.15 Hz to about 0.4 Hz with the addition of 0.6 μg/ml epinephrine. We found a dose dependent increase in frequency as the bath epinephrine concentration was varied in between 0 and 0.6 μg/ml. The process was completely reversible and removal of epinephrine from the testing batch resulted in the cardioids returning to baseline spontaneous contractility.

8. Conclusions

In this chapter, we describe an *in vitro* method for the formation of contractile 3-D cardiac muscle, which we have termed cardioids. Cardioids are formed from the spontaneous delamination of a confluent monolayer of primary cardiac myocytes. One of the most attractive features of the cardioid model is that isolated cardiac cells self-organize to form 3-D cardiac muscle. This eliminates the need for synthetic scaffolding material in the contractile region of cardioids and allows cardioids to exhibit uninhibited contractions. Cardioids have been shown to exhibit several physiologically relevant metrics of function. Cardioids can be electrically stimulated to generate active force and can be electrically paced at frequencies of 1-7 Hz. In addition, cardioids are responsive to calcium and various cardio-active drugs. The cardioid model has several potential applications in basic research and may provide viable cardiac tissue for clinical applications.

9.   Acknowledgments

The author would like to thank Dr. Krystyna Pasyk for obtaining transmission electron micrographs. Dr. Robert G. Dennis provided scientific and financial support towards the development of the cardioid model. This work was supported by a grant from the Defense Advanced Research Projects contract #N66001-02-C-8034.

10.   References

1. 2002 Heart and Stroke Statistical Update, American Heart Association. 2002.
2. Miniati DN, Robbins RC. Heart transplantation: a thirty-year perspective. [Review] [74 refs]. Annual Review of Medicine. 2002;53:189–205.
3. Goldstein S. Heart failure therapy at the turn of the century. [Review] [53 refs]. Heart Failure Reviews. 2001;6:7–14.
4. Stevenson LW, Kormos RL. Mechanical cardiac support 2000: current applications and future trial design. [Review] [111 refs]. Journal of Heart & Lung Transplantation. 2001;20:1–38.
5. Stevenson LW, Warner SL, Steimle AE, Fonarow GC, Hamilton MA, Moriguchi JD, Kobashigawa JA, Tillisch JH, Drinkwater DC, Laks H. The impending crisis awaiting cardiac transplantation. Modeling a solution based on selection. Circulation 89(1):450–7. 1994.
6. Eschenhagen T, Fink C, Remmers U, Scholz H, Wattchow J, Weil J, Zimmermann W, Dohmen HH, Schafer H, Bishopric N, Wakatsuki T, Elson EL. Three-dimensional reconstitution of embryonic cardiomyocytes in a collagen matrix: a new heart muscle model system. FASEB Journal. 1997;11:683–694.
7. Akins RE. Can tissue engineering mend broken hearts? [letter; comment.]. Circulation Research. 2002;90:120–122.
8. Eschenhagen T, Didie M, Heubach J, Ravens U, Zimmermann WH. Cardiac tissue engineering. [Review] [21 refs]. Transplant Immunology. 2002;9:315–321.
9. Papadaki M. Cardiac muscle tissue engineering. [Review] [13 refs]. IEEE Engineering in Medicine & Biology Magazine. 2003;22:153–154.
10. Shimizu T, Yamato M, Kikuchi A, Okano T. Cell sheet engineering for myocardial tissue reconstruction. [Review] [38 refs]. Biomaterials. 2003;24:2309–2316.
11. Zimmermann WH, Eschenhagen T. Cardiac tissue engineering for replacement therapy. [Review] [79 refs]. Heart Failure Reviews. 2003;8:259–269.
12. Fedak PW, Weisel RD, Verma S, Mickle DA, Li RK. Restoration and regeneration of failing myocardium with cell transplantation and tissue engineering. [Review] [78 refs]. Seminars in Thoracic & Cardiovascular Surgery. 2003;15:277–286.
13. Carrier RL, Papadaki M, Rupnick M, Schoen FJ, Bursac N, Langer R, Freed LE, Vunjak-Novakovic G. Cardiac tissue engineering: cell seeding, cultivation parameters, and tissue construct characterization. Biotechnology & Bioengineering. 1999;64:580–589.
14. Bursac N, Papadaki M, Cohen RJ, Schoen FJ, Eisenberg SR, Carrier R, Vunjak-Novakovic G, Freed LE. Cardiac muscle tissue engineering: toward an in vitro model for electrophysiological studies. American Journal of Physiology. 1999;277:t-44.

15. Papadaki M, Bursac N, Langer R, Merok J, Vunjak-Novakovic G, Freed LE. Tissue engineering of functional cardiac muscle: molecular, structural, and electrophysiological studies. American Journal of Physiology-Heart & Circulatory Physiology. 2001;280:H168–H178.
16. Carrier RL, Rupnick M, Langer R, Schoen FJ, Freed LE, Vunjak-Novakovic G. Perfusion improves tissue architecture of engineered cardiac muscle. Tissue Engineering. 2002;8:175–188.
17. Carrier RL, Rupnick M, Langer R, Schoen FJ, Freed LE, Vunjak-Novakovic G. Effects of oxygen on engineered cardiac muscle. Biotechnology & Bioengineering. 2002;78:617–625.
18. Zimmermann WH, Fink C, Kralisch D, Remmers U, Weil J, Eschenhagen T. Three-dimensional engineered heart tissue from neonatal rat cardiac myocytes. Biotechnology & Bioengineering. 2000;68:106–114.
19. Zimmermann WH, Schneiderbanger K, Schubert P, Didie M, Munzel F, Heubach JF, Kostin S, Neuhuber WL, Eschenhagen T. Tissue engineering of a differentiated cardiac muscle construct. [see comments.]. Circulation Research. 2002;90:223–230.
20. Zimmermann WH, Didie M, Wasmeier GH, Nixdorff U, Hess A, Melnychenko I, Boy O, Neuhuber WL, Weyand M, Eschenhagen T. Cardiac grafting of engineered heart tissue in syngenic rats. Circulation. 2002;106:Suppl-7.
21. Eschenhagen T, Didie M, Munzel F, Schubert P, Schneiderbanger K, Zimmermann WH. 3D engineered heart tissue for replacement therapy. Basic Research in Cardiology. 2002;97:Suppl-52.
22. Fink C, Ergun S, Kralisch D, Remmers U, Weil J, Eschenhagen T. Chronic stretch of engineered heart tissue induces hypertrophy and functional improvement. FASEB Journal. 2000;14:669–679.
23. Okano T, Yamada N, Sakai H, Sakurai Y. A novel recovery system for cultured cells using plasma-treated polystyrene dishes grafted with poly(N-isopropylacrylamide). Journal of Biomedical Materials Research. 1993;27:1243–1251.
24. Shimizu T, Yamato M, Kikuchi A, Okano T. Two-dimensional manipulation of cardiac myocyte sheets utilizing temperature-responsive culture dishes augments the pulsatile amplitude. Tissue Engineering. 2001;7:141–151.
25. Okano T, Yamada N, Okuhara M, Sakai H, Sakurai Y. Mechanism of cell detachment from temperature-modulated, hydrophilic-hydrophobic polymer surfaces. Biomaterials. 1995;16:297–303.
26. Shimizu T, Yamato M, Akutsu T, Shibata T, Isoi Y, Kikuchi A, Umezu M, Okano T. Electrically communicating three-dimensional cardiac tissue mimic fabricated by layered cultured cardiomyocyte sheets. Journal of Biomedical Materials Research. 2002;60:110–117.
27. Shimizu T, Yamato M, Isoi Y, Akutsu T, Setomaru T, Abe K, Kikuchi A, Umezu M, Okano T. Fabrication of pulsatile cardiac tissue grafts using a novel 3-dimensional cell sheet manipulation technique and temperature-responsive cell culture surfaces. Circulation Research. 2002;90:e40.
28. Akins RE, Boyce RA, Madonna ML, Schroedl NA, Gonda SR, McLaughlin TA, Hartzell CR. Cardiac organogenesis in vitro: reestablishment of three-dimensional tissue architecture by dissociated neonatal rat ventricular cells. Tissue Engineering. 1999;5:103–118.
29. Li RK, Yau TM, Weisel RD, Mickle DA, Sakai T, Choi A, Jia ZQ. Construction of a bioengineered cardiac graft. Journal of Thoracic & Cardiovascular Surgery. 2000;119:368–375.

30. Ozawa T, Mickle DA, Weisel RD, Koyama N, Wong H, Ozawa S, Li RK. Histologic changes of nonbiodegradable and biodegradable biomaterials used to repair right ventricular heart defects in rats. Journal of Thoracic & Cardiovascular Surgery 124(6):1157–64. 2002.
31. Ozawa T, Mickle DA, Weisel RD, Koyama N, Ozawa S, Li RK. Optimal biomaterial for creation of autologous cardiac grafts. Circulation. 2002;106:Suppl-82.
32. Li RK, Jia ZQ, Weisel RD, Mickle DA, Choi A, Yau TM. Survival and function of bioengineered cardiac grafts. Circulation. 1999;100:Suppl-9.
33. Sakai T, Li RK, Weisel RD, Mickle DA, Kim ET, Jia ZQ, Yau TM. The fate of a tissue-engineered cardiac graft in the right ventricular outflow tract of the rat. Journal of Thoracic & Cardiovascular Surgery. 2001;121:932–942.
34. Akhyari P, Fedak PW, Weisel RD, Lee TY, Verma S, Mickle DA, Li RK. Mechanical stretch regimen enhances the formation of bioengineered autologous cardiac muscle grafts. Circulation. 2002;106:Suppl-42.
35. Leor J, Aboulafia-Etzion S, Dar A, Shapiro L, Barbash IM, Battler A, Granot Y, Cohen S. Bioengineered cardiac grafts: A new approach to repair the infarcted myocardium? Circulation. 2000;102:Suppl-61.
36. Dar A, Shachar M, Leor J, Cohen S. Optimization of cardiac cell seeding and distribution in 3D porous alginate scaffolds. Biotechnology & Bioengineering. 2002;80:305–312.
37. Baar K, Birla R, Boluyt MO, Borschel GH, Arruda EM, Dennis RG. Heart muscle by design: Self-organization of ratcardiac cells into contractile 3-D cardiac tissue. FASEB Journal. 4 A.D..
38. Dennis RG, Kosnik PE. Excitability and isometric contractile properties of mammalian skeletal muscle constructs engineered in vitro. In Vitro Cellular & Developmental Biology Animal. 2000;36:327–335.
39. Dennis RG, Kosnik PE, Gilbert ME, Faulkner JA. Excitability and contractility of skeletal muscle engineered from primary cultures and cell lines. American Journal of Physiology -Cell Physiology. 2001;280:C288–C295.
40. Kosnik PE, Faulkner JA, Dennis RG. Functional development of engineered skeletal muscle from adult and neonatal rats. Tissue Engineering. 2001;7:573–584.
41. Kosnik PE, Dennis RG. Mesenchymal Cell Culture: Functional Mammalian Skeletal Muscle Constructs. In: Methods of Tissue Engineering. Anthony Atala RPL, ed. 2002. Academic Press.
42. Dennis RG, Kosnik PE. Mesenchymal Cell Culture: Instrumentation and Methods for Evaluating Engineered Muscle. In: Methods of Tissue Engineering. Anthony Atala RPL, ed. 2002. Academic Press.
43. Layland J, Young IS, Altringham JD. The effect of cycle frequency on the power output of rat papillary muscles in vitro. Journal of Experimental Biology. 198;1035–1043.
44. Friedman WF. The intrinsic physiologic properties of the developing heart. Progress in Cardiovascular Diseases 15(1):87–111. 1972;-Aug.

Functional and Electrophysiological Assessment after Cell Tranplantation

17
The Role of Pet Scan in Stem Cell Therapy

UCHECHUKWU SAMPSON, ATUL LIMAYE, SHARMILA DORBALA, AND MARCELO F. DI CARLI[*]

1. Introduction

Chronic heart failure is a pandemic disease entity of significant economic burden, given its major contribution to morbidity and mortality.[1] It represents the final common pathway for most forms of heart disease of which coronary artery disease is the most frequent contributor. In this context, the advent of revascularization, and advances in pharmacologic treatment such as angiotensin-converting enzyme (ACE) inhibitors,[2,3] beta-blockers[4-12] and spironolactone[13] have not sufficed in curbing the impact of chronic heart failure on morbidity and mortality.

The concept of newer therapies like cell transplantation for the repair or replacement of damaged tissue following myocardial infarction is becoming increasingly attractive in the battle to prevent post-infarct congestive heart failure (CHF), as well as end-stage heart failure of other etiologies. Furthermore, the imbalance in demand and supply of transplant organs makes cellular therapy a welcome alternative to whole organ transplantation and the problems that attend chronic immunosuppression. However, the translation of cell therapy from bench to bedside has been met with challenges that stem from gaps in our understanding regarding specific cells to be used, dosage and method of delivery. Of equal significance is our limited understanding on cell survival and the difficulties with *in vivo* tracking of cell survival.

Thus far, studies of animal models have required the harvest of tissue samples to demonstrate the success of cellular therapy by imunohistochemistry analysis.[14] However, the latter is limited by the inability for *in vivo* monitoring, three-dimensional evaluation and serial assessment. Successful cellular therapy should entail the demonstration of improvement in myocardial

[*]Marcelo F. Di Carli, M.D., Brigham and Women's Hospital, Division of Nuclear Medicine,75 Francis Street, Boston, MA 02115, Telephone: (617) 732-6291, Fax: (617) 582-6056, E-mail: mdicarli@partners.org

function presumably by improving myocardial blood flow and metabolism. This chapter will discuss the potential role of positron emission tomography (PET) in clinical studies for evaluating perfusion, metabolism, and function in humans following cell therapy.

2.   Methods for Assessing Cell Viability with Pet

The most commonly used protocol for the evaluation of tissue viability with PET includes the assessment of regional myocardial perfusion with [^{13}N]-ammonia, ^{82}Rubidium or [^{15}O]-water, followed by the delineation of regional glucose uptake with [^{18}F]-FDG (a marker of exogenous glucose uptake), thereby providing an index of myocardial metabolism and, thus, cell viability.

2.1.   Physiologic Basis

Normal myocardium uses a variety of energy-producing substrates to fulfill its energy requirements.[15] In the fasting state, free fatty acids (FFA) are mobilized in relatively large quantities from triglycerides stored in adipose tissue. Thus, the increased availability of FFA in plasma makes them the preferred energy-producing fuel in the myocardium.[15] In the fed state, however, the increase in plasma glucose and the subsequent rise in insulin levels significantly reduce FFA release from adipose tissue and, consequently, its availability in plasma. In addition, the increased insulin levels mobilize glucose transporters (especially GLUT 4) onto the cell membrane, resulting in an increased transport and utilization of exogenous glucose by the myocardium.[16]

FFA metabolism via beta-oxidation in the mitochondria is highly dependent on oxygen availability and, thus, it declines sharply during myocardial ischemia.[17,18] Under this condition, studies in animal experiments[17] and in humans[19] have shown that the uptake and subsequent metabolism of glucose by the ischemic myocardium is markedly increased. This shift to preferential glucose uptake plays a critical role in the survival of functionally compromised myocytes (i.e., stunned and hibernating), as glycolytically-derived, high-energy phosphates are thought to be critical for maintaining basic cellular functions. Consequently, noninvasive approaches that can assess the magnitude of exogenous glucose utilization play an important role in the evaluation of tissue viability in patients with myocardial dysfunction due to CAD. For these metabolic adaptations to occur, sufficient nutrient perfusion is required to supply energy-rich substrates (e.g., glucose) and oxygen, and for removal of the byproducts of glycolysis (e.g., lactate and hydrogen ion). A prolonged and severe reduction of myocardial blood flow rapidly precipitates depletion of high-energy phosphate, cell membrane disruption and cellular death. Therefore, assessment of regional blood flow also provides important information regarding the presence of tissue viability within dysfunctional myocardial regions.

2.2. Protocols

Because dysfunctional myocardium that improves functionally after revascularization must retain sufficient blood flow and metabolic activity to sustain myocyte viability, the combined assessment of regional blood flow and glucose metabolism appears most attractive for delineating myocardial viability. With this approach, regional myocardial perfusion is first evaluated following the administration of [13N]-ammonia, [82]Rubidium or [15O]-water; regional glucose uptake is then assessed with FDG (a marker of exogenous glucose uptake), providing an index of myocardial metabolism and, thus, cell viability (Figure 1). After intravenous administration, FDG traces the initial transport of glucose across the myocyte membrane and its subsequent hexokinase-mediated phosphorylation to FDG-6-phosphate (Figure 2).[20] Since the latter is a poor substrate for further metabolism and is rather impermeable to the cell membrane, it becomes virtually trapped in the myocardium.

2.3. Patient Preparation for FDG Imaging

As mentioned above, utilization of energy-producing substrates by the heart muscle is largely a function of their concentration in plasma

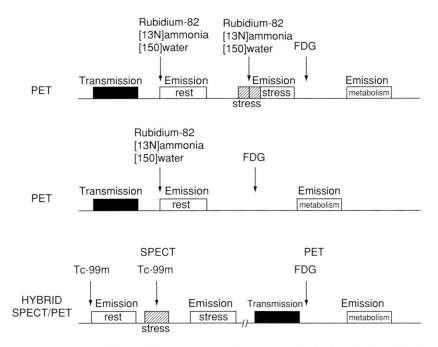

FIGURE 1. Myocardial viability protocols using PET and the hybrid SPECT/PET approach.

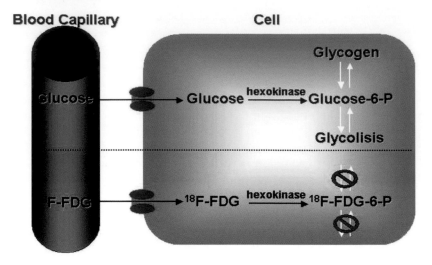

FIGURE 2. Metabolic fate of [^{18}F]deoxyglucose as a marker of exogenous glucose utilization.

and hormone levels (especially plasma insulin, insulin/glucagon ratio, growth hormone, and catecholamines) and oxygen availability for oxidative metabolism. For a detailed, step-by-step description of the available methods for FDG imaging, the reader should review the Guidelines for PET Imaging published by the American Society of Nuclear Cardiology and the Society of Nuclear Medicine.[21] These approaches for FDG imaging include:

2.3.1.   Fasting

This is the simplest method because it does not require any substrate manipulation. With this approach, ischemic but viable tissue shows as a "hot spot" due to the preferential FFA utilization by normal (non-ischemic) myocardium. While imaging interpretation would seem straight forward, the lack of tracer uptake in normal (reference) myocardium may occasionally lead to an overestimation of the amount of residual viability within a dysfunctional territory. Indeed, the predictive accuracy of this approach is lower than with the glucose-loaded approach.

2.3.2.   Glucose Loading

This is the most commonly used approach to FDG imaging. The goal of glucose loading is to stimulate the release of endogenous insulin in order to decrease the plasma levels of FFA, and to facilitate the transport and utilization of FDG. Patients are usually fasted for at least six hours and then receive an oral or intravenous glucose load. Most patients require the administration of IV insulin to maximize myocardial FDG uptake. With this approach, images are generally of diagnostic quality and the reported diagnostic accuracy very good.[22]

2.3.3. Hyperinsulinemic-Euglycemic Clamp

This approach is technically demanding and time-consuming. However, it provides the highest and most consistent image quality.[23] Based on the reported predictive accuracies, however, this does not necessarily translate in improved predictions of functional outcome.[24] Because it is technically demanding, most laboratories reserve this approach for challenging conditions (e.g., diabetes and severe congestive heart failure).

2.3.4. Acipimox

It is a nicotinic acid derivative that inhibits peripheral lipolysis, thereby reducing plasma FFA levels and, indirectly, forcing a switch to preferential myocardial glucose utilization. The drug is usually given in combination with a glucose load 60 minutes prior to FDG administration. The approach is practical and provides consistent image quality.[23] However, Acipimox is not available for clinical use in the US.

2.4. PET Patterns of Myocyte Viability

Using the sequential perfusion-FDG approach, four distinct perfusion-metabolism patterns (Figure 3) can be observed in dysfunctional myocardium:

(1) Normal perfusion associated with normal FDG uptake;
(2) Reduced perfusion associated with preserved or enhanced FDG uptake (so-called perfusion-metabolism mismatch), reflecting myocardial viability;
(3) Proportional reduction in perfusion and FDG uptake (so-called perfusion-metabolism match), reflecting non-viable myocardium; and
(4) Normal or near-normal perfusion with reduced FDG uptake (so-called reversed perfusion-metabolism mismatch).[25,26]

The patterns of normal perfusion and metabolism or of a PET mismatch identify cell viability and potentially reversible myocardial dysfunction; whereas, the PET match pattern identifies irreversible myocardial dysfunction. The reversed perfusion-FDG mismatch has been described in the context of repetitive myocardial stunning,[25] and in patients with left bundle branch block.[26] Quantitation of regional myocardial perfusion and FDG tracer uptake, and their difference can be helpful to objectively assess the magnitude of viability.

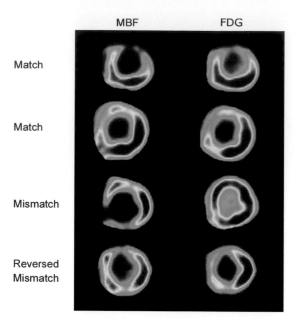

FIGURE 3. Patterns of myocardial viability using FDG PET imaging.

3.   Evidence Supporting the Use of Pet for Evaluating Cell Viability

3.1.   *Myocardial Perfusion*

Since timely restoration of nutritive perfusion to ischemic myocardium is crucial for cell survival, estimates of regional perfusion have been used for predicting functional recovery of dysfunctional myocardium. The experience using PET tracers of blood flow, including [^{15}O]-water, [^{11}C]-acetate and [^{13}N]-ammonia, for predicting recovery of function has been documented in six studies including 182 patients with LV dysfunction.[27] Contractile dysfunction was predicted to be reversible after revascularization when regional blood flow was only mild or moderately reduced (>50% of normal) and irreversible when regional blood flow was severely reduced (<50% of normal). Using these criteria, the average positive predictive accuracy of blood flow estimates for predicting functional recovery after revascularization is 63% (range, 45% to 78%); whereas, the average negative predictive accuracy is 63% (range, 45% to 100%).

While normal or near-normal blood flow in a dysfunctional region served by a stenosed coronary artery indicates tissue viability and that function can be improved with revascularization, a severe blood flow deficit generally (although not always) reflects mostly nonviable myocardium that is unlikely to show improved function with revascularization. However, blood flow deficits of intermediate severity are more difficult to interpret. They may represent the coexistence of extensive subendocardial necrosis with normal myocardium, a condition unlikely to show improved function with revascularization. Alternatively, they may reflect the coexistence of extensive areas of ischemic but viable with normal and/or scar tissue, a condition likely to show improved function with revascularization. In this situation, FDG imaging adds significant independent information for distinguishing reversible from irreversible myocardial dysfunction.[28] Patients with low ejection fraction and relatively normal perfusion at rest should undergo stress imaging to determine whether reversible ischemia (followed by stunning) is the likely cause of LV dysfunction.

3.2. Predicting Improvement in Regional and Global LV Function

The experience with the combined perfusion-FDG approach using PET or the PET-SPECT hybrid technique (Figure 1: SPECT perfusion with PET FDG imaging) has been extensively documented in 17 studies including 462 patients.[29] Using the patterns described above, the average positive predictive accuracy for predicting improved regional function after revascularization is 76% (range, 52% to 100%); whereas, the average negative predictive accuracy is 82% (range, 67% to 100%). Several studies using different PET approaches have shown that the gain in global left ventricular systolic function after revascularization is related to the magnitude of viable myocardium assessed preoperatively.[27] These data demonstrate that clinically meaningful changes in global LV function can be expected after revascularization only in patients with relatively large areas of hibernating and/or stunned myocardium ($\geq 17\%$ of the left ventricular mass). Similar results have been reported using estimates of myocardial scar with PET.[30] These results are in agreement with those obtained with SPECT,[31] dobutamine echocardiography[32] and contrast-enhanced MRI.[33]

3.3. Predicting Improvement in Symptoms

In keeping with the observed changes in LV function post-revascularization, the magnitude of improvement in heart failure symptoms also correlates with the preoperative extent of viable myocardium.[34] Patients with large areas of PET mismatch ($\geq 18\%$ of the left ventricle) appear to show the greatest clinical benefit. In these patients, exercise capacity is expected to improve significantly after CABG compared to patients without significant viability ($<5\%$ of the left ventricle). The concept that noninvasive imaging of viability can predict the degree of symptomatic improvement in heart failure patients have been confirmed in studies involving PET[35] and SPECT imaging of Tl-201 or Tc-99m sestamibi,[36] as well as identification of contractile reserve by dobutamine echocardiography.[37] Taken together, these data suggest that the extent of dysfunctional ischemic viable myocardium in heart failure patients can be used as a potential marker of the symptomatic benefit that will occur as a result of revascularization.

3.4. Predicting a Reduction in Hospital Re-Admissions for CHF

The notion that pre-operative viability imaging may be able to identify patients with a high likelihood of improvement in LV function and CHF symptoms is of great clinical importance, as it would decrease morbidity and also prevent costly hospitalizations for CHF. In a recent study, Rohatgi et al found that among patients with relatively large areas of viable myocardium pre-operatively, high-risk revascularization provided a significant reduction in hospital re-admissions for CHF as compared to medical therapy alone (3% vs 31%, respectively).[38] In contrast, hospital admissions for CHF were similarly high regardless of the mode of treatment in patients without significant amounts of viability by PET (50% vs 48% for revascularization and medical therapy, respectively).

3.5. Stratifying Risk and Predicting Improvement in Survival

An issue of even greater clinical relevance is whether viability imaging may help identify patients with low ejection fraction for whom revascularization may offer a survival advantage. Early PET reports showed that patients with viable myocardium treated medically had a consistently higher event rate than those without viability. These data also suggested that the poor, event-free survival of patients with viable myocardium undergoing medical therapy was improved significantly and consistently by early referral to revascularization. These initial findings with FDG PET have been confirmed by virtually all subsequent studies using noninvasive imaging with either nuclear testing or echocardiography.[39,40] Together, these findings imply that, despite an increasing clinical risk of revascularization with worsening LV dysfunction, non-invasive imaging evidence of preserved viability may provide information on clinical benefit to balance against that risk, allowing informed clinical decision making.

4. Noninvasive Imaging for in Vivo Assessment of Cell Therapy

The objective and ultimate proof of successful cell therapy usually requires demonstration of improved regional and global LV function. There may be other unexpected, yet beneficial, effects of cell therapy beyond restoration of contractile function. For example, cell transplantation within areas of prior infarction may lead to beneficial changes in LV geometry that can affect LV remodeling. Most of these changes require a demonstration of changes in LV size and volumes, and/or improvement in regional and global LV function. Metabolic imaging with PET may help understand the changes in regional myocardial perfusion (reflecting angiogenesis) and/or metabolism (reflecting cell viability) that ultimately will mediate changes in LV function and/or remodeling. This may help understand, *in vivo,* the mechanism of success or failure following cell therapy (Figures 4 and 5).

The quest for the application of PET imaging in the *in vivo* monitoring of cell transplantation has not been limited to the field of cardiovascular disease. Following basic science experience involving the evaluation of neural transplants in dopamine-deficient animal models,[41] PET has been utilized in gaining further insights on functional recovery in humans following transplantation of neural cells.[42-47] A recent review by Mode et al[14] provides a detailed discussion on the current status of *in vivo* monitoring of cellular therapy in neurobiology, and is replete with evidence supporting the utility of PET imaging for functional assessment following cell transplantation.

However, in the field of cardiovascular medicine, there are few clinical studies that have addressed the use of nuclear imaging for the *in vivo* quantification of stem cell viability in patients. Ozbaran et al recently reported that stem cell therapy in six patients with clinical, radiological and echocardiographic signs of heart failure, and reduced left ventricular ejection

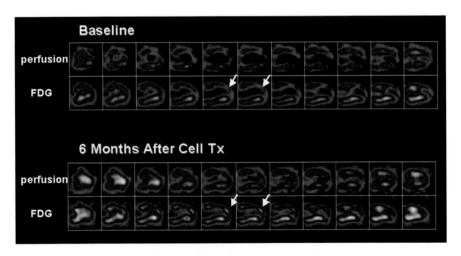

FIGURE 4. Myocardial perfusion SPECT and corresponding FDG PET images of a patient with prior MI and severe LV dysfunction before and 6 months after surgical implantation of autologous myoblasts. The baseline FDG images (Top Panel) demonstrate concordant reduction in perfusion and FDG uptake in the anterior wall and the LV apex (PET match). After myoblast implantation, the FDG images demonstrate increase FDG uptake relative to perfusion (PET mismatch), suggesting the presence of cell viability at the site of implantation.

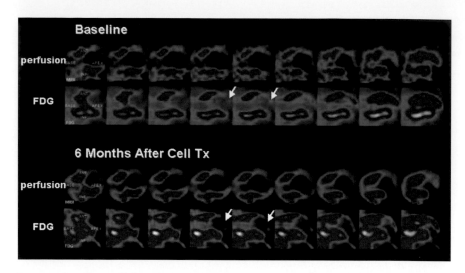

FIGURE 5. Myocardial perfusion SPECT and corresponding FDG PET images of a patient with prior MI and severe LV dysfunction before and 6 months after surgical implantation of autologous myoblasts. The baseline FDG images (Top Panel) demonstrate concordant reduction in perfusion and FDG uptake in the anterior wall and the LV apex (PET match). After myoblast implantation, the FDG images are essentially unchanged compared to the baseline study demonstrate increase FDG uptake relative to perfusion (PET match), suggesting the absence of cell viability at the site of implantation.

fraction (LVEF ≤ 25%) was associated with significant improvement in quality of life and NYHA class; some beneficial increase in viability was documented with the aid of PET imaging.[48] In another recent report, Herreros et al applied PET imaging to demonstrate an increase in metabolic activity following intramyocardial injection of cultured autologous skeletal muscle-derived stem cells in patients with chronic myocardial infarction.[49] Menasche and colleagues incorporated the use of FDG PET in demonstrating new-onset contraction of akinetic and nonviable segments following autologous skeletal myoblast transplantation for severe postinfarction left ventricular dysfunction.[50]

In a prospective, nonrandomized open-label study of 21 patients involving the use of transendocardial autologous bone marrow cell transplantation for severe chronic ischemic heart failure, Perin et al documented a statistically significant reduction in total reversible perfusion defect (as assessed by SPECT imaging) within the treatment group, and between the treatment and control groups plus an increase in global LV function.[51] Similarly, Strauer et al utilized SPECT imaging in the evaluation of a 46 year-old man who underwent intracoronary autologous stem cell transplantation following myocardial infarction; they demonstrated a reduction in transmural infarct area from 24.6% to 15.7%, ten weeks after stem cell transplantation.[52] The recently reported MAGIC cell randomized clinical trial employed SPECT to demonstrate improved cardiac function and angiogenesis in patients with prior myocardial infarction following intracoronary infusion of peripheral blood stem-cells.[53]

These studies, involving the use of nuclear imaging in the evaluation of patients following cellular therapy, have generally involved small number of patients with short periods of follow-up. However, they clearly provide the initial clinical evidence for the potential utility of PET/SPECT imaging in the context of cellular therapy. The superior spatial and contrast resolution of PET and its ability to quantify myocardial perfusion and metabolism makes it ideal to study the effects of cell therapy. Ideally, studies designed to evaluate the effects of cell therapy post-infarction should include paired imaging studies before and after treatment, making each patient serve as his/her own control. Such design should help control for the between-individual variability in myocardial perfusion and metabolism. The establishment of baseline studies may help tackle the current problem of documenting the differential effect of treatments, given the frequent superimposition of cell transplants on areas of prior/or simultaneous revascularization; however, on this point, it will be appropriate to have control subjects in order to ensure correct attribution of treatment benefit.

5.   Conclusions and Future Directions

As the efforts at translating cellular therapy to bedside continue, some of the current controversies may be resolved as answers to some questions become evident. Noninvasive imaging with PET should help to demonstrate changes in regional blood flow and metabolism that may ultimately account for the observed improvement in LV function and/or remodeling. PET imaging may be able to provide mechanistic insights to understand the causes of success and failure of cell therapy, and ultimately help improve the design of this promising, novel form of therapy for this difficult group of patients

6.   References

1. Berry C, Murdoch DR, McMurray JJ. Economics of chronic heart failure. Eur J Heart Fail 2001;3:283–91.
2. Pitt B, Poole-Wilson PA, Segal R, et al. Effect of losartan compared with captopril on mortality in patients with symptomatic heart failure: randomised trial–the Losartan Heart Failure Survival Study ELITE II. Lancet 2000;355:1582–7.
3. Effects of enalapril on mortality in severe congestive heart failure. Results of the Cooperative North Scandinavian Enalapril Survival Study (CONSENSUS). The CONSENSUS Trial Study Group. N Engl J Med 1987;316:1429–35.
4. Leizorovicz A, Lechat P, Cucherat M, Bugnard F. Bisoprolol for the treatment of chronic heart failure: a meta-analysis on individual data of two placebo-

controlled studies–CIBIS and CIBIS II. Cardiac Insufficiency Bisoprolol Study. Am Heart J 2002;143:301–7.

5. Eichhorn EJ, Bristow MR. The Carvedilol Prospective Randomized Cumulative Survival (COPERNICUS) trial. Curr Control Trials Cardiovasc Med 2001;2: 20–23.

6. Waagstein F, Caidahl K, Wallentin I, Bergh CH, Hjalmarson A. Long-term beta-blockade in dilated cardiomyopathy. Effects of short- and long-term metoprolol treatment followed by withdrawal and readministration of metoprolol. Circulation 1989;80:551–63.

7. Engelmeier RS, O'Connell JB, Walsh R, Rad N, Scanlon PJ, Gunnar RM. Improvement in symptoms and exercise tolerance by metoprolol in patients with dilated cardiomyopathy: a double-blind, randomized, placebo-controlled trial. Circulation 1985;72:536–46.

8. Pollock SG, Lystash J, Tedesco C, Craddock G, Smucker ML. Usefulness of bucindolol in congestive heart failure. Am J Cardiol 1990;66:603–7.

9. Andersson B, Blomstrom-Lundqvist C, Hedner T, Waagstein F. Exercise hemodynamics and myocardial metabolism during long-term beta-adrenergic blockade in severe heart failure. J Am Coll Cardiol 1991;18:1059–66.

10. Eichhorn EJ, Bedotto JB, Malloy CR, et al. Effect of beta-adrenergic blockade on myocardial function and energetics in congestive heart failure. Improvements in hemodynamic, contractile, and diastolic performance with bucindolol. Circulation 1990;82:473–83.

11. Eichhorn EJ, Heesch CM, Barnett JH, et al. Effect of metoprolol on myocardial function and energetics in patients with nonischemic dilated cardiomyopathy: a randomized, double-blind, placebo-controlled study. J Am Coll Cardiol 1994;24:1310–20.

12. Packer M, Coats AJ, Fowler MB, et al. Effect of carvedilol on survival in severe chronic heart failure. N Engl J Med 2001;344:1651–8.

13. Pitt B, Zannad F, Remme WJ, et al. The effect of spironolactone on morbidity and mortality in patients with severe heart failure. Randomized Aldactone Evaluation Study Investigators. N Engl J Med 1999;341:709–17.

14. Modo M, Roberts TJ, Sandhu JK, Williams SC. In vivo monitoring of cellular transplants by magnetic resonance imaging and positron emission tomography. Expert Opin Biol Ther 2004;4:145–55.

15. Opie LH. The Heart. Physiology and Metabolism. Second ed. New York: Raven Press, 1991.

16. Young LH, Coven DL, Russell RR, 3rd. Cellular and molecular regulation of cardiac glucose transport. J Nucl Cardiol 2000;7:267–76.

17. Opie LH. Effects of regional ischemia on metabolism of glucose and fatty acids. Circ Res 1976;38:152–74.

18. Liedtke AJ. Alterations of carbohydrate and lipid metabolism in the acutely ischemic heart. Progr Cardiovasc Dis 1981;23:321–36.

19. Camici P, Araujo LI, Spinks T, et al. Increase uptake of 18F-fluorodeoxyglucose in postischemic myocardium of patients with exercise-induced angina. Circulation 1986;74:81–88.

20. Phelps ME, Hoffman EJ, Selin C, et al. Investigation of [18F]2-fluoro-2-deoxyglucose for the measure of myocardial glucose metabolism. J Nucl Med 1978;19:1311–9.

21. Bacharach SL, Bax JJ, Case J, et al. PET myocardial glucose metabolism and perfusion imaging with 18FDG, 13NH3 and 82Rb. Part 1-Guidelines for data acquisition and patient preparation. J Nucl Cardiol 2003;10:543–56.
22. Schoder H, Campisi R, Ohtake T, et al. Blood flow-metabolism imaging with positron emission tomography in patients with diabetes mellitus for the assessment of reversible left ventricular contractile dysfunction. J Am Coll Cardiol 1999;33:1328–37.
23. Bax JJ, Veening MA, Visser FC, et al. Optimal metabolic conditions during fluorine-18 fluorodeoxyglucose imaging; a comparative study using different protocols. Eur J Nucl Med 1997;24:35–41.
24. Pagano D, Bonser RS, Townend JN, Ordoubadi F, Lorenzoni R, Camici PG. Predictive value of dobutamine echocardiography and positron emission tomography in identifying hibernating myocardium in patients with postischaemic heart failure. Heart 1998;79:281–8.
25. Di Carli MF, Prcevski P, Singh TP, et al. Myocardial blood flow, function, and metabolism in repetitive stunning. J Nucl Med 2000;41:1227–34.
26. Nowak B, Sinha AM, Schaefer WM, et al. Cardiac resynchronization therapy homogenizes myocardial glucose metabolism and perfusion in dilated cardiomyopathy and left bundle branch block. J Am Coll Cardiol 2003;41:1523–8.
27. Di Carli MF. Predicting improved function after myocardial revascularization. Curr Opin Cardiol 1998;13:415–24.
28. Di Carli MF, Asgarzadie F, Schelbert HR, Brunken RC, Rokhsar S, Maddahi J. Relation of myocardial perfusion at rest and during pharmacologic stress to the PET patterns of tissue viability in patients with severe left ventricular dysfunction. J Nucl Cardiol 1998;5:558–66.
29. Di Carli MF, Maddahi J, Rokhsar S, et al. Long-term survival of patients with coronary artery disease and left ventricular dysfunction: implications for the role of myocardial viability assessment in management decisions. J Thorac Cardiovasc Surg 1998;116:997–1004.
30. Beanlands RS, Ruddy TD, deKemp RA, et al. Positron emission tomography and recovery following revascularization (PARR-1): the importance of scar and the development of a prediction rule for the degree of recovery of left ventricular function. J Am Coll Cardiol 2002;40:1735–43.
31. Ragosta M, Beller, GA, Watson, DD, Kaul, S, Gimple, LW. Quantitative planar rest-redistribution 201Tl imaging in detection of myocardial viability and prediction of improvement in left ventricular function after coronary bypass surgery in patients with severely depressed left ventricular function. Circulation 1993;87:1630–1641.
32. Perrone-Filardi P, Pace L, Prastaro M, et al. Dobutamine echocardiography predicts improvement of hypoperfused dysfunctional myocardium after revascularization in patients with coronary artery disease. Circulation 1995;91:2556–65.
33. Kim RJ, Wu E, Rafael A, et al. The use of contrast-enhanced magnetic resonance imaging to identify reversible myocardial dysfunction. N Engl J Med 2000;343:1445–53.
34. Di Carli MF, Asgarzadie F, Schelbert HR, et al. Quantitative relation between myocardial viability and improvement in heart failure symptoms after revascularization in patients with ischemic cardiomyopathy. Circulation 1995;92:3436–44.

35. Marwick TH, Zuchowski C, Lauer MS, Secknus MA, Williams J, Lytle BW. Functional status and quality of life in patients with heart failure undergoing coronary bypass surgery after assessment of myocardial viability. J Am Coll Cardiol 1999;33:750–8.
36. Senior R, Kaul S, Raval U, Lahiri A. Impact of revascularization and myocardial viability determined by nitrate-enhanced Tc-99m sestamibi and Tl-201 imaging on mortality and functional outcome in ischemic cardiomyopathy. J Nucl Cardiol 2002;9:454–62.
37. Bax JJ, Poldermans D, Elhendy A, et al. Improvement of left ventricular ejection fraction, heart failure symptoms and prognosis after revascularization in patients with chronic coronary artery disease and viable myocardium detected by dobutamine stress echocardiography. J Am Coll Cardiol 1999;34:163–9.
38. Rohatgi R, Epstein S, Henriquez J, et al. Utility of positron emission tomography in predicting cardiac events and survival in patients with coronary artery disease and severe left ventricular dysfunction. Am J Cardiol 2001;87:1096–9, A6.
39. Allman K, Shaw, LJ, Hachamovitch, R, Udelson, JE. Myocardial viability testing and impact of revascularization on prognosis in patients with coronary artery disease and left ventricular dysfunction: a meta-analysis. J Am Coll Cardiol 2002;39:1151–8.
40. Udelson JE, Bonow RO, Dilsizian V. The historical and conceptual evolution of radionuclide assessment of myocardial viability. J Nucl Cardiol 2004;11:318–34.
41. Chen YI, Brownell AL, Galpern W, et al. Detection of dopaminergic cell loss and neural transplantation using pharmacological MRI, PET and behavioral assessment. Neuroreport 1999;10:2881–6.
42. Bachoud-Levi AC, Remy P, Nguyen JP, et al. Motor and cognitive improvements in patients with Huntington's disease after neural transplantation. Lancet 2000;356:1975–9.
43. Bachoud-Levi A, Bourdet C, Brugieres P, et al. Safety and tolerability assessment of intrastriatal neural allografts in five patients with Huntington's disease. Exp Neurol 2000;161:194–202.
44. Piccini P, Brooks DJ, Bjorklund A, et al. Dopamine release from nigral transplants visualized in vivo in a Parkinson's patient. Nat Neurosci 1999;2:1137–40.
45. Piccini P, Lindvall O, Bjorklund A, et al. Delayed recovery of movement-related cortical function in Parkinson's disease after striatal dopaminergic grafts. Ann Neurol 2000;48:689–95.
46. Hagell P, Schrag A, Piccini P, et al. Sequential bilateral transplantation in Parkinson's disease: effects of the second graft. Brain 1999;122 (Pt 6):1121–32.
47. Hagell P, Piccini P, Bjorklund A, et al. Dyskinesias following neural transplantation in Parkinson's disease. Nat Neurosci 2002;5:627–8.
48. Ozbaran M, Omay SB, Nalbantgil S, et al. Autologous peripheral stem cell transplantation in patients with congestive heart failure due to ischemic heart disease. Eur J Cardiothorac Surg 2004;25:342–50; discussion 350–1.
49. Herreros J, Prosper F, Perez A, et al. Autologous intramyocardial injection of cultured skeletal muscle-derived stem cells in patients with non-acute myocardial infarction. Eur Heart J 2003;24:2012–20.
50. Menasche P, Hagege AA, Vilquin JT, et al. Autologous skeletal myoblast transplantation for severe postinfarction left ventricular dysfunction. J Am Coll Cardiol 2003;41:1078–83.

51. Perin EC, Dohmann HF, Borojevic R, et al. Transendocardial, autologous bone marrow cell transplantation for severe, chronic ischemic heart failure. Circulation 2003;107:2294–302.
52. Strauer BE, Brehm M, Zeus T, et al. [Intracoronary, human autologous stem cell transplantation for myocardial regeneration following myocardial infarction]. Dtsch Med Wochenschr 2001;126:932–8.
53. Kang HJ, Kim HS, Zhang SY, et al. Effects of intracoronary infusion of peripheral blood stem-cells mobilised with granulocyte-colony stimulating factor on left ventricular systolic function and restenosis after coronary stenting in myocardial infarction: the MAGIC cell randomised clinical trial. Lancet 2004;363:751–6.

18
The Measurement of Systolic Function in the Mammalian Heart

Blasé A. Carabello[*]

1. Introduction

The heart is a muscular pump that generates pressure in order to deliver a flow of blood to the body. The ability of the heart to perform this function is widely recognized as a critical factor in predicting the outcome of heart disease. To this end, scores of investigations over the past five decades have sought to define measures of cardiac function that would give the patient and his/her physician the ability to predict the outcome of heart disease and also to measure the impact of therapy. Because the heart is a muscle, and because muscles generate force that enables them to do perform their function, efforts were directed toward measurement of contractility: the innate ability of the heart muscle to generate force. In general, such measures are constructed from the two most observable properties of the heart, changes in pressure and changes in volume during the cardiac cycle. The ideal index of contractility would be (1) sensitive to changes in inotropy, (2) independent of loading conditions, (3) independent of cardiac volume and mass, (4) effective in assessing both acute and chronic changes in contractility and (5) easy to apply. Literally dozens of such indexes were conceived and investigated and even proven to be useful but none met all of the above criteria. Thus despite all efforts at more sophistication, the simple index of ejection fraction (EF) became the mainstay of clinical cardiac assessment. Its general acceptance stems from its easy applicability and relative accuracy in predicting heart disease outcome. Although extremely load dependent, EF has been a good indicator of function because in most conditions, load is relatively normal. However in some notable exceptions such as valvular and congenital heart disease, EF may either over or under-estimate contractility. In fact these conditions are rare enough in adult cardiology that they didn't force a change away from EF in the clinical assessment of ventricular function.

[*]Baylor College of Medicine, Department of Medicine and the Michael E. DeBakey Veterans Affairs Medica Center, Houston, Texas 77030

Although dormant for the last decade, the topic of ventricular function has again been brought to the forefront by the advent of molecular cardiology. One of the mainstays of basic cardiology research today is the investigation of gene function in genetically altered mice (and other mammals). In such experiments, the expression of a candidate gene is increased or diminished in an effort to determine the phenotype that such manipulation causes, in turn imputing the biologic role of that specific gene. When such manipulations cause death or overt cardiomyopathy, a sophisticated measuring stick for contractility is unnecessary. However in other experiments specifically designed to alter cardiac load in an effort to induce hypertrophy, both load and more subtle changes in function may need to be measured. In concert with these needs, development of high-resolution echocardiography together with miniaturized pressure catheter systems allow for the construction of virtually all of the indexes of function available in man, now to be used in mice.

More recently the availability of cell and gene therapy in man and experimental animals has become a topic of intense interest. Especially at the current stage of development, these therapies are likely to produce subtle rather than dramatic changes in contractility requiring sensitive global and regional measures of function with small enough variability in measurement that small changes in function can be relied upon as significant. To this end the following is a review of the uses and limitations of indexes on contractility and their applications in the mammalian heart. In general the chapter will deal with left ventricular function because most indexes were developed for that chamber and because the complex geometry of the right ventricle has made it less easily studied.

2.   Definitions

2.1.   Afterload

Afterload is the force opposing cardiac contraction. Only when the force that the myocardium generates exceeds this force can systolic volume diminish and ejection occur. Making an analogy to skeletal muscle, the weight of a dumbbell in an athlete's hand during biceps flexion is the afterload on the biceps. While easy to assess in the case of the biceps and the dumbbell, measuring this force in the left ventricle (LV) is much more difficult. Common measures of afterload include systolic blood pressure, total peripheral resistance, systolic wall stress, and aortic impedance. Each has its own limitations in the assessment of afterload.

2.1.1.   Pressure

Pressure is defined as force/area, thus force = pressure × area. Therefore, simple measurement of pressure does not account for the area over which the force is distributed and is imprecise as a measure of afterload. Indeed a large ventricle must develop more force to reach the same pressure than does a smaller chamber. As such, systolic pressure as a measure of afterload is suspect when comparing chambers of different sizes.

2.1.2.   Wall Stress

Wall stress (σ) for a sphere = p × r/2th, where p = pressure, r = radius and th = wall thickness. Several modifications of this formula have been made to make it applicable to the prolate ellipsoid shape of the left ventricle.[1,2] Stress normalizes pressure for the existing ventricular geometry. This measure has been very useful in investigation of cardiac function but the need to simultaneously measure its three component terms has limited its use in clinical medicine. Further most investigations assume a homogeneous distribution of the three component terms, a false assumption when regional hypertrophy or wall motion abnormalities intervene.

2.1.3.   Total Peripheral Resistance (TPR)

TPR = mean arterial pressure/cardiac output. During the cardiac cycle, blood flow is pulsatile in the great vessels but becomes more continuous as vessel caliber diminishes. Because mean arterial pressure = 2DP+SP/3, where DP = diastolic pressure and SP = systolic pressure, mean pressure is derived more from a diastolic property (reflecting diastolic flow through the arterioles and capillaries) than it is from a systolic property. This problem is especially manifest in older patients with stiff vessels and a wide pulse pressure. In such a patient with a blood pressure of 150/60, afterload is almost certainly increased but the mean arterial pressure is normal (90mm Hg) and TPR would not be elevated.

2.1.4.   Aortic Impedance

In words, aortic impedance is that portion of peripheral resistance that occurs during systole and represents the resistance met by the ventricle when the semi-lunar valve opens. This measure is obtained by computer analysis of pressure-flow velocity data obtained by a catheter specially designed to simultaneously record those parameters.[3] Thus obtaining aortic impedance requires the hardware and software necessary to obtain and analyze the pressure and flow inputs. While usually it is a reliable measure of afterload, it becomes unreliable in the presence of mitral regurgitation or other conditions in which all the LV output does not exit via the aortic valve.

2.2.   Preload

Preload is end diastolic sarcomere stretch that is responsible for the degree of actin-myosin crossbridge interaction that occurs during systole according to the sliding filament theory. Greater stretch exposes more of the actin filament for myosin interaction, in turn increasing the force of contraction. This property cannot be measured clinically but sarcomere length can be measured experimentally.[4] In the intact beating heart, preload can only be inferred from left ventricular volume (or dimension) or pressure data. Acute increases in either diastolic pressure or volume must surely be associated with increased preload. However the extent of this increase is dependent upon ventricular compliance and volume. Thus in stiff (non-compliant) ventricles, a given increase in diastolic pressure will increase preload less than would occur for the same change in a compliant ventricle. Since compliance data is almost never known clinically, there is no way to equate a change in filling pressure with a known change in preload.

Likewise, an acute increase in diastolic volume must be due to an increase in preload. However nothing can be inferred about preload from end diastolic volume when comparing individuals or in cases of volume overload where eccentric hypertrophy has increased myocyte sarcomere number (Figure 1).[5]

In such cases, increased LV volume could be due more to increased sarcomere number rather than due to increased sarcomere stretch.

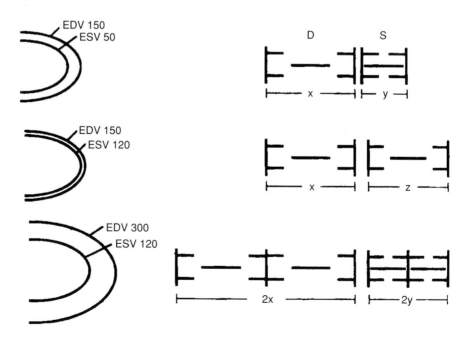

FIGURE 1. The effect of sarcomere number on end diastolic and end systolic volume is depicted. Either volume can be affected both by sarcomere length and by sarcomere number. Taken from Carabello and Spann, ref. 5, with permission.

3.   Measures of Contractility

3.1.   Isovolumic indexes

As the name implies, Isovolumic indexes are derived during that portion of systole when volume is not changing. Such indexes rely on examination of pressure development between mitral valve closure and aortic valve opening. Most are developed from the rate of pressure change, dP/dt. These indexes measure global ventricular function but cannot measure differences in regional function. Although Doppler-derived pressure has been used to obtain these indexes non-invasively,[6] for the most part cardiac catheterization is employed to insert a high fidelity pressure catheter into the ventricle and dP/dt is derived electronically from the catheter output.

3.1.1.   Maximum dP/dt and its Derivatives

Changes in maximal dP/dt have been quite useful in examining acute changes in inotropic state.[7] Although this index is modestly affected by afterload and preload, it has accurately reflected changes in inotropic state caused by a wide variety of pharmacologic agents in a given individual. Load dependence is further reduced by examining peak dP/dt at a systolic pressure well below that which occurs at aortic valve opening such as dP/dt_{40mmHg}. Unfortunately, dP/dt has been much less useful in comparing individuals to each other or in comparing the same individual to itself at different points in time.[8] While not entirely understood, the discrepancy between the index's efficacy in acute assessment and its failure in chronic assessment appears multifactorial. One problem is the wide range of normal values reported in the literature. Subjects with as much as a 100% variation in peak dP/dt might not differ from one another.[9] Second in comparing individuals to themselves over time, dP/dt fails to account for changes in ventricular geometry that might have developed chronically. Increases in wall thickness increase dP/dt.[10] Thus for a subject whose dP/dt was the same at two observation points but in whom concentric hypertrophy also developed intercurrently, it is likely that inotropic state decreased yet was not reflected by this measure of contractility. Third, as noted below, dP/dt is affected by heart rate[11] and comparisons of individuals should be made at comparable heart rates but this is not always the case.

In summary, dP/dt is useful index in assessing acute changes in inotropic state in a given individual. However, it has significant limitations in comparing groups of individuals or in comparing individuals to themselves at different points in time.

3.1.2.   Force-Frequency Relationship

Although dP/dt is only modestly affected by load, it is very dependent upon heart rate.[12] Indeed this forms the basis for using dP/dt to assess the myocardial force frequency relationship. In normal subjects the force of contraction increases with heart rate (frequency). Using dP/dt as a surrogate for force, a heart rate-maximal dP/dt relationship is developed as shown in Figure 2.[11]

In disease states, the heart rate at which peak dP/dt occurs is lower than it is in normals and further increases in heart rate cause a fall rather than an increase in dP/dt.[13] These findings seem a reliable way to separate normal from pathologic myocardial function. The major drawbacks of the method are the need for invasive catheterization to place catheters for pressure measurement and for varying heart rate by temporary pacemaker installation.

3.2.   Ejection Phase Indexes

Ejection phase indexes are derived from assessing the way in which the ventricle ejects blood. Most are based on some measure of ventricular motion and some incorporate simultaneous measurement of pressure.

3.2.1.   Ejection Fraction and Shortening Fraction

Ejection fraction is simply that portion of end diastolic volume (EDV) that is ejected during systole and = EDV-ESV/EDV or stroke volume (SV)/EDV. When obtained echocardiographically, % minor axis shortening, end diastolic dimension (EDD) minus end systolic dimension (ESD) divided by end diastolic dimension (or EDD-ESD/EDD) is substituted for volume. As noted

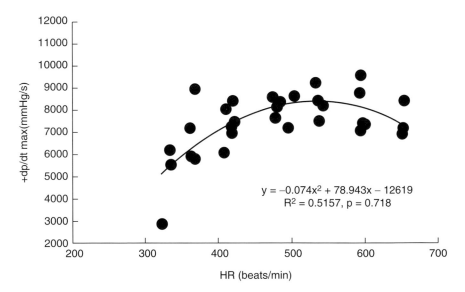

FIGURE 2. The force-frequency curve for the normal intact murine heart is demonstrated. Taken from Nemoto et al., ref. 11, with permission.

above these measures are easily obtained and understood and are relatively accurate in assessing function, facts accounting for their widespread usage. Significant load dependency and relative insensitivity to changes in both global and regional function limit use in situations of abnormal load or when there are only modest changes in inotropic state.[11] Another often unrecognized confounder in the use of these measures is the presence on concentric left ventricular hypertrophy (LVH).[14] Average sarcomere shortening is about 10%. The way in which this modest degree of shortening is transformed into an ejection fraction of 60% is by ventricular thickening. If the myocardium were only one sarcomere thick, ejection fraction would be only 10%. However as sarcomeres shorten, because mass is conserved, they also thicken. The effect of stacking millions of sarcomeres on top of one another is to sum this thickening, which is the major impetus for expelling blood from the ventricle. This factor is magnified in LVH where yet more sarcomeres exist in parallel. As such, subnormal shortening can still cause the same amount of thickening and the same ejection fraction.[15] In fact many subjects with so-called pure diastolic dysfunction may have a normal ejection fraction but also have systolic dysfunction because most such patients also have LVH.

3.2.2.   Corrected Ejection Phase Indexes

Several efforts have focused on making ejection phase indexes less load dependent. Division by ejection time reduces preload dependence probably partially by coincidence and partially because ejection time (et) increases with preload.[16] Thus dividing shortening fraction by ejection time (EDD-ESD/EDD × et) yields mean velocity of fiber shortening (VCF) a relative preload measure of function. Similarly EF divided by et yields mean normalized systolic ejection rate (MNSER) also a relative preload independent index. While corrected for preload, both VCF and MNSER remain afterload dependent. One strategy to make ejection phase indexes yet more load independent is to plot VCF (or MNSER) against systolic wall stress (Figure 3).[17]

Thus a relative preload index is corrected for afterload. Once the relationship is established for normal subjects, experimental subjects can be plotted against this relationship. Subjects whose plot falls down and to the left of the confidence bands of the normal population show reduced shortening rate for any given afterload, indicating contractile dysfunction. This concept has been vetted against an independent gold standard of contractile function, i.e. the contractility of individual myocytes taken from the ventricle for which the MNSER-stress relationship was developed (Figure 4).[18]

Because of variation in measurement techniques from laboratory to laboratory, the relationship and its confidence intervals must be developed from normal subjects in each venue and the position of the test subject is then plotted against this relationship. The cumbersome nature of developing this index limits its use to that of an investigational tool. It is impractical for clinical use.

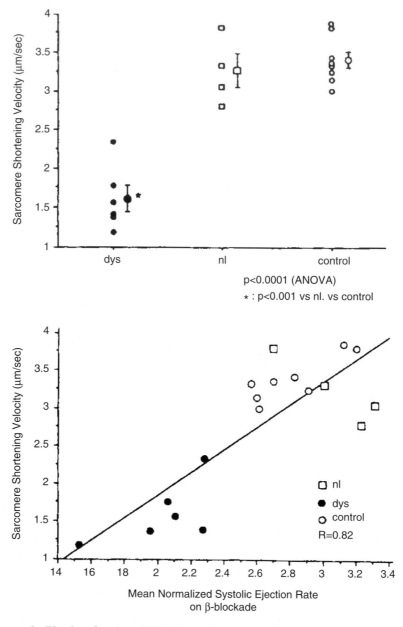

FIGURE 3. Ejection fraction (EF, left panel) and mean velocity of circumferential fiber shortening (V_{cf}) is plotted against end systolic stress (ESS) for patients with valvular heart disease. Patients whose plot falls down and to the left have reduced contractility and a higher incidence of a poor outcome at surgery (closed triangles). Patients with normal contractility had better surgical outcome (open circles). Taken from Carabello, ref. 17, with permission.

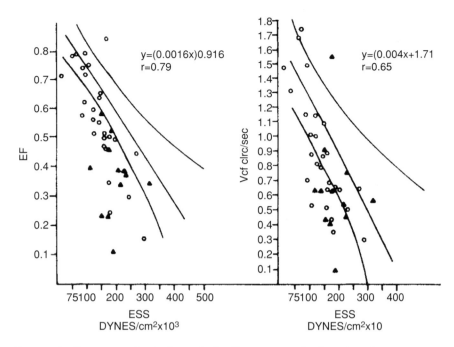

FIGURE 4. Sarcomere shortening velocity for myocytes is plotted against mean normalized ejection velocity of the ventricle from which the myocytes were taken for normal dogs (con), for aortic stenosis dogs with normal contractility (nl) and for dogs with LV dysfunction (dys). There is excellent correlation between the index of myocyte contractility and that of the chamber from which the myocytes were removed. Taken from Koide et al., ref. 18, with permission.

3.2.3.   Tissue Doppler Imaging, Strain Rate Imaging and MRI Tagging

Doppler interrogation of left ventricular movement (tissue Doppler imaging, TDI) can measure segmental differences in myocardial velocities addressing differences in regional function.[19,20] However in assessing viability, TDI cannot distinguish between active contraction versus nonviable myocardium moved passively by tethering to adjacent viable tissue.

Strain is defined as a change in length/reference length (akin in some respects to regional shortening fraction). Strain rate imaging (SRI) is a refinement of TDI that employs an algorithm that calculates differences in velocities of adjacent areas of myocardium to derive strain and strain rate. SRI appears superior to TDI in assessing myocardial function.[21] Strain is both preload and afterload sensitive while strain rate is primarily afterload sensitive in a manner similar to VCF. The advantages of strain imaging are the ease with which regional measurements can be made echocardiographically and the ability to examine regional function.

Magnetic resonance imaging (MRI) tagging also affords rapid assessment of regional and global wall motion.[22,23] In this process, specific portions of the myocardium are "tagged" using localized magnetic resonant frequency pulses placed perpendicular to the myocardium. Tagging is following by an imaging sequence that records wall motion in relation to a superimposed grid. The technique's major limitation compared to Doppler interrogation is cost.

3.3.   End Systolic Volume and Dimension

The volume to which the ventricle contracts at end systole is preload independent.[24] Like a rubber band, irrespective of what length the ventricle (or rubber band) is stretched to passively in diastole, it finishes at the same length when contraction is finished. On the other hand, end systolic volume and dimension are afterload sensitive. The higher the afterload, the greater the resistance to contraction and the larger is end systolic volume. End systolic volume and dimension have been explored as markers of LV dysfunction in a variety of diseases, most prominently in valvular regurgitation.[25-27] In these diseases, increased preload causes indexes like ejection fraction to overestimate contractile function; hence use of a preload-independent index improves accuracy.

3.3.1.   Pressure-Volume Relationships

Ejection phase indexes based on changes in ventricular volume fail to measure the fundamental function of muscles: force generation. By introducing pressure measurement into the index, force (p=force/area) is also incorporated. Stroke work is one such measure. Stroke work is the area surrounded by the pressure volume trajectory of the ventricle (Figure 5).[28]

Work = f × d where d = distance. In examining the ventricle's pressure volume area, Work = d3 (volume) × f/d2 (pressure) or f × d. Preload-recruitable stroke work (PRSW) is the augmentation of stroke work produced by augmenting preload.[29] By examining the change in stroke work produced by rapidly changing volume (such as with balloon occlusion of the inferior vena cava), the slope of the change in work vs. the change in EDV can be developed. Preload-recruitable stroke work is sensitive to changes in inotropy and is load independent. Its biggest potential draw back is in comparing different hearts of different sizes and weights. Presumably a hypertrophied heart should be able to generate more work for any given preload. Thus if comparison is made at two different time points and LVH has developed in the interim, the slope of this relationship should probably increase. However the relationship has not been compared to an independent gold standard such as papillary muscle function or sarcomere function of muscle from the same ventricle from which PRSW was developed.

Time varying elastance makes use of the principle that during systole the myocardium gets progressively stiffer as contractile element interaction

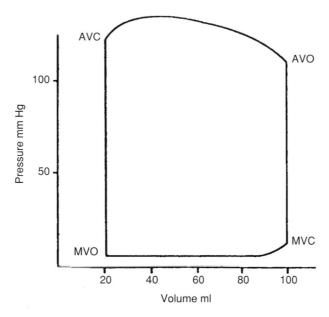

FIGURE 5. The trajectory of left ventricular pressure and volume during the cardiac cycle is shown. The area of the enclosed loop is stroke work. At mitral valve opening, volume begins to increase until the beginning of systole (mitral valve closure, MVC). Pressure then increases until high enough to force aortic valve opening (AVO). Volume is expelled and lessens until aortic valve closure (AVC). Taken from Carabello, ref. 28, with permission.

increases until maximum elastance (E_{max}) is reached just at the end of systole.[30] As the heart becomes more contractile throughout systole, for any change in pressure there is a lesser change in volume and the slope of the pressure-volume relationship increases throughout (Figure 6).

Development of the whole time-varying elastance framework for a given ventricle requires multiple pressure and volume points be plotted at given times (isochrones) after the QRS to develop the slopes of the elastance relationship. Fortunately, because E_{max} occurs at the end of systole, the end systolic pressure-volume relationship (ESPVR, Figure 7)[24] closely approximates E_{max}.

This linear relationship based upon end systolic volume (ESV) and pressure is preload independent because as noted above, end systolic volume is preload independent. It is based on the principle that for stronger ventricles, a given increase in afterload causes a smaller increase in end systolic volume than does the same change in afterload for a weaker ventricle. Thus when contractility is high any given change in end systolic pressure (or wall stress) creates less of a change in volume resulting in a greater slope (e_{es}) than would occur when contractility is reduced.

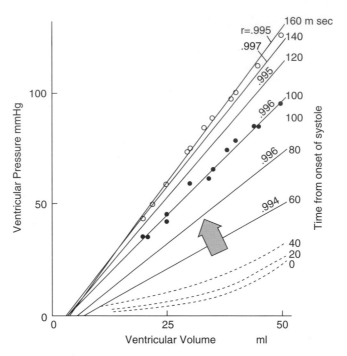

FIGURE 6. Left ventricular pressure-volume relations for progressive time points (isochrones) throughout systole are shown. As systole progress, the slope of the relationship steepens indicating progressively increasing strength of contraction. Taken from Sagawa, ref. 30, with permission.

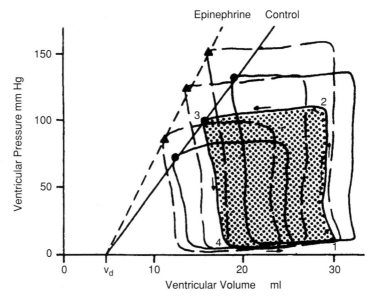

FIGURE 7. The slope of the left ventricular end systolic pressure volume relationship is shown for a canine ventricle. This slope increases with infusion of a known positive inotrope. Taken from Suga et al., ref. 24, with permission.

ESPVR and E_{max} are load independent and are sensitive to changes in inotropy.[30,31] They are excellent measures of acute changes in ventricular function. The major limitation of these indexes is that they do not account for either eccentric or concentric LVH. Because most mammalian hearts operate as roughly similar LV pressures but have widely differing volumes, e_{es} differs from species to species and differs among ventricles of different volumes in the same species.[32-34] That is, because slope = $\Delta y/\Delta x$ where y = pressure and x = volume, a change in end systolic pressure of 10 mm Hg in a rat might cause a change of end systolic volume of 0.1 cc yielding a slope of 100. In man this same change in pressure might cause a change in volume of 3 cc giving a slope of 3.33. It is highly unlikely that contractility in a rat is 30× that of man. Rather it is size dependence that causes this discrepancy. Indeed correction for size among species and within the same species must be made but is often neglected.[32-34] Likewise pressure change is not an accurate descriptor of afterload when either concentric or eccentric LVH has developed (see above). Thus stress rather than pressure should be employed on the y-axis if the intent is to evaluate muscle rather than chamber function.

A way around these limitations is to evaluate end systolic stiffness (stress vs. strain) instead of pressure vs. volume.[35] Because strain is dimensionless (see above), it is unaffected by changes in heart size, and because stress accounts for concentric LVH, it is a better measure of afterload than is pressure. In fact, end systolic stiffness is not only an excellent theoretic measure of contractility, it has been vetted against independent measures of isolated myocyte function.[36] Unfortunately this index, like E_{max}, requires variation in pressure and volume for its construction and extensive mathematics are needed to create the index, both factors acting in concert to limit its usefulness to the experimental laboratory.

Table 1 lists the characteristics of various measures of systolic function.

4. Summary

The heart is a muscular pump that generates force in order to do work and pump volume. The major determinants of its ability to perform these functions are its size, mass, innate strength or contractility, preload and afterload. While all of these parameters should be kept in mind when assessing cardiac function, assessment of most pathologies and therapies rely on measuring contractility. Despite major advances in our understanding of cardiac function over the past 50 years, a simple, easily applied and accurate measure of contractility still eludes us. Easily applied measures lack sensitivity and accuracy while complex measures are cumbersome and difficult to apply. These principles must be kept in full view in order to avoid errors in assessing cardiac function.

5. References

1. Mirsky I: Assessment of passive elastic stiffness of cardiac muscle: Mathematical concepts, physiologic and clinical considerations, directions of future research. Prog Cardiovasc Dis 1976;18:277–308.
2. Yin FCP. Ventricular wall stress. Circ Res 1981:49;829.
3. MurgeJP, Westerhof N, Giolma JP, Altobelli SA. Aortic input impedance in normal man: relationship to pressure wave forms. Circ 62:105–116, 1980.
4. Gordon AM, Huxley AF, Julian FJ. The variation in isometric tension with sarcomere length in vertebrate muscle fibers. J. Physiol. (Lond.) 184:170–192, 1966.
5. Carabello BA, Spann JF: 1988. The uses and limitations of end-systolic stress-volume relationships in chronic aortic regurgitation. In Gaasch WH, Levine JH, eds. Chronic Aortic Regurgitation. Boston, Kluwer, pp 33–49.
6. Chen C, Rodriguez L, Lethor JP, Levine RA, Semigran MS, Fifer MA, Weyman AE, Thomas JD. Continuous wave Doppler echocardiography for noninvasive assessment of left ventricular dP/dt and relaxation time constant from mitral regurgitant spectra in patients. J Am Coll Cardiol. 1994 Mar 15;23(4):970–6.
7. Grossman W, Mclaurin LP, Saltz S, et al. Changes in inotropic state of the left ventricle during isometric exercise. Br Heart J 1973;35:697, 1973.
8. Peterson KL, Skloven D, Ludbrook P, Uther JB, Ross J Jr. Comparison of isovolumic and ejection phase indices of myocardial performance in man. Circ. 1974;49:1088–1101.
9. Gleason WL, Braunwald E. Studies on the first derivative of the ventricular pressure pulse in man. J Clin Invest 1962;41:80, 1962.
10. Fifer MA, Gunther S, Grossman W, et al. Myocardial contractile function in aortic stenosis as determinted from the rate of stress development during isovolumic systole. Am J Cardiol. 1979;44:1318–1325.
11. Nemoto S, Defreitas G, Mann DL, Carabello BA. Effects of changes in left ventricular contractility on indexes of contractility in mice. Am J Physiol Circ Physiol 283:H2504–H2510, 2002;10.1152/ajpheart.00765.2001.
12. Parakodeti V, Oh S, Oh BH, Mao L, Hongo M, Peterson K, Ross J Jr. Force-frequency effect is a powerful determinant of myocardial contractility in the mouse. Am J Physiol Heart Circ Physiol 273:H1283–H1290, 1997.
13. Alpert Nr, Leavitt BJ, Ittleman FP, Hasenfuss G, Pieske B, Mulieri LA. A Mechanistic analysis of the force-frequency relation in non-failing and progressively failing human myocardium. Basic Res Cardiol. 1998;93 Suppl 1:23–32.
14. Shimizu G, Hirota Y, Kita Y, Kawamura K, Saito T, Gaasch WH. Left ventricular midwall mechanics in systemic arterial hypertension. Myocardial function is depressed in pressure-overload hypertrophy. Circ. 1991 May;83(5):1676–84.
15. de Simone G, Devereux RB. Rationale of echocardiographic assessment of left ventricular wall stress and midwall mechanics in hypertensive heart disease. Eur J Echocardiogr. 2002 Sep;3(3):192–8.
16. Nixon JV, Murray RG, Leonard PD, Mitchell JH, Blomqvist CG. Effect of large variations in preload on left ventricular performance characteristics in normal subjects. Circ. 1982;65:698–703.
17. Carabello BA, Williams H, Gash AK, Kent R, Belber D, Maurer A, Siegel J, Blasius K, Spann JF: Hemodynamic predictors of outcome in patients undergoing valve replacement. Circ. 1986;74 (6):1309–1316.

18. Koide M, Nagatsu M, Zile MR, Hamawaki M, Swindle MM, Keech G, DeFReyte G, Tagawa H, Cooper G 4th, Carabello BA. Premorbid determinants of left ventricular dysfunction in a novel model of gradually induced pressure overload in the adult canine. Circ. 1997 Mar 18;95(6):1601–10. Comment in: Circ. 1997 Mar 18;95(6):1349–51.

19. Sutherland GR, Stewart MJ, Groundstroem KWE, et al. Color Doppler myocardial imaging: a new technique for assessment of myocardial function. J Echocardiogr 1994;7:441–58.

20. Miyatake K, Yamagishi M, Tanaka N, et al. New method of evaluating left ventricular wall motion by color-coded tissue Doppler imaging: in vitro and in vivo studies. J Am Coll Cardiol 1995;25:717–24.

21. Hoffmann, R, Altiok E, Nowak B, Heussen N, Kuhl H, Kaiser HJ, Bull U, Hanrath P. Strain rate measurement by Doppler echocardiography allows improved assessment of myocardial viability in patients with depressed left ventricular function. JACC Vol. 39, No. 3, 2002.

22. Lima JA, Jeremy R, Guier W, Bouton S, Zerhouni EA, McVeigh E, Buchalter MB, Weisfeldt ML, Shapiro EP, Weiss JL. Accurate systolic wall thickening by nuclear magnetic resouance imaging with tissue tagging: correlation with sonomicrometers in normal and ischemic myocardium. J Am Coll Cardiol. 1993 Jun;21(7):1741–51.

23. Yeon SB, Reichek N, Tallant BA, Lima JA, Calhoun LP, Clark NR, Hoffman EA, Ho KK, Axel L. Validation of in vivo myocardial strain measurement by magnet resonance tagging with sonomicrometry. J Am Coll Cardiol. 2001 Aug;38(2): 555–61.

24. Suga H, Sagawa K, Shoukas AA. Load independence of the instantaneous pressure-volume ratio of the canine left ventricular and effects of epinephrine and hear rate on the ratio. Circ Res. 1973;32:314–322.

25. Henry WL, Bonow RO, Borer JS, et al. Observations on the optimum time for operative intervention for aortic regurgitation: I. Evaluation of the results of aortic valve replacement in symptomatic patients. Circ. 1980;61:471–483.

26. Zile Mr, Gaasch WH, Carroll JD, Levine HF: 1984. Chronic mitral regurgitation: predicative value of preoperative echocardiographic indexes of left ventricular function and wall stress. J Am Coll Cardiol 3:235–242.

27. Wisenbaugh T, Skudicky D, Sareli P. Prediction of outcome after valve replacement for rheumatic mitral regurgitation in the era of chordal preservation. Circ. 1994 Jan;89(1):191–7.

28. Carabello BA. Cardiac Catheterization. Cardiology Vol 1 Physiology, Pharmacology, Diagnosis. 1988.

29. Glower D, Spratt J, Snow N, et al. Linearity of the Frank-Starling relationship in the intact heart: the concept of preload recruitable stroke work. Circ. 1985;71: 994–1009.

30. Sagawa K, Suga H, Shoukas AA, Bakalar KM: 1977. End-systolic pressure/volume ration: a new index of ventricular contractility. Am J Cardiol 40:748–753.

31. Suga H, Sagawa K. Instantaneous pressure-volume relationships and their ratio in the excised, supported canine left ventricle. Circ Res 1974;35:117–126.

32. Belcher P, Boerboom LE, Olinger GN: Standardization of end-systolic pressure-volume relation in the dog. Am J Physiol 1985;249:H547–H553.

33. Suga H, Yamada O, Goto Y, Igarashi Y, Yasumura Y, Nozawa T: Reconsideration of normalization of E_{max} for heart size. Heart Vessels 1986;2:67–73.

34. Suga H, Hisano R, Goto Y, Yamada O: Normalization of end-systolic pressure-colume relation and E_{max} of different sized hearts. Jpn Circ J 1984;48:136–143.
35. Nakano K, Sugawara M, Ishihara K, Kanazawa S, Corin WJ, Denslow S, Biderman RWW, Carabello BA. Myocardial stiffness derived from end-systolic wall stress and logarithm of reciprocal of wall thickness: contractility index independent of ventricular size. Circ. 1990;82:1352–1361.
36. Urabe Y, Mann DL, Kent RL, Nakano K, Tomanek RJ, Carabello BA, Cooper G 4th. Cellular and ventricular contractile dysfunction in experimental canine mitral regurgitation. Circ Res. 1992 Jan;70(1):131–47.

19
Electrophysiological Aspects of Cell Transplantation

NICHOLAS S. PETERS, NICOLAS A. F. CHRONOS AND FERNANDO TONDATO*

1. Introduction

Of the approximate 550,000 new cases of congestive heart failure per year in United States,[1] epidemiologic studies indicate that more than half of these patients die suddenly,[2] mostly related to occurrence of malignant ventricular arrhythmias.

Several pharmacologic and non-pharmacologic approaches have been developed in the last years to treat myocardial dysfunction. Most recently, the use of cell therapy emerged as an attempt to regenerate myocardium or augment blood supply to ischemic areas in the heart, ultimately addressing the reversion of the damage induced to the cardiac tissue, regardless of its etiology. Preliminary clinical and preclinical studies have been performed worldwide, with promising initial results, showing improvement in cardiac function. However, the electrophysiological effects of the cell transplantation and the interaction with the host myocardium have been modestly investigated to date, and there remains some concern as to whether the net result is to improve or worsen arrhythmic tendency.

Adequate analysis of arrhythmic events related to cell therapy presents a challenge. The recruited population most likely will have a substantial arrhythmic tendency secondary to myocardial dysfunction (~10-30% per annum for NYHA Class III/IV) and it is therefore difficult to discern whether an arrhythmic event represents the natural history of the underlying disease or a consequence of the cell treatment.

Experimental studies have shown that all three basic mechanisms of arrhythmia can potentially be present in transplanted cells: creation of zones of slow conduction, facilitating reentrant circuits; triggered activity or abnormal automaticity.

---
*Nicholas S. Peters, Imperial College London, United Kingdom. Fernando Tondato, Nicolas A.F. Chronos & Nicholas S. Peters: American Cardiovascular Research Institute, Atlanta, Georgia, 30071

There have been documented arrhythmic events and arrhythmic deaths in the early clinical studies in cell therapy. The consensus appears to be that there may be an early window of perhaps 30 days after intramyocardial injection (of at least some of the precursor cell types used in clinical trials to date) in which there may be enhanced arrhythmic tendency, but whether this is the case, and whether it relates to physical trauma and healing from the injections, or the injectate, remains unclear.

2. Mechanisms of Arrhythmia and Potential Interaction with Cell Therapy: Antiarrhythmic or Proarrhythmic?

In both animal models and in clinical settings, transplantation of different types of cells have been tested, such as bone marrow derived mononuclear and mesenchymal cells, skeletal myoblast, fibroblasts, embryonic stem cells, fetal cardiomyocytes, smooth muscle cells, among others. These various cell types possess a wide variety of intrinsic electrical behavior. Regardless of the type of cell used, the electrophysiological properties of the transplanted cells and their interaction with the host tissue will need to be well characterized for rational interpretation of the clinical arrhythmic events, their prediction, avoidance and treatment.

Because current will tend to flow, and the action potential propagate, between cells and regions of myocardium displaying different voltages at different phases of the action potential, particularly if interspersed with anatomical obstacles interrupting the myocardial syncytium and slowing conduction, heterogeneity of electrophysiological properties of the failing hearts is considered a principal cause of lethal arrhythmias. Fibrous tissue can be focally distributed, as commonly seen in ischemic cardiac disease or have a patchy distribution, typically found in diffuse cardiomyopathy. Common to both of these pathologies, surviving cardiac fibers amongst fibrotic tissue can be related to slow conduction and consequently lead to reentrant arrhythmias.

Theoretically speaking, transplanted cells might be expected to suppress an arrhythmic tendency, by restoring greater uniformity of healthy tissue architecture and function, or, by adding further to the heterogeneity, enhance any arrhythmic tendency and increase the risk of arrhythmias. Alternatively, it may be suggested that transplanted cells not thought to become incorporated electrically, may act to isolate preexisting arrhythmogenic electrical pathways and circuits.

The presence of gap junctions, the membrane specializations responsible for electrical coupling of cardiac myocytes, provides the basis for the behavior of myocardium as an electromechanical syncytium. Gap junctional channel subunits are called connexons, of which connexin43 is the principle constituent protein in ventricular myocardium, tissue, and it is known that ischaemia, hypertrophy and inflammation can affect the expression of connexin43 in the cell membrane, therefore interfering with this electromechanical syncytium and electrical conduction velocity through the affected myocardium.[3-5] Gap junctional cell-to-cell coupling between native (possible healthy and diseased) cardiac myocytes and transplanted cells, which may or may not express connexin43, would be expected to be fundamental to the resulting electromechanical function and arrhythmic tendency.

Myocardial stretch secondary to left ventricular dilatation can also generate electrical instability by affecting the function of ionic channels in the cell membrane. If transplanted cells can alter left ventricular remodeling and reduce wall stress, it could reduce arrhythmic tendency.

What must also be considered is that the injections itself can induce transitory inflammatory response and facilitate the occurrence of arrhythmic episodes.[6] Also, the media used for culture or cell transportation might also elicit an immune response after intramyocardial injection and induce inflammation and ventricular arrhythmias.[7]

3. *Invitro* Studies

3.1. *Action Potential Characterization*

Of the few studies have focused on electrophysiologic aspects of progenitor cells *in vitro*, embryonic cells are the most commonly studied. Zang et al.[8] showed that cultured pluripotent embryonic stem cell and embryonal carcinoma cells extracted from rats can differentiate into at least three different types of action potential indicative of atrial, nodal and ventricular-like cells. These cells characteristically had prolonged action potential duration and triggered arrhythmia could be easily induced by both early and late afterdepolarization. Jia-Qiang He et al.[9] showed very similar results with human embryonic stem cells. It is not known if any change in the electrophysiologic properties of these cells can take place after their interaction with the host tissue. These results, however, raise concern about the potential arrhythmogenicity of these cells.

3.2. *Engraftment and Electromechanical Incorporation: Cell-to-Cell Coupling*

The identification of viable transplanted cells in an injected area is enough to demonstrate engraftment but it does not necessarily represent the presence of electrical interaction with the host tissue. Cell-to-cell coupling is essential to have electromechanical incorporation of the transplanted cells; therefore adequate expression of connexins would appear necessary to form gap junctions. Intrinsic expression of connexin43 is extremely variable between the different types of progenitor cells.

Clinical and experimental studies have shown that autologous skeletal myoblasts can engraft in ischemic tissue and improve cardiac function.[10,11]

However, this type of cell is able to express connexin43 only in its early myoblast stage of development, losing this capacity through the transformation to myotube, and then myocyte.[9,12] It has been suggested that this property of skeletal myoblasts is causative of ventricular arrhythmias in clinical trials, but this is entirely unproven.[6,9,12]

By contrast, Rubart et al.,[13] using syngeneic mice, elegantly demonstrated that donor fetal cardiomyocytes can couple with the host myocardium after transplantation. This author described the presence of calcium transients in the donor myocardium, synchronous with neighboring host tissue, which can be considered reliable evidence of formation of a functional syncytium. Ruhparwar et al.[14] showed morphological and functional integration of transplanted fetal canine atrial cardiomyocytes (including sinus node cells) into the free wall of the left ventricle of adult canines. The author could demonstrate the presence of ventricular escape rhythm after ablation of atrioventricular node and electrophysiological mapping showed that the escape rhythm was originated at the site of injections. Histological analysis revealed expression of connexin43 by the transplanted cells. These studies support the evidence that transplanted cells of some origins can interact electrically with the host myocardium.

4.   Initial Lessons from Clinical Trials

Several studies in cell therapy have been conducted worldwide, mostly related to efficacy and safety of the use of autologous skeletal myoblasts and bone marrow derived stem cells. The use of autologous cells is preferable for not requiring use of immunosuppression and lack of risk of transmitting infectious diseases. For legal and ethic reasons, the use of embryonic cells has been restricted to preclinical studies.

In the study by Menasche et al.,[6] varying doses of autologous skeletal myoblasts were injected in the epicardial surface of infarcted hearts concomitant to coronary artery bypass surgery. The results show promising indications of improved cardiac function. However, four patients presented with ventricular tachycardia after 11 to 22 days of postoperative period. The mechanism of these arrhythmic events is not clear but it may relate to poor electromechanical incorporation of transplanted cells into host myocardium, generating areas of conduction slowing and block, or it could be related to the trauma of the injections themselves, inducing healing and an inflammatory response. It is interesting to notice that these events did not recur after several months of follow-up, suggesting the existence of a window of arrhythmic potential following the cell injections.

Wollert et al.[15] studied the effects of intracoronary transfer of autologous bone marrow cells in patients after acute myocardial infarction and successful percutaneous coronary intervention (BOOST trial). The cells were infused in the treated coronary artery four to eight days after the percutaneous revascularization. The main focus of the study was on cardiac function but safety aspects related to arrhythmogenesis were also included, and this is the only clinical trial in cell therapy in which programmed ventricular stimulation has been performed at follow-up. More than 90% of the population agreed to undergo electrophysiologic study and no difference in inducibility of ventricular arrhythmias was found between control and treated groups, with induction of non-sustained ventricular tachycardia in one patient from each group and ventricular fibrillation in one patient in control group. Holter analysis was performed before discharge, at six weeks, three months and six months follow-up, and no difference was noted between groups with regard to number of premature ventricular complexes per hour and number of episodes of non-sustained ventricular tachycardia.

In the study by Schachinger et al.,[16] intracoronary injections of either circulating progenitor cells or bone marrow derived progenitor cells after acute myocardial infarction (TOPCARE-AMI trial) was shown to have favorable effects on left ventricular remodeling after one-year follow up. It was considered safe from the arrhythmic standpoint despite little monitoring of these patients, restricted to telemetry during the first 24 hours after the cell injections and Holter analysis 12 months later in only 80% of the population. It must be emphasized, though, that no patient had symptoms compatible with ventricular arrhythmia and no episode of sudden death was registered during follow-up.

Perin et al.[17] performed intramyocardial injections of autologous bone marrow-derived mononuclear cells, guided by electromechanical mapping (NOGA system), in patients with severe ischemic left ventricular dysfunction and were ineligible for surgical or percutaneous myocardial revascularization. The authors described improvement in cardiac function and no occurrence of arrhythmias monitored by Holter analysis at two, six and 12 months. This is the only study that used signal average electrocardiogram (SAECG), which would indicate the presence of areas in the ventricles of slow conduction and no difference was observed during the follow-up, indicating that no new area of slow conduction was created after the cell injections.

Most of these studies were performed as a combination of cell transplantation and coronary artery bypass grafting. It remains difficult to confirm whether any findings were secondary to the surgical revascularization, to cell transplantation or a combination of both.

5. Arrhythmia Assessment: Determining the Gold Standard

The interpretation of data related to cardiac arrhythmias is a challenge. Firstly, it is important to acknowledge that while enrollment to cell therapy trials remains restricted to patients with significant LV dysfunction, the occurrence of ventricular arrhythmias may simply represent the natural history of the underlying disease, and is not necessarily related to the cell therapy. Secondly, the tools commonly used to evaluate the risk of arrhythmias (ambulatory ECG monitoring, programmed stimulation, SAECG, microvolt T-wave alternans) are not adequately sensitive to provide definitive grading of arrhythmic risk.

In the era of the implantable cardioverter-defibrillator (ICD), and in an attempt to improve patient selection for the device, the question of the best way to predict patients at major risk of arrhythmia has been constantly raised. Lessons learned from ICD trials show that, although programmed ventricular stimulation can be safely performed, its sensitivity and specificity is limited, and indicative principally of reentrant arrhythmogenesis. It has been observed that patients with no inducible arrhythmias at programmed stimulation had a higher number of ICD therapy for ventricular fibrillation (which is typically not related to reentrant mechanism) when compared to patients with induced ventricular tachycardia.[2] The sensitivity of programmed ventricular stimulation in predicting future events is less than 5% in non-coronary cause of heart failure and it declines with the progression of the heart disease.[18] Nonetheless, electrophysiologic testing may still have a role in identifying modification of reentrant arrhythmogenesis after cell transplantation in the phase of adequately powered randomized multicenter clinical studies of cell transplantation.

The Holter system provides information about occurrence of spontaneous arrhythmias. However, it is known that the occurrence of ectopic beats and sustained or non-sustained ventricular arrhythmias can vary significantly on a daily basis. Therefore, the sporadic monitoring may not reflect the actual prevalence of arrhythmic episodes and continuous monitoring is not practical for long periods of time in clinical studies. It is known that patients with previous myocardial infarction with frequent episodes of non-sustained ventricular tachycardia have an increased risk of sudden cardiac death.[19] However, there is no information about the prognostic value of spontaneous arrhythmias after cell injections. These episodes, if present, can represent only a transitory electrical instability related to the engraftment or can be simply related to inflammatory or healing response to the injections itself, with no prognostic implication in a long term. Since the biological substrate is being modified in a dynamic fashion, it will be necessary to revisit the concepts of arrhythmic risk stratification in the realm of cell therapy.

Once the arrhythmic issue became apparent, the use of implantable cardioverter-defibrillator was established as mandatory in some clinical studies, especially those involving the use of autologous myoblast transplantation. Having ICDs in situ presents the advantage of combining diagnostic and therapeutic features-records from arrhythmic events can be retrieved from the memory of these devices for diagnostic purposes after appropriate therapeutic shock has been applied. Large randomized studies may enable addressing the arrhythmic question from the stored ICD data, but previous large studies of these devices have illustrated the pitfalls in this approach, since the "uncertainty principal" dictates that ICD therapies interfere with the prognostic implication of any particular arrhythmic episode. In that the clinical profile of candidates for cell transplantation will clearly overlap almost completely with the criteria for prophylactic ICD implantation (as per the MADIT II study), it is difficult to envision a clinical setting in which any patient will receive cell therapy without also having an ICD.

6.   Future Directions

Despite the promising results obtained in the preclinical and early phase clinical studies, it is imperative to have better characterization of transplanted cells with respect to their electrophysiolgical incorporation and optimization of electromechanical functioning before clinical use in large scale.

The normal heart has a complex variety of regionally distinct electrophysiological properties. Cardiac myocytes showing inherent automaticity are responsible for pacemaker, Purkinje fibers have distinct action potentials and rapid conduction velocity, and three different types of action potential can be found in the left ventricular wall, from endocardial to epicardial cells, going through the mid portion of the wall (M cells). Ideally, the electrical properties of the transplanted cells should match the ones of the recipient area. In this way, it may be possible to replace specific structures of the heart using cells with the appropriate properties, such as intrinsic automaticity for sinus node disease or rapidly conducting Purkinje-type cells to resynchronize the ventricles in case of bundle branch block. Whether the appropriate conditions and cell treatment can promote transdifferentiation of the implanted cells to match the electromechanical properties of the host myocardium at the site of implantation, and whether this change would be desirable or simply additive to the electrophysiological instability, remains to be seen.

7.   References

1. Levy D, Kenchaiah S, Larson MG et al. Long-term trends in the incidence of and survival with heart failure. *N Engl J Med*. 2002;347:1397–1402.
2. Moss AJ. MADIT-I and MADIT-II. *J Cardiovasc Electrophysiol*. 2003;14:S96-S98.
3. Yao JA, Hussain W, Patel P et al. Remodeling of gap junctional channel function in epicardial border zone of healing canine infarcts. *Circ Res*. 2003;92:437–443.
4. Peters NS, Coromilas J, Severs NJ et al. Disturbed connexin43 gap junction distribution correlates with the location of reentrant circuits in the epicardial border zone of healing canine infarcts that cause ventricular tachycardia. *Circulation*. 1997;95:988–996.
5. Peters NS, Green CR, Poole-Wilson PA et al. Reduced content of connexin43 gap junctions in ventricular myocardium from hypertrophied and ischemic human hearts. *Circulation*. 1993;88:864–875.

6. Menasche P, Hagege AA, Vilquin JT et al. Autologous skeletal myoblast transplantation for severe postinfarction left ventricular dysfunction. *J Am Coll Cardiol.* 2003;41:1078–1083.
7. Chachques JC, Herreros J, Trainini J et al. Autologous human serum for cell culture avoids the implantation of cardioverter-defibrillators in cellular cardiomyoplasty. *Int J Cardiol.* 2004;95 Suppl 1:S29–S33.
8. Zhang YM, Hartzell C, Narlow M et al. Stem cell-derived cardiomyocytes demonstrate arrhythmic potential. *Circulation.* 2002;106:1294–1299.
9. He JQ, Ma Y, Lee Y et al. Human embryonic stem cells develop into multiple types of cardiac myocytes: action potential characterization. *Circ Res.* 2003;93:32–39.
10. Dib N, Diethrich EB, Campbell A et al. Endoventricular transplantation of allogenic skeletal myoblasts in a porcine model of myocardial infarction. *J Endovasc Ther.* 2002;9:313–319.
11. Scorsin M, Hagege A, Vilquin JT et al. Comparison of the effects of fetal cardiomyocyte and skeletal myoblast transplantation on postinfarction left ventricular function. *J Thorac Cardiovasc Surg.* 2000;119:1169–1175.
12. Reinecke H, MacDonald GH, Hauschka SD et al. Electromechanical coupling between skeletal and cardiac muscle. Implications for infarct repair. *J Cell Biol.* 2000;149:731–740.
13. Rubart M, Pasumarthi KB, Nakajima H et al. Physiological coupling of donor and host cardiomyocytes after cellular transplantation. *Circ Res.* 2003;92:1217–1224.
14. Ruhparwar A, Tebbenjohanns J, Niehaus M et al. Transplanted fetal cardiomyocytes as cardiac pacemaker. *Eur J Cardiothorac Surg.* 2002;21:853–857.
15. Wollert KC, Meyer GP, Lotz J et al. Intracoronary autologous bone-marrow cell transfer after myocardial infarction: the BOOST randomised controlled clinical trial. *Lancet.* 2004;364:141–148.
16. Schachinger V, Assmus B, Britten MB et al. Transplantation of progenitor cells and regeneration enhancement in acute myocardial infarction: final one-year results of the TOPCARE-AMI Trial. *J Am Coll Cardiol.* 2004;44:1690–1699.
17. Perin EC, Dohmann HF, Borojevic R et al. Improved exercise capacity and ischemia 6 and 12 months after transendocardial injection of autologous bone marrow mononuclear cells for ischemic cardiomyopathy. *Circulation.* 2004;110:II213–II218.
18. Stevenson WG, Epstein LM. Predicting sudden death risk for heart failure patients in the implantable cardioverter-defibrillator age. *Circulation.* 2003;107:514–516.
19. Huikuri HV, Makikallio TH, Raatikainen MJ et al. Prediction of sudden cardiac death: appraisal of the studies and methods assessing the risk of sudden arrhythmic death. *Circulation.* 2003;108:110–115.

Regulatory Perspective

20

Regulatory Considerations in Manufacturing, Product Testing, and Preclinical Development of Cellular Products for Cardiac Repair

ELLEN AREMAN, KIM BENTON AND RICHARD MCFARLAND[*]

1. Introduction

In the US, administration of cellular products for cardiac repair remains investigational, and must be conducted under an Investigational New Drug application (IND) that has been reviewed and allowed to proceed by the Food and Drug Administration (FDA). The Office of Cellular, Tissue, and Gene Therapies (OCTGT) in the Center for Biologics Evaluation and Research (CBER), US Food and Drug Administration (FDA), has review responsibilities for cellular products. Because no catheters have yet been approved for delivery of cellular products to the myocardium or coronary circulation, all catheters are considered investigational when used for these purposes. The review of catheters for these investigational uses is performed by the Center for Devices and Radiological Health (CDRH) concurrently with the IND review.

The successful initiation of a clinical trial with an investigational cellular therapy for cardiac repair requires not just a thorough knowledge of clinical medicine and clinical trial design, but also a working knowledge of the other disciplines inherent to prudent product development for any cellular therapy, namely manufacturing and preclinical testing. Frequently, academic cardiologists with previous experience as clinical investigators, but limited experience in the manufacturing or preclinical testing aspects of product development, serve as the sponsor-investigators for trials of cellular therapies for cardiac repair. A sponsor-investigator must fulfill the obligations of both the sponsor and investigator under the IND regulations (21 CFR 312). The

---

[*]Richard McFarland, Ph.D, M.D., FDA/CBER/OCTGT, 1401 Rockville Pike, HFM-760, Rockville, MD 20852. E-mail: mcfarlandr@cber.fda.gov

role of the sponsor includes ultimate responsibility for all aspects of the clinical investigation, including manufacturing and preclinical testing. This chapter will outline the current expectations for product manufacturing controls for the different types of cellular products under investigation, general product testing requirements and expectations, and general design characteristics for preclinical studies capable of generating a sufficient safety database to permit clinical trials of cellular products for cardiac repair to proceed.

2.   Product Manufacturing and Testing

2.1.   Product Considerations for Cardiac Cellular Therapies

Whether the mechanism of the cells involved in repair of cardiac damage is cardiomyocyte generation/regeneration, angiogenesis/revascularization, production of cytokines or other secreted factors, or a combination of these actions, is still being explored. Until these mechanisms are elucidated, many types of cells, alone or in combination, and prepared by a variety of methods will be candidates for clinical trials in the US and worldwide.

The FDA evaluates the data submitted in INDs to determine if an adequate safety profile has been demonstrated to support the administration of a given cellular product to human subjects. From the initiation of clinical investigation, product safety is the primary concern. During manufacturing, safety is ensured through the implementation of and adherence to a controlled process, combined with testing of the cellular product, before administration to subjects. Investigators must demonstrate that all devices and materials used for processing or administration of the cellular product are compatible with the cell suspension components; a subject that will be discussed further in the section on preclinical studies.

In addition to safety, parameters of product characterization such as the source, phenotype, purity, number and proliferative potential of the cells should be considered early in product development to anticipate issues that may become important in the translation and scale-up from an investigational to a licensed product. For example, a cell number equivalent to an effective murine dose may be impossible to achieve for a human recipient. Purification and selection of specific cell types based on phenotypic markers may be problematic until the time that the actual mechanisms and associated cellular phenotypes affecting cardiac function are known. In addition, interaction of two or more cell populations may be necessary for optimal therapeutic benefit. Product characterization is encouraged from the initiation of early clinical trials to determine product safety, and increases in importance as subsequent trials are conducted to evaluate product efficacy. Appropriate identity and potency tests must also be developed and validated so that if and when the product is shown to be safe and effective, each commercial lot of that product can be properly tested to assure its safety, purity and potency.

2.2.   Sources and Collection of Cellular Products for Cardiac Repair

2.2.1.   Bone Marrow-Derived Cellular Products

2.2.1a   Hematopoietic Progenitor Cells (HPCs)

Pluripotent HPCs capable of restoring hematopoiesis in a myeloablated individual are found in the marrow cavities of the bones. These cells may also be capable of repopulating other tissues and organs in the body, including damaged myocardium.[1] These HPCs can be identified by expression of CD34, a surface glycophosphoprotein appearing on 2-4% of normal bone marrow cells. Another surface marker, CD133, is expressed on a subset of CD34[+] cells including immature myeloid and monocytic progenitors.[3] The exact functions of these molecules are not yet well defined, although there is some evidence that CD34 is involved in cell adhesion and migration. CD133 is expressed not only on CD34[+] hematopoietic stem and progenitor cells, but also on endothelial progenitors and some CD34[-]negative nonhematopoietic progenitors, such as neural stem cells, embryonic stem cell lines, and adult pluripotent stem cells (MAPC). If administered to the heart vessels or tissue, these undifferentiated cells may have the potential to differentiate *in vivo* into angioblasts and/or cardiomyocytes[1] or into cells that produce factors instrumental in restoring function to damaged myocardium.[3]

These HPCs can be collected directly from the bone marrow, from the peripheral blood of hematopoietic growth factor-mobilized individuals, and from umbilical cord blood. Cellular products composed of HPCs will vary in cell number and phenotype due to inherent variability in donors and source tissue, as well as differences in the processing that is performed. Although some investigators administer unfractionated bone marrow to the heart immediately after collection and filtration, the products usually undergo additional processing steps to yield a more homogeneous preparation. This processing may consist of one or more of the following procedures: concentration, isolation, immunomagnetic selection, culture expansion or differentiation, and cryopreservation. The classic method of recovering mononuclear cells from a heterogeneous bone marrow harvest is a post-filtration isolation procedure in which the diluted bone marrow is layered on a density gradient medium such as Ficoll-Hypaque. After centrifugation the light-density cell layer is harvested. However, although large numbers of red blood cells and neutrophils are removed, the remaining cell suspension still contains an assortment of diverse cell populations at various levels of development. In addition, even though the cellular material is processed under aseptic conditions, the procedure is not performed in a totally closed system. Therefore there is some risk of microbial contamination from environmental sources.

Hematopoietic progenitor cells can also be mobilized from the bone marrow into the peripheral blood by administration of a recombinant human growth factor, such as granulocyte colony-stimulating factor (rhG-CSF).

Cells are then collected by a leukapheresis (apheresis) procedure using a con-tinuous flow cell separator and a citrate-based anticoagulant. The apheresis process permits harvesting of a light-density mononuclear cell population from circulating blood, while reinfusing most of the donor's red blood cells, neutrophils, platelets and plasma. Using this technique, as many as 4 times the volume of the donor's blood can be processed for optimal recovery of HPCs with minimum loss of other blood components. Growth factor-mobilized peripheral blood, like bone marrow, contains a variety of cell populations, although in different proportions. HPC products collected by apheresis do not require density gradient separation, as the apheresis procedure itself pref-erentially collects mononuclear cells such as lymphocytes and monocytes as well as HPCs.

Umbilical cord blood (UCB) is another source of hematopoietic and endothelial cell progenitors and is just beginning to be explored as a cellular therapy for cardiac repair.[4] Because these cells can be collected, processed, tested, cryopreserved and stored in advance, they are a potential source of readily available HLA-matched allogeneic progenitor cells.

Hematopoietic stem and progenitor cells from any of these sources can be further purified by immunomagnetic selection using monoclonal antibodies to the progenitor cell antigens (CD34 or CD133) and paramagnetic micros-pheres, resulting in a highly enriched progenitor cell product. Use of these selection systems to manufacture cells for cardiovascular therapy is currently investigational and requires an IND for use in clinical trials.

2.2.1b   Endothelial Progenitor Cells (EPCs)

The source (or sources) of EPCs required for new blood vessel formation in damaged myocardial tissue is still not entirely clear. Expression of the CD34 and CD133 antigens suggests that they may be derived from hematopoietic progenitors or from an earlier progenitor common to HPCs and EPCs. Endothelial cells (EC) have also been generated from umbilical cord blood,[5] from CD14+/CD34– myeloid cells[6] and from non-hematopoietic mesenchy-mal stem cells (MSC).[7]

2.2.1c   Mesenchymal Stem Cells (MSCs)

MSCs can be grown from non-hematopoietic stromal cells from bone mar-row and can be induced to differentiate into a cardiomyogenic cell type under appropriate culture conditions.[8] They can then be expanded, treated with enzymes, pooled and cryopreserved. Cells from allogeneic donors can be stored as cell banks, aliquots of which can be used to prepare individual MSC products. The cells are reportedly easy to culture and can be cryopreserved, making them available for immediate administration after myocardial infarction.[9] There is some evidence that these cells lack the immunogenicity found in allogeneic hematopoietic progenitor cells, and may, therefore, permit administration without the need for the immune suppression normally required for successful transplantation of allogeneic grafts.[1]

To participate in the regeneration of cardiac function, bone marrow-derived cells must be able to participate in a variety of activities not usually associated with their tissue of origin including revascularization, muscle regeneration, and electrical conduction. Although the marrow-derived cells described above may not normally perform these functions, they can be induced to expand and differentiate into a variety of cell types when cultured *ex vivo* with cytokines and growth factors.[10] For example, unfractionated bone marrow cells, which do not normally secrete measurable amounts of vascular endothelial growth factor (VEGF), can do so after 4 weeks in culture,[11] indicating the existence of a cell population with the potential to facilitate angiogenesis when introduced into myocardium.

2.2.2. Muscle-Derived Cellular Products

Because skeletal muscle is easily obtained from biopsy material, and contains muscle precursor cells (myoblasts or satellite cells) that proliferate in culture and are capable of regeneration, this tissue was an early candidate for a source of cells for cardiac repair. *In vitro* studies have shown that these myoblasts can take on the characteristics and functions of cardiomyocytes.[9] The cell suspension is usually prepared from quadriceps muscle biopsies, and the cells isolated from the tissue are expanded in culture with growth factors until the desired cell number is reached.[12]

2.2.3. Embryo-Derived Cellular Products

Embryonic stem cells, derived from the inner cell mass of early embryos, have the potential to expand and differentiate into large numbers of cardiomyocytes. If it were possible to direct and control the differentiation and growth of these cells *in vitro*, they would be likely candidates for study as a cellular therapy for cardiac repair.[9]

2.2.4. Tissue Stem Cells

Adult stem cells in various tissues are potential sources of regenerative cell populations. For example, cells capable of differentiating into endothelial cells have recently been isolated from cardiac tissue.[13] Adipose (fat) tissue[14] and lipoaspirates[15] contain a variety of multipotent progenitor cells that could be isolated from autologous donors and administered to injured myocardium.

2.3.   Testing of Cellular Products for Cardiac Repair

Regardless of the type of product and the manufacturing process, a variety of parameters must be evaluated by adequate and appropriate testing to ensure administration of a safe product.

2.3.1. Infectious Disease Testing

Although most cellular products currently used in clinical trials for cardiac repair are autologous, other allogeneic cell types such as bone marrow, mobilized peripheral blood and umbilical cord blood are being explored. In accordance with the donor eligibility rule [21 CFR 1271.1(a)] allogeneic donors, including the mothers of umbilical cord blood donors, must be tested and screened for communicable diseases. Testing and screening of autologous donors for infectious diseases, although not required, is recommended, particularly if there is a risk that the processing could expand any infectious disease agents present in the source material.

2.3.2. Microbiological Safety

Many of the cellular preparations used in clinical trials for cardiac repair are collected, processed, and administered in a matter of hours. Processes should be designed to minimize the risk of microbial contamination and appropriate product testing should be performed on each lot of the cellular product to ensure its safety for clinical use. Those products collected and processed in systems that are open or partially open to the environment are at the greatest risk for contamination with adventitious agents. Strict aseptic processing techniques must be employed when working with these products, using sterile disposable materials and reagents. Whenever possible, manufacturing steps should be performed in a system that is closed and protected from sources of possible contamination. Devices are available that provide sterile welds of transfer tubing so that cellular products can be transferred from container to container without breaking the sterile product pathway.

Because many of these products are stored for a few hours, at most, between preparation and administration, it is not possible to complete conventional 14-day microbial safety testing. Therefore, Gram staining or newer and more sensitive rapid tests for microbial detection should be performed and reported as negative before issuing the product. In addition, sterility cultures should still be performed on samples of the final product, results monitored, and positive results reported promptly. Even with the use of aseptic techniques, microbiological cultures may become positive days after the recipient has received the product. Therefore, each study must include a comprehensive action plan for physician and patient notification, patient monitoring (and treatment, if necessary), organism identification, and investigation of contamination source, should a positive culture of an infused product be reported. Cryopreservation and storage of products for at least 14 days permits availability of final sterility culture results prior to administration.

Depending on the way the cells are processed in preparation for administration, other testing may be required to ensure that the product has not been exposed to microbial agents. If manipulations are performed in a system that is open to the environment, the final product should be tested for the presence of endotoxin. Even without contamination of the final cellular product with live bacteria, endotoxin can be introduced into the product in various ways and pose a serious risk to the recipient. Ancillary materials that are used in the collection, processing, or formulation of cells should be documented to be free of endotoxin and pyrogens.

For cellular products that are expanded or otherwise cultured, a test for the presence of mycoplasma should be performed at the end of the culture period. To maximize detection of potential contamination, we recommend obtaining samples containing both culture supernatants and cells prior to final wash procedures. Ancillary materials such as bovine sera should be documented to be free of mycoplasma.

2.3.3. Cell Dose and Viability

The cell dose of each lot should be accurately measured and its viability determined for product safety and consistency. The most popular viability assays make use of the live cells' ability to exclude a nuclear stain or dye to enable discrimination of live and dead cells. Detection systems are available using bright light and fluorescent microscopy as well as flow cytometry. The FDA generally recommend that the manufacturing process maintain viability of at least 70% of total cells, unless data are available that support a lower criterion. *In vitro* testing of the cellular product in conjunction with the delivery system that will be used for the infusion should be part of the preclinical product development process. This testing should show, at a minimum, that the initial cell number and viability are not significantly reduced by passage through the catheter.

2.3.4. Product Characterization

Few if any of the products currently in clinical trials consist of a pure population of well-characterized cells. Even those preparations prepared by immunoselection with CD34 or CD133 monoclonal antibodies may contain as many as 50% contaminating cells of various phenotypes. Some or all of these other cell populations may be important to the success or failure of a particular cellular preparation and investigations of cellular therapies for cardiac repair should explore methods of identifying and quantifying the cell populations in each type of product. *In vitro* analysis of such features as immunophenotype, viability, proliferative potential, colony formation, cytokine production, gene and protein expression, and morphology can help determine whether certain cells in a heterogeneous population may have a positive or negative effect on the therapeutic product. Although some characteristics of these cells may be altered when placed in the cardiac environment, investigators need to find or develop assays that can correlate safety and efficacy with specific *in vitro* product characteristics. Once these characteristics can be identified and quantified using available and reproducible assays, then product specifications should be developed for use as product release criteria.

2.3.4a   Product Identity

Because most of the cellular products in development for cardiac therapy are prepared for a specific recipient, it is critical that the identity of the product be confirmed before it is issued and administered. Whether autologous or allogeneic, the product may undergo a variety of manipulations, some or all of which may be performed by different manufacturing personnel in different locations. In addition, cellular products for more than one patient may be in process at the same time. Therefore the product in its final form must be tested by an assay that will distinguish it from other products prepared in the facility as well as adequately identifying it as the product designated on the container label. Immunophenotyping and molecular histocompatibility typing are some of the techniques used in identity testing.

2.3.4b   Product Potency

As product development progresses and cellular products for use in cardiac repair become better defined and characterized, an assay or combination of assays that demonstrate product potency must be implemented. An assay or group of assays should be designed to demonstrate that the cellular product possesses biologic activity indicative of its intended effect.

2.3.4c   Product Purity

The type(s) of purity testing that should be developed and performed on cellular products for cardiac repair will depend on the nature of the product, the manufacturing process, and the ancillary materials used. For example, if immunogenic or toxic materials are used in collection or processing, their removal by washing or other steps must be validated. Alternatively, testing must be developed and performed on each lot to demonstrate safe levels for administration.

2.4.   *Product Testing During Clinical Development*

In all investigational phases and post licensure, product safety testing must be performed on each lot of cellular product. Testing and screening of allogeneic donors should be performed. Microbiological safety testing is necessary to ensure administration of a sterile product. Endotoxin and/or mycoplasma testing should be performed if the manufacturing process uses an open system or culture step, respectively, or otherwise presents risks of contamination. The cell dose and viability should be measured to ensure safety and consistency.

The requirements for additional product characterization and testing are dependent on the risks posed by the cellular product and route of administration, and also on the stage of clinical investigation. In general, purity, identity, and potency testing of each lot are recommended from early phases but fully validated assays are not required until phase 3 clinical trials. The development and implementation of testing for these parameters in early phases will allow the investigator to obtain data that will be useful for establishing release criteria for pivotal clinical trials.

3.   Preclinical Studies

3.1.   General Toxicological Principles as Applied to Cellular Products

Preclinical data derived from *in vitro* experiments, bench testing, and *in vivo* animal models can support the safety and suggest potential benefits of innovative therapies. Cellular products are complex and preclude a standard design of preclinical studies, as sponsors might use in the development of small molecule pharmaceuticals. The major sources of a cellular product's complexity include: the inherent biological heterogeneity (in terms of both phenotypic and functional characteristics), potential safety concerns posed by novel routes of administration, cell-device interactions, and the effects of an immune response to the product.

Studies performed in animal models of disease provide insight regarding dose/activity and dose/toxicity relationships. Standard animal models of disease are frequently modified to generate the preclinical toxicity data needed for regulatory decisions on trials of cellular therapies. The key design modification needed to ensure the collection of sufficient safety data is the inclusion of endpoints in studies to collect sufficient toxicology data to support the proposed clinical trial. These endpoints will vary depending on the animal models used, the product tested, and the clinical trial design, but generally include, at a minimum, routine clinical chemistry, cardiac enzymes, hematology, in-life observations, and full necropsy. In addition to providing toxicity data, preclinical studies may provide useful data regarding a cellular product's mechanism of action by collecting data on a product's effects on cardiac function, electrical activity, and histology. Knowledge of a product's mechanism of action that is acquired in preclinical trials can be beneficial in the design and conduct of the clinical trials. It can guide clinical trial design in terms of mirroring dosing regimens, clinical monitoring modalities and monitoring intervals as well as inform critical product quality parameters such as potency. Without detailed preclinical studies, clinical trial design decisions are frequently based on hypotheses supported largely by *in vitro* data, limited animal studies, and/or anecdotal clinical experience. Early phase clinical trial design can be constrained by inadequate preclinical testing of the investigational product.

The desire to obtain *in vivo* preclinical data on products that are composed of human cells poses a particular complication, as these cells are xenogeneic to all animal species, and therefore at risk for xenotransplant rejection. The immunological reactions to the human product in animals often necessitate that preclinical studies be performed with animal cellular products that are analogous to the intended clinical product, rather than the actual human product. The determination that a specific animal cell is analogous is often made on the basis of similar phenotype, ontogeny, or function. Ideally this determination would be multifaceted and involve not just *in vitro* measures of cell identity, but also detailed understanding of the *in vivo* activity of both the animal analog and putative human correlate cell. This approach is similar to an approach that is frequently used during preclinical testing of monoclonal antibodies directed against epitopes expressed only in humans, a situation in which an immune response or lack of an applicable epitope limit the adequacy of the clinical product in the preclinical model. Implicit in the use of analogous animal cells as a means to assess biological activity and/or safety of a human cellular product is the assumption that cells from the two species will respond sufficiently similarly to provide data from which to make a risk/benefit analysis. The degree of understanding of the relationship between an animal cell and its human correlate is an important factor in determining the strength of the extrapolations from findings in animals to human risk assessment.

3.2. Preclinical Testing of Cellular Products for Cardiac Repair

Most, if not all, cellular products presently in clinical trials for cardiac repair can be traced to either of two major sites of origin: bone marrow (hematopoietic and mesenchymal lineages) or skeletal muscle. The manufacturing processes of the harvested cells to produce the ultimate cellular products for administration represent a very broad range of processes as described above. Several routes of administration are presently under experimentation, namely (1) direct, syringe-and-needle injection of cellular products through the exposed epicardial surface into the subjacent myocardium during concomitant thoracic surgery; (2) infusion of cellular products into coronary arteries; and (3) intramyocardial injection of cell suspensions through cardiac catheters. The diversity inherent in the combination of a specific cellular product, route of administration and clinical indication results in an extensive array of combinational possibilities. Each of these possibilities presents a somewhat different spectrum of pharmacological opportunities, toxicological concerns, and regulatory challenges. Insufficient information exists in the published literature to serve as the sole basis for allowing clinical trials to proceed due to the multitude of specific combinations that are possible, the novelty of both the investigational cellular products and catheters, and the variability in their activity and interactions.

4.   Advisory Committee Discussions and Recommendations

In order to provide a venue for public discussion and advice to the FDA concerning the manufacturing, preclinical and clinical issues involved with cellular therapies for cardiac disease, the FDA CBER OCTGT convened its advisory committee, the Biological Response Modifiers Advisory Committee (BRMAC; hereafter referred to as the 'Committee') on March 18th-19th, 2004. The minutes, transcript, and additional materials from this meeting are available on the CBER website.[16] Much of the discussion involved the state of research in the field and the characteristics of the preclinical studies that should be included in an IND application. The Committee generally agreed that it is critical to perform preclinical safety studies with each specific cellular therapy prior to initiating clinical studies. However, the Committee also agreed that there is no single species that can serve as a sole model for generation of data to support clinical trials of cellular therapies for cardiac diseases. In light of these conclusions, the Committee recommended a conservative approach to clinical studies of cellular products for cardiac diseases that includes both *in vitro* and *in vivo* preclinical studies prior to initiation of clinical trials. Although recognizing that data from varied models and sources, including the published literature, could be combined in an IND application to support a particular clinical trial, the Committee recommended that investigators perform studies in large animal models of disease that mimic the clinical situation as closely as possible. Given the novelty of the therapeutic approaches and the inherent risks to subjects, the Committee agreed that requiring such large animal studies to support a clinical trial would not be unreasonable.

4.1.   Small Animal Models

However, it was also suggested that small animal models (e.g., immunocompromised rodents) can provide information regarding the ability of the human cellular product to target the myocardium, as well as insight into potential safety issues. These models provide the ability to study the potential of cellular products to survive and transdifferentiate in the myocardium following infarction. However, they do not lend themselves to sensitive assessment of overall cardiac function or toxicities related to catheter administration of cellular products due to constraints of anatomy and physiology related mainly to body size.

4.2.   Use of in vitro Data

The Committee suggested that *in vitro* data, i.e., immunophenotype or functional assays, generated during processing and manufacture of cellular products could be taken into consideration when designing preclinical studies because of the inferences that can be made about potential activities of the cells of different immunophenotypes. These data can be used to direct the design and extent of the bench and animal testing needed to support a clinical trial.

4.3.   Catheter Testing

Quantification of the changes in viability and cell count of cellular subpopulations by passage through specific catheters during bench testing can provide insight into potential deleterious interactions between the catheter and the cellular product during clinical use, especially if the bench testing is designed to simulate the extended dwell times, infusion rates, viscosity of the cell suspension, and other conditions to be expected during suboptimal clinical administration. FDA expects data from bench testing for each unique cellular product/catheter combination prior to proceeding with a clinical trial of that combination. In addition to bench testing the Committee recommended *in vivo* testing of cellular products with experimental catheters and catheters cleared for other indications. Further, the Committee's consensus was that preclinical or clinical data derived with any specific catheter-cellular product combination cannot be broadly applied because of the numerous potentially important differences between two specific combinations that could result in significantly different performance and clinical safety concerns. In addition to the complexities related directly to the cellular product there are numerous components of catheter design that limit a broad applicability of the data. These include: (1) the potential for cytotoxicity due to interactions of the cellular product with catheter materials or due to excessive shear forces during administration through small-bore delivery lumens and (2) failure to accurately deliver the cellular product due to clogging of the catheter with cells and cellular debris, or frank engineering failure. Additionally the Committee stated that any *in vivo* model used should be sensitive to potential toxicities related to the formation of microemboli and arrhythmogenesis.

4.4.   Large Animal Models

It was generally accepted that large animal models such as pigs, sheep, and dogs can provide information on the safety and effectiveness of cellular products and the delivery systems, leading to the selection of a potentially safe starting dose for the Phase 1 clinical trial. In contrast, it was generally accepted that these data cannot be generated using small animal models due to the inability to directly test catheters for clinical use and the limited ability to monitor cardiac function. While the Committee generally endorsed the use of large animal models of ischemia to evaluate the activity and safety of cellular products following myocardial infarction, there was no consensus reached regarding the specific method that should be used to generate the ischemic myocardium in the animals. The resulting pathologies from the commonly used methods for cardiac ischemia (ligation, ameroid constriction and bead embolization) are not fully representative of the predominant mechanism of ischemia in humans, which is atherosclerotic coronary heart disease. However, these procedures are useful for modeling acute, subacute and chronic myocardial infarction in animals because they allow assessment of cellular products in ischemic microenvironments and ischemia-damaged tissues. Intramyocardial injection of cellular products may necessitate additional animal studies to explore potential factors contributing to arrhythmogenesis such as: the specific composition of the cellular product, the dose of cells (absolute cell number and volume administered), and the site of cell implantation (with respect to anatomic features such as major conduction pathways or valves and to location within a scarred, ischemic area of myocardium). Members of the Committee recognized that models for non-ischemic congestive heart failure are somewhat more limited than models of ischemic disease.

4.5. Study Duration

Although a consensus recommendation for a specific study duration in animals was not reached by the Committee, it was stressed that the preclinical data package should include studies of sufficient duration to assess both potential acute toxicities within days of product administration and potential toxicities that occur several weeks or months later, due to the biological activity of the cellular product as it resides in the myocardium. In practice a study of 6 weeks duration with an interim sacrifice is frequently used to address both acute and late effects on cardiac function. Ultimately the choice of the particular model(s) and overall preclinical study design should reflect the intended clinical situation that the data are intended to support, and are left to the investigator's discretion, although final assessment of applicability rests with FDA. Therefore early consultation with FDA to discuss applicability of a particular experimental approach is prudent.

5.   Concluding Comments

This chapter outlined the authors' current perspective on the complexities of general product testing requirements and design characteristics for preclinical studies involved in investigational use of cellular products for cardiac repair. The IND process is intended to balance the potential benefit of novel therapies to society with the need to generate data for prudent product development, to increase scientific knowledge, to protect subject safety, and to benefit the public health. This chapter represents an introduction to the regulation of these cellular products and investigator/sponsors are encouraged to contact FDA CBER OCTGT for more specific information on the conduct of clinical trials.

6.   References

1. Orlic D, Hill JM, Arai AE. Stem cells for myocardial regeneration. Circ Res. 2002 Dec 13;91(12):1092–102
2. Wognum AW, Eaves AC, Thomas TE. Identification and isolation of hematopoietic stem cells. Arch Med Res. 2003 Nov-Dec;34(6):461–75.
3. Rehman J, Li J, Orschell CM, March KL. Peripheral blood "endothelial progenitor cells" are derived from monocyte/macrophages and secrete angiogenic growth factors. Circulation. 2003 Mar 4;107(8):1164–9.
4. Hirata Y, Sata M, Motomura N, Takanashi M, Suematsu Y, Ono M, Takamoto S. Human umbilical cord blood cells improve cardiac function after myocardial infarction. Biochem Biophys Res Commun. 2005 Feb 11;327(2):609–14.
5. Murohara T, Ikeda H, Duan J, Shintani S, Sasaki K, Eguchi H, Onitsuka I, Matsui K, Imaizumi T. Transplanted cord blood-derived endothelial precursor cells augment postnatal neovascularization. J Clin Invest. 2000 Jun;105(11):1527–36.
6. Schmeisser A, Garlichs CD, Zhang H, Eskafi S, Graffy C, Ludwig J, Strasser RH, Daniel WG. Monocytes coexpress endothelial and macrophagocytic lineage markers and form cord-like structures in Matrigel under angiogenic conditions. Cardiovasc Res. 2001 Feb 16;49(3):671–80.
7. Oswald J, Boxberger S, Jorgensen B, Feldmann S, Ehninger G, Bornhauser M, Werner C. Mesenchymal stem cells can be differentiated into endothelial cells in vitro. Stem Cells. 2004;22(3):377–84.
8. Pittenger MF, Mackay AM, Beck SC, Jaiswal RK, Douglas R, Mosca JD, Moorman MA, Simonetti DW, Craig S, Marshak DR. Multilineage potential of adult human mesenchymal stem cells. Science. 1999 Apr 2;284(5411):143–7.
9. Hassink RJ, Brutel de la Riviere A, Mummery CL, Doevendans PA. Transplantation of cells for cardiac repair. J Am Coll Cardiol. 2003 Mar 5;41(5):711–7.
10. Gunsilius E, Gastl G, Petzer AL. Hematopoietic stem cells. Biomed Pharmacother. 2001 May;55(4):186–94.
11. Fuchs S, Satler LF, Kornowski R, Okubagzi P, Weisz G, Baffour R, Waksman R, Weissman NJ, Cerqueira M, Leon MB, Epstein SE. Catheter-based autologous bone marrow myocardial injection in no-option patients with advanced coronary artery disease: a feasibility study. J Am Coll Cardiol. 2003 May 21;41(10): 1721–4.
12. Pagani FD, DerSimonian H, Zawadzka A, Wetzel K, Edge AS, Jacoby DB, Dinsmore JH, Wright S, Aretz TH, Eisen HJ, Aaronson KD. Autologous skeletal myoblasts transplanted to ischemia-damaged myocardium in humans. Histological analysis of cell survival and differentiation. J Am Coll Cardiol. 2003 Mar 5;41(5):879–88
13. Beltrami AP, Barlucchi L, Torella D, Baker M, Limana F, Chimenti S, Kasahara H, Rota M, Musso E, Urbanek K, Leri A, Kajstura J, Nadal-Ginard B, Anversa P. Adult cardiac stem cells are multipotent and support myocardial regeneration. Cell. 2003 Sep 19;114(6):763–76.
14. Miranville A, Heeschen C, Sengenes C, Curat CA, Busse R, Bouloumie A. Improvement of postnatal neovascularization by human adipose tissue-derived stem cells. Circulation. 2004 Jul 20;110(3):349–55. Epub 2004 Jul 06.

15. Zuk PA, Zhu M, Mizuno H, Huang J, Futrell JW, Katz AJ, Benhaim P, Lorenz HP, Hedrick MH. Multilineage cells from human adipose tissue: implications for cell-based therapies. Tissue Eng. 2001 Apr;7(2):211–28.
16. US Food and Drug Administration. Transcripts of the meeting of the Biological Response Modifiers Advisory Committee: Discussion of Cellular Therapies of Cardiac Disease. 18-19 March 2004. Available at http://www.fda.gov/ohrms/dockets/ac/cber04.html#BiologicalResponseModifiers

Appendix:
Catheter Descriptions

Catheter Systems

1. Biocardia Helical Infusion Catheter System

BioCardia's Helical Infusion System combines two device platforms:

BioCardia's Morph® Deflectable Guide Catheter is a thin walled guide catheter that provides for single direction deflection with a tight radius of curvature with a large lumen. It is used to advance and maneuver BioCardia's Helical Infusion Catheters for local delivery as well as place other devices and delivery catheters into the arterial and venous system. This catheter has been cleared for market release by the FDA.

BioCardia's Helical Infusion Catheter is a catheter with a small hollow, distal corkscrew needle which may be rotated into tissue to provide active fixation during drug delivery, similar to the active fixation electrodes used in cardiac pacing. This catheter is under investigational use in multiple ongoing clinical trials.

This system provides a means to have fixation to the beating heart wall, uses simplified fluoroscopic imaging, crosses the aortic arch and valve safely over a guide wire with BioCardia's unique steerable guide, and provides the operator with three degrees of freedom to maximize operator control.

The Morph® Deflectable Guide Catheter can be used to steer a guide wire across the aortic valve for transendocardial delivery from within the left ventricle, and is believed to be the safest and quickest way to enter the left ventricular chamber. For transendocardial delivery the Morph® Deflectable Guide Catheter is advanced over the wire and the wire is removed to allow for advancement and navigation of the Helical Infusion Catheter.

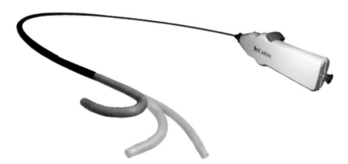

FIGURE 1. The BioCardia Morph® Deflectable Guide Catheter is a thin walled 8F guide catheter that enables significant deflection of its distal end upon pulling of a lever on the handle controlled with the thumb. This commercially available device is intended to serve as a conduit for access into the chambers and coronary vasculature and has been cleared for market release by the FDA.

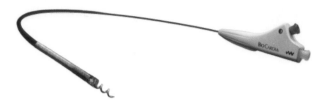

FIGURE 2. The BioCardia Helical Infusion Catheter has two fluid ports, one for therapeutic and one for contrast. These are identified by the red helix for the drug lumen and the black and white contrast droplet on the handle. The first drug port discharges through the distal tip of the helical needle. The second discharges through the base of the helix for contrast imaging.

2.   Sr200 Myocath™ Percutaneous Catheter Delivery System

The MyoCath™ Percutaneous Catheter Delivery System is indicated for assisting in the percutaneous delivery and controlled myocardial injections of biologic solutions to a desired endoventricular treatment site. It provides for multiple injections to a pre-determined needle insertion depth with a single core needle that can be advanced and retracted from the tip of the catheter. This system is an Investigational Device, limited by Federal (or United States) law to investigational use.

The MyoCath™ consists of a steerable catheter comprised of an outer shaft that encases a flexible core needle sub assembly. The flexible core needle subassembly possesses a standard, beveled needle top at its distal end and runs the full length of the catheter to serve as the injection lumen. The entire core needle subassembly can be controlled to advance and retract its needle tip from the distal end of the catheter. The radiopaque tip of the catheter serves as a marker to aid in proper positioning of the device. The steerable catheter portion of the device attaches to the proximal handle that allows the device user to both maneuver and position the catheter, as well as control the injection capabilities of the device. The handle possesses controls for the catheter tip deflection, the needle insertion depth, and needle advancement/retraction. The catheter is available in both a medium and large curvature configuration.

3.   Myostar™ Cordis-biosense Webster Needle Injection Catheter

The Myostar™ Injection Catheter, (Biosense Webster, Inc.) is a multi-electrode, percutaneous catheter with a deflectable tip and injection needle designed to inject soluble agents or cells transendocardially into the myocardium.

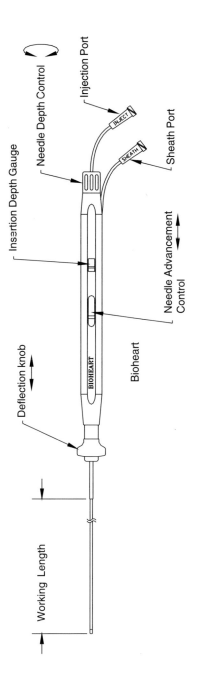

SR200 MyoCath™ Percutaneous Catheter Delivery System
Features and benefits

- Minimally invasive (8F) approach to delivering injectate in tissue
- Customized needle advancement and depth control (3mm – 6mm)
- Deflecting tip with long working length for precise injection
- Minimize exposure time and trauma to the patient

TABLE 1. Technical features and specifications

Feature	Specification
Syringe Compatibility	1cc Luer Lock
Usable Catheter Length	115 cm
Core Needle Diameter	25 gauge
Core Needle Extended Length	3-6 mm
Sheath Compatibility	8F

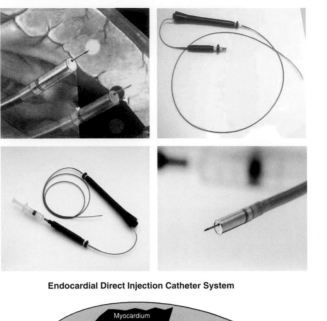

Endocardial Direct Injection Catheter System

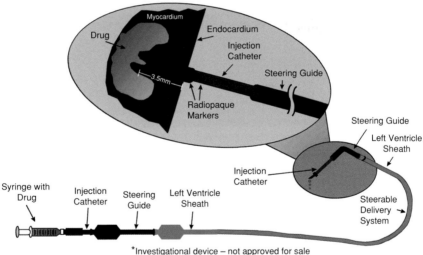

*Investigational device – not approved for sale

5. Stiletto™ Endocardial Direct Injection Catheter System (Boston Scientific Corporation)*

The tip of the Injection Catheter is equipped with a location sensor and a retractable, hollow 27-gauge nitinol needle for fluid delivery. Tip deflection is controlled at the proximal end by a tubular hand piece holding a piston and pull-wire mechanism. The high-torque shaft allows for controlled rotation of the curved tip to facilitate accurate positioning towards the desired site for agent injection. A second handle located at the proximal end of the catheter allows for controlled needle extension from the distal tip. The extended length of the needle is adjustable. The handle has a standard Luer lock fitting for connection to a syringe. The catheter interfaces with the NOGA^R 3-dimentional electromagnetic cardiac mapping system for facilitation of navigated local agent delivery into the myocardium.

4. Transaccess® Microlume™ Intramyocardial Injection System

Applications:

- Angiogenisis, myogenesis and restinosis
- Multple therapeutic agents

Venous approach:

- Accurate, stable targetıng
- Flouoroscopic guidance
- Epicardial, tangential access to myocardium
- Increased efficiency
- Reduced risk of embolization

4.1. TransAccess®

Tracks over 0.014 guide wire
Preshaped 24G Nitinol needle
6.2F catheter with integrated JOMED IVUS

4.2. MicroLume™

27G injection catheter
Delivered through TransAccess needle
Radiopaque beveled tip
Tested for compatibility with viral. Protein and cellular injectates
Single or dual lumen (dual lumen for injection site qualification)

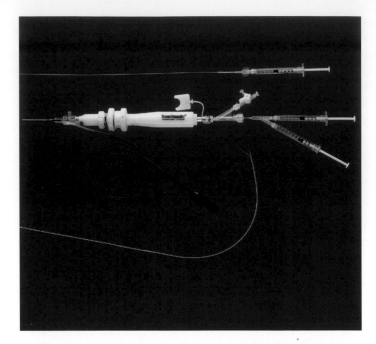

FIGURE 3. The TransAccess® MicroLume™ Intramyocardial Injection System.

Index

AC133+ cells, 87, 88, 126–127, 180
Acipimox, 261
Action potential, *in vitro* studies, 291
Acute phase treatment, MI, 196–197, 203–208
Adipose tissue cells, 128, 141, 303
Administration routes: *see* Delivery modes/routes
Adult stem cells, 122–123, 128, 303
  cardiac primitives as, 45–46
  regulatory considerations, 301
  types of cells, 124–125
Adverse effects: *see* Arrhythmias; Complications/adverse effects
Afterload, 274–275
Aging, and cardiac stem cells, 49
Algorithm, bone-marrow derived stem cell transplantation, 194
Angina, 180, 181
Angiogenesis, 16, 29–30, 180, 182
  endothelial progenitor cells, 303
  myocardial infarction sequelae, 172
  repair process, 85, 89
Angiogenesis factors, 29–30
Angiography
  bone marrow-derived stem cell transplantation, 195
  porcine model of MI, 232, 233, 235
Angiotensin coverting enzyme (ACE) inhibitors, 14–15, 178
Animal models, 17, 25–26, 101, 126–127, 307; *see also* Preclinical studies
  bone marrow-derived stem cell transplantation, 145–146, 164, 165
  delivery modes/routes, 174–175

Animal models (*cont.*)
  labeling cells, 142-145
  history of transplantation, 61–71
  PET studies, 264
  porcine model of MI, 231–238
  regulatory considerations, 307, 309
  ventricular remodeling, 5, 7, 8
Antigens, surface markers: *see* Surface markers/antigens
Aortic impedance, 275
Apheresis, 128, 302
Arrhythmias
  bone marrow-derived stem cell transplantation, 196
  electrophysiology, 289–295
    assessment, gold standard determination, 293–295
    future directions, 295
    initial lessons, 292–293
    mechanisms of arrhythmias and potential interactions with cell therapy, 290–291
    in vitro studies, 291–292
    skeletal myoblast transplantation and porcine model of MI, 235–236
    unresolved clinical issues, 98–99
    U.S. experience, 113
  steps in research, 225
Assessment
  clinical trials, 96–97, 98
  posttransplantation: *see* Posttransplantation assessment
  risk-benefit, 192–193
Atrial cardiomyocytes, 292
Autologous transplantation, 123
  bone marrow-derived stem cells, 145

Autologous transplantation (*cont.*)
  myoblasts, 213–229
    histological studies, 235–236
    isolation of, 234, 234–235
    steps in translational research,
      223–228
Autonomic compensation, 6
Azacytidine, 29, 145

Balloon catheters, 177–178
Bench testing, 307
Beta adrenergic receptor density, 14
Beta blockers, 14–15, 178, 281
BioCardia Helical Infusion System,
  317, 318
BioCardia Helical Injection Catheter™,
  214
Bioheart injection (delivery) catheter, 214
Biological Response Modifiers Advisory
  Committee (BRMAC)
  recommendations, 309–311
  catheter testing, 310
  large animal models, 310–311
  small animal models, 309
  study duration, 311
  in vitro data, 309–310
Biopsy
  cell procurement, 107–108
  steps in research, flow chart, 227
Bio-Z, 227
Blood flow, bone marrow-derived stem
  cell transplantation and, 149, 150
Bone marrow-derived stem cells, 27, 29,
  128, 213
  clinical experience, surgical delivery,
    159–165
    cell types, identification of,
      162–163
    delivery modes/routes, 163–164
    mechanisms of action, 164–165
    scarred myocardium, effects on,
      160–162
  clinical trials, 126–127
  comparisons of cell types, 87, 88,
    101–102
  electrophysiology, 292–293
  mesenchymal stem cells, 302–303
  mobilizing cells for repair after
    myocardial infarction, 203–208

Bone marrow-derived stem cells (*cont.*)
  myocardial cell formation and
    integration with myocardium,
      41–44
  myocardial infarction
    German experience, 169–182
    Spanish experience, 187–198
  myocardial infarction, acute phase
    management, 203–208
    controversies, 208
    initial human experience, 207
    mobilizing stem cells, 204–207
    risks, potential, 208
  preclinical experience, 137–153
    allogeneic implantation, 147
    angiogenesis, vascular
      repair/regeneration, 149–152
    cell labeling, 142–145
    characterization, 139–142
    expansion, 138–139, 140
    immunology, 142
    mesenchymal stem cells, 137–138
    tracking and quantification,
      147–149
    types of cells, 137
    in vivo cardiomyoplasty, 145–147
  regulatory considerations, 301–302,
    301–303
    infectious disease testing, 304
    types of cells, 124–125
BOOST trial, 292

Calcium flow, remodeling process, 11
Calcium sensitivity, 17
  cardioids, 250
  remodeling process, 11
Cancer risk, 128
Canine model of heart failure, 5, 7, 8
Cardiac index, 227
Cardiac output, 227
Cardiac stem cells, 39–52, 87
  aging and, 49
  bone marrow-derived stem cells,
    formation of myocardial
    cells and myocardial integration,
      41–44
  comparisons of cell types, 88
  distribution of, 48–49
  homeostasis, role in, 49–50, 51

Cardiac stem cells (*cont.*)
identification of cardiac primitive
cells, 44–45
myocyte death and regeneration,
40–41
primitive cells in adult heart as true
stem cells, 45–46
prospects for regeneration in humans,
50–52
regeneration of functional
myocardium, 46–48
types of cells, 123
Cardioids, tissue engineering
contractility metrics, 248–249
delamination process, 246–247
formation method, 244–246
histological studies, 247–248
physiological metrics, 249–251
strategies for, 242–244
Cardiomyocytes, 26–27
embryonic stem cells, 30–31
fetal, 26, 27
Catheters, 128
Biocardia Helical Infusion System,
317, 318
bone marrow-derived stem cell
delivery, 174–175, 180, 181
descriptions of commercial products,
317–321
percutaneous myoblast
transplantation, steps in
translational research
bioretention and distribution of
cells, 221, 223
catheter-cell biocompatibility, 217
cell types, 213
delivery modes/routes, 213–215
feasibility of cell delivery, 221–222
flow chart, 227
instrumentation, 214, 215–217, 218,
219
porcine animal model, 219–220, 221
safety and efficacy, 223–228
preclinical studies, 308
regulatory considerations, 310
SR200 MyoCath™ Percutaneous
Catheter Delivery System, 318,
319
TransAccess® MicroLume™, 321

CD antigens, 302
identification of bone marrow stem
cells, 301
mesenchymal stem cells, 141
Cell-cell coupling, 16, 26
electrophysiology, 291–292
repair process, 102
Cell culture
cardioids, tissue engineering, 241–252
mesenchymal stem cells, 138–142
porcine model of MI, 234
skeletal myoblasts
early experiments, 62–64
primary culturing, 108, 109
propagation, 111
Cell death
immunology: *see* Immune reaction
ischemia and: *see* Pathophysiology
unresolved clinical issues, 99–100
Cell dose and volume, 223
Cell harvest and processing for culture
bone marrow-derived stem cells, 189,
190, 192
regulatory considerations, 301
skeletal muscle cells, 107–108, 109,
111
Cells, catheter biocompatibility, 217–218
Cell therapy, 15–16
Cell types, 25–31, 121–129
adult stem cells, 124–125
animal models, 25–26
bone marrow-derived stem cells, 29,
160–162
cardiac stem cells, 123
cardiomyocytes, 26–27
choices, 121–123
clinical trials, 126–128
comparisons of, 87–88, 101–102
embryonic stem cells, 30–31, 123–124
endothelial cells, 38–39
future directions, 128–129
myoblasts, 27–28
smooth muscle cells, 29–30
transdifferentiation versus fusion,
125–126
Cellular homeostasis in heart, 39, 40–41
Cellular remodeling, 11–12, 13
Center for Biologics Evaluation and
Research (CBER), 299

Center for Devices and Radiological
    Health (CDRH), 299
Chemoattractants, cardiac stem cells,
    48
Chronic ischemic heart disease, 128
Circumferential fiber shortening, 280,
    281
Clinical development, regulatory
    considerations, 306–307
Clinical experience/trials
    bone marrow-derived stem cells,
        126–127, 160–162
    Germany, 169–182
    Spain, 187–198
    Spanish studies, 194–196
    surgical delivery, 159–165
    history of transplantation, 65–66,
        69–70
    initial lessons from clinical trials,
        292–293
    regulatory considerations, 299–300,
        307
    skeletal myoblast transplantation
        European experience, 95–102
        U.S. experience, 105–117
    types of cells, 126–128
Cloning, therapeutic, 31
Coil placement, porcine model of MI,
    232
Complications/adverse effects: *see also*
    Arrhythmias
    blood-derived progenitor cells, 127
    bone marrow-derived stem cell
        transplantation, 181, 196
    embryonic stem cells, 123–124
    skeletal myoblast transplantation
        European experience, 98–99
        U.S. experience, 113–114, 115–116,
            117
Concentric hypertrophy, 279
Congestive heart failure (CHF),
    cardioid tissue engineering
    cardioid formation method,
        244–246
    contractility metrics, 248–249
    delamination process, 246–247
    histological studies, 247–248
    physiological metrics, 249–251
    strategies for, 242–244

Connexin 43, 116
    cell design, 89
    electrophysiology, 292
    ischemia, hypertrophy and
        inflammation effects, 290, 291
Connexins, 290
Contractility
    bone marrow-derived stem cells, 146
    cardioids, 244–245, 248–249, 250
    remodeling process, 11
    repair process, 102
    systolic function assessment,
        posttransplantation, 277–285
        ejection phase indexes, 278–282
        end systolic volume and dimensions,
            282–285
        isovolumic indexes, 277–278
    ventricular remodeling and, 12–14
Cord blood, 128, 182, 302
Cordis MyoStar™ systems, 215, 216,
    217, 221
Coronary artery bypass grafting
    (CABG), 180
    cells delivered during, 127
    comparison of cell transplantation
        with, 105–117

Defibrillators, 116, 294–295
Delamination, cardioid tissue
    engineering, 244, 246–247
Delivery modes/routes, 128, 308
    bone marrow-derived stem cells,
        188
        acute phase treatment prospects,
            197
        German studies, 174–176, 181–182
        Spanish studies, 190, 191
        surgical, 159–165, 163–164
    catheters, commercial, 317–321
    clinical trials, 127
    preclinical studies, 308
    skeletal myoblasts, 213–215
        porcine model of MI for evaluation
            of, 231–238
        steps in translational research,
            213–229
Demographics, U.S. experience with
    skeletal myoblasts, 110–111
Detection of cells: *see* Tracking cells

Differentiation, bone marrow-derived
  stem cells, 142–143, 145–146
Dosage testing, regulatory requirements,
  305
Dose/activity relationships, 307
Dose/toxicity relationships, 307
Drug therapies, 14–15
Duration of preclinical studies, 311

Echocardiography, 264
  bone marrow-derived stem cell
    transplantation, 193, 195–196
  clinical trials, 96
  porcine model of MI, 232, 233
  steps in research, 227, 228
Ejection fraction
  bone marrow-derived stem cell
    transplantation, 180
  derivation of, 278–279
  patient evaluation, 107
  porcine model of MI, 232
  remodeling process, 5, 6
  steps in research, 220, 228
  systolic function assessment,
    posttransplantation, 273
Ejection phase
  corrected indices, 279, 280, 281
  derivation of, 278–279
  systolic function assessment,
    posttransplantation, 278–282
Ejection rate, beta-blockade, 281
Elastance
  maximum, 283, 285
  time-varying, 282–283, 284
Electrocardiography
  bone marrow-derived stem cell
    transplantation, 191–192
  patient monitoring, 111
  porcine model of MI, 232, 233,
    235
  steps in research, flow chart, 227
Electromechanical mapping: see
  Mapping
Electrophysiology
  arrhythmias, 289–295
    assessment, gold standard
      determination, 293–295
    future directions, 295
    initial lessons, 292–293

Electrophysiology (cont.)
  mechanisms of, potential
    interactions with cell therapy,
    290–291
  in vitro studies, 291–292
  cardioid tissue engineering, 249–251
  repair process, 89, 102
Embolization, cell injection and, 221
Embryonic carcinoma cells, 291
Embryonic stem cells, 26, 27, 30–31,
  121–122, 128, 182, 213, 303
  electrophysiology, 291
  regulatory considerations, 301
  types of cells, 123–124
Emergent setting, bone marrow-derived
  stem cells, 145
End diastolic pressure-volume
  relationships (EDPVRs), 5, 6,
  7–11, 17
Endothelial cells, 28–29
Endothelial progenitor cells (EPCs), 27,
  126, 302
Endoventricular delivery of cells
  porcine model, 231–238
  steps in research, 213–229
End systolic pressure-volume
  relationship (ESPVR), 5, 6, 7, 17,
  283, 285
End systolic stress (ESS), 281
End systolic volume and dimensions,
  276, 282–285
Engraftment
  bone marrow-derived stem cells
    homing, 151–152
    labeling for tracking, 147–149
  skeletal myoblasts, porcine model,
    231
  steps in research, 221, 223–228
Epinephrine, cardioid sensitivity, 251
Escape rhythm, 292
European experience
  bone marrow stem cell mobilization
    for repair
    Germany, 169–182
    Spain, 187–198
  skeletal myoblast transplantation,
    95–102
Evaluation: see Assessment
Extracellular milieu, 146, 147

Fasting, 260
Fetal cells, 25–26, 27
Fiber shortening, velocity of (VCF),
    280, 281
Fibroblasts, comparisons of cell types,
    87, 88
Fluorescent labels, bone marrow-derived
    stem cells, 143
Fluoroscopic guidance system, catheter
    delivery, 214, 215, 224, 226
Follow-up
    bone-marrow derived stem cell
        transplantation, 190–194
    initial lessons from clinical trials, 293
Food and Drug Administration (FDA),
    299, 300, 308, 311
Force-frequency relationship, 11,
    277–278
    remodeling process, 13–14
Fusion, bone marrow-derived stem cells,
    165
Fusion, transdifferentiation versus, types
    of cells, 125–126

Gamma imaging, bone marrow-derived
    stem cells, 147, 148
Gap junctions, 16, 26, 290–291
Gene expression
    physical treatments and, 15
    remodeling process, 11–12
Gene therapy, 182
Genetic labeling
    bone marrow-derived stem cells,
        143–144
    bone marrow-derived stem cell
        transplantation, 176
Germany, bone-marrow derived stem
    cell transplantation experience,
    169–182
    cardiomyoplasty, 173–174
    clinical data, 177–181
        endogenous bone marrow cells, 177
        exogenous bone marrow cells,
            177–181
    delivery modes/routes, 174–176
    detection of transplanted cells, 176–177
    future directions and unresolved
        issues, 181–182
    regeneration after MI, 170–173

Glucose loading, PET, 260–261
Granulocyte colony-stimulating factor
    (G-CSF), 127, 194–196, 301–302
Granulocyte-macrophage colony-
    stimulating factor (GM-CSF), 179
Growth factors, 301–302, 303
    blood-derived progenitor cells, 127
    bone marrow-derived stem cells, 179
    mode of action, 164
    cardiac stem cells and, 48
    mesenchymal stem cell receptors, 141
    smooth muscle cell response, 29–30
Guidance systems, catheter delivery,
    214, 215, 226

Heart failure, myocardial infarction
    sequelae, 170–174
Helical Infusion Catheter, 317, 318
Helical Injection Catheter™, 214
Hematopoietic stem cells, 213
    comparisons of, 101–102
    regulatory considerations, 301–302
    transdifferentiation versus fusion,
        126
Hemodynamics, remodeling process,
    7–11
Histocompatibility complexes, 31
Histological studies, 151–152
    atrial cardiomyocytes, 292
    bone marrow-derived stem cells, 149,
        150
    cardioid tissue engineering, 247–248
    porcine model of MI, 221, 222, 231,
        235–236, 237
    U.S. experience with skeletal
        myoblasts, 112
History of skeletal myoblast
    transplantation, 61–71
    cardiovascular disease application,
        70–71
    muscle disease applications
        cell culture, 62–64
        early clinical trials, 65–66
        immune response/rejection, 67–68
        improvements of process, 66–67
        pioneer transplantation
            experiments, 64–65
        preclinical and clinical progress,
            68–70

Holter analysis, 191–192, 293, 294
Homeostasis, myocardium, 40–41,
    49–50, 51
Homing, mesenchymal stem cells,
    151–152, 175–176
Hyperinsulinemic-euglycemic clamp, 261
Hypertrophy
    concentric, 279
    connexin43 effects, 290

Identity, product, 306
Immune reaction
    bone marrow-derived stem cells, 182
    embryonic stem cells, 30–31, 124
    history of transplantation, 67–68
    mesenchymal stem cells, 142,
        302–303
    porcine model of MI, 236, 241–252
    types of cells, 122
    unresolved clinical issues, 99–100
Immunosuppression, 26
Implantable cardioverter-defibrillator
    (ICD) therapy, 116, 294–295
Infectious disease testing, regulatory
    considerations, 304
Inflammation, connexin43 effects, 290
Infusion procedures: see Delivery
    modes/routes
Instrumentation
    percutaneous transplantation of
        skeletal myoblasts, 214, 215–217,
        218, 219
    regulatory considerations, 310
Intramyocardial administration, clinical
    trials, 127
Intravenous administration, bone
    marrow-derived stem cells, 175–176
Investigational New Drug (IND)
    application, 299
In vitro studies
    arrhythmias, 291–292
    regulatory considerations, 309–310
        product manufacturing and testing,
        305
        toxicology, 307–308
In vivo studies
    catheter testing, 310
    PET, preoperative use of, 257–267
    regulatory considerations, 307, 308

Iridium labeled myoblasts, 223
Ischemia
    cardiac stem cell tropism, 48
    connexin43 effects, 290
Ischemic cardiomyopathy, 128
    clinical trials, 127
    remodeling in: see Remodeling in
        ischemic cardiomyopathy
Isochrones, time-varying elastance, 283,
    284
Isoprotereneol, 15
Isovolumic indexes, 277–278

Labeling
    bone marrow-derived stem cells, 176
        preclinical experience, 142–145
        for tracking, 147–149
    myoblasts, 223
Large animal models, 101
    porcine model of MI, 231–238
    regulatory considerations, 310–311
Left ventricular assist devices (LVAD)
    remodeling process, 7–14
    U.S. experience, 105–117
Length-force relationships, cardioids,
    250
Leukapheresis, 302
Lipoaspirates, 128, 303
Loop recorder, 227

MADIT II study, 295
MAGIC (Myoblast Autologous
    Grafting in Ischemic
    Cardiomyopathy), 98–99, 267
Magnetic field sensor, mapping catheter,
    216
Magnetic resonance imaging (MRI),
    114
    bone marrow-derived stem cell
        transplantation, 148, 176, 180
    skeletal myoblast transplantation
        monitoring, 112–113, 114
        patient selection, 107
        systolic function measurement,
        281–282
Major histocompatibility complex
    (MHC) proteins
    embryonic stem cells, 124
    mesenchymal stem cells, 142

Manufacturing, regulatory
  considerations, 300–306
  product considerations for cellular
    therapies, 300
  sources and collection of cellular
    products, 301–303
Mapping, 128, 174
  bone marrow-derived stem cell
    transplantation, 163–164, 293
  porcine model of MI, 235
Mapping catheters, 215, 216, 225, 226,
  227, 228
Match, perfusion-metabolism, 261, 262
Maximal dP/dt, 277–278
Maximum elastance, 283, 285
Mean velocity of fiber shortening
  (VCF), 279, 280, 281
Mechanism of cell repair, 100–101, 300
Mesenchymal stem cells, 28, 29, 213; see
    also Bone marrow-derived stem cells
  comparisons of cell types, 87, 88,
    101–102
  harvesting and processing, 302–303
  preclinical experience, 137–138
Methylene blue, 221
Microbiological safety, regulatory
  considerations, 304–305
Mismatch, perfusion-metabolism, 261,
  262
MNSER (mean normalized systolic
  ejection rate), 280
Mode of delivery: see Delivery modes
Molecular and cellular remodeling,
  11–12, 13
Monitoring
  cell distribution: see Tracking cells
  follow-up: see Follow-up
  PET, preoperative use of, 257–267
Morph® Deflectable Guide Catheter,
  317
Muscle biopsy for cell procurement,
  107–108
Myoblast Autologous Grafting in
  Ischemic Cardiomyopathy
  (MAGIC), 98–99, 267
Myoblasts, 27–28
  autologous, 213; see also Autologous
    transplantation
  skeletal: see Skeletal myoblasts

Myocardial function: see Ventricular
  function
Myocardial infarction, 128, 208
  bone marrow-derived stem cells
    acute phase treatment study,
      203–208
    German studies, 169–182
    Spanish studies, 187–198
  clinical trials, 126–127
  porcine model, 231–238
    animal preparation, 232–233
    bone marrow stem cell mobilization
      for repair, 203–208
    induction of infarct, 233
    myoblast isolation, 234–235
  regeneration after, 170–174
Myocardial perfusion, 262–263
Myocardial regeneration, 25–31; see also
  Regeneration
Myocardial remodeling: see Remodeling
  in ischemic cardiomyopathy
Myocardial viability, 258–261, 262
Myocardial wrap, 15
MyoCath™ Percutaneous Catheter
  Delivery System, 214, 318, 319
Myocytes
  PET, preoperative use of, 261
  remodeling process, 10
  skeletal: see Skeletal myoblasts
Myofilaments, 17
Myogenesis, 85, 89
Myosin 32-beta, 115–116
MyoStar™ system, 214, 215, 216, 217,
  221, 226, 227, 318, 320
Myotube formation, 115
  cardioid tissue engineering, 244, 245
  swine model, 221, 222

Neurohormonal activation, 17
  drug treatments, 15
  remodeling process, 5, 6, 9
Nitric oxide, 30
NOGASTAR® Mapping Catheter, 225,
  226, 227, 228
NOGA systems, 215, 217, 226, 321
  electrophysiology, 293
  porcine model of MI, 232, 237
  steps in research, flow chart, 227
Nuclear transfer techniques, 31, 124

Office of Cellular, Tissue, and Gene
    Therapies (OCTGT), 299

Pacing, 16
Pathophysiology
    drug treatments, 14–15
    myocardial infarction sequelae,
        170–174
    regeneration after MI, 181–182
    repair process, 85
    ventricular remodeling, 3–7, 8
Patient preparation, PET, 259–261
Patient selection
    PET, preoperative use of, 263–264
    U.S. experience with skeletal
        myoblasts, 106
Percutaneous transplantation, 17
    bone marrow-derived stem cells, 177
    clinical trials, 127
    porcine model of MI for evaluation
        of, 231–238
    preclinical studies, 308
    steps in research, 213–229
        bioretention and distribution of
            cells, 221, 223
        catheter-cell biocompatibility, 217
        cell types, 213
        delivery modes/routes, 213–215
        feasibility of cell delivery, 221–222
        flow chart, 227
        instrumentation, 214, 215–217, 218,
            219
        porcine animal model, 219–220, 221
        safety and efficacy, 223–228
Perfusion-metabolism match, 261
Perfusion-metabolism mismatch, 261,
    262
Peripheral blood cells
    clinical trials, 127
    comparisons of cell types, 87
    regulatory considerations, infectious
        disease testing, 304
PET: see Positron emission tomography
    (PET)
Physiological metrics, cardioids,
    249–251
Physiology
    cardioid tissue engineering, 251
    PET, preoperative use of, 258

Placebo effect, 180
Porcine model of myocardial infarction,
    231–238
    animal preparation, 232–233
    induction of infarct, 233
    myoblast isolation, 234–235
    percutaneous transplantation, steps in
        research, 213–229
Positron emission tomography (PET),
    257–267
    bone marrow-derived stem cell
        transplantation
        German studies, 176–177
        Spanish studies, 193, 195, 196
    cell viability assessment, 258–261
        patient preparation, 259–261
        physiology, 258
        protocols, 259
    European experience, 96–97, 98
    noninvasive imaging for in vivo
        assessment of cell therapy,
        264–267
    patterns of myocyte variability, 261
    preoperative use, evidence supporting,
        261–264
        candidate selection, 264
        myocardial perfusion, 262–263
        predicting regional and global LV
            function, 263
        predicting symptom improvement,
            263–264
        risk stratification and survival
            prediction, 264
    U.S. experience with skeletal
        myoblasts, 112–113, 114
Post mortem studies, skeletal myoblast
    transplantation, 177
Posttransplantation assessment
    arrhythmias, electrophysiology,
        289–295
    future directions, 295
    gold standard determination,
        293–295
    initial lessons, 292–293
    mechanisms of, 290–291
    in vitro studies, 291–292
    bone marrow-derived stem cell
        tracking, 142–145
    PET, 257–267

Posttransplantation assessment (*cont.*)
  skeletal myoblast transplantation
    European experience, 96, 97, 98
    U.S. experience with, 107
  systolic function measurement, 273–285
    contractility metrics, 277–285
    definitions, 274–276
Potency, product, 306
Preclinical studies
  bone marrow-derived stem cells,
    137–153
  history of transplantation, 69
  regulatory considerations, 307, 307–308
  skeletal myoblast transplantation, 81–90
    comparisons of cell types, 87–88
    early experiments, 82–85
    future directions, 88–89
    present role, 85–87
Preload, 275–276
Premature ventricular contractions
  (PVCs), 225, 226
Pressure, afterload measures, 274–275
Pressure change, measures of
  contractility, 277–278
Pressure-volume relationships
  end systolic volume and dimensions,
    282–285
  remodeling process, 5, 6, 7, 7–11
Primitives, cardiac
  in adults, 45–46
  identification of, 44–45
Product manufacturing and testing:
  see Manufacturing
Progenitor cells, 121–129
Protein expression, bone marrow-
  derived stem cells, 146
Purity, product, 306

Radiolabeled cells, 147, 148
Rat model, 25–26
Recombinant granulocyte colony-
  stimulating factor (G-CSF), 301–302
Reduced perfusion, 261, 262
Regeneration, myocardial
  cardiac stem cells for, 39–52
    aging and, 49
    bone marrow stem cells, formation
      of myocardial cells and
      myocardial integration, 41–44

Regeneration, myocardial (*cont.*)
    distribution of, 48–49
    homeostasis, role in, 49–50, 51
    identification of cardiac primitive
      cells, 44–45
    myocyte death and regeneration,
      40–41
    primitive cells in adult heart as true
      stem cells, 45–46
    prospects for regeneration in
      humans, 50–52
    regeneration of functional
      myocardium, 46–48
  cell types, 25–31
    animal models, 25–26
    bone marrow-derived stem cells,
      29
    cardiomyocytes, 26–27
    embryonic stem cells, 30–31
    endothelial cells, 38–39
    myoblasts, 27–28
    smooth muscle cells, 29–30
  tissue engineering, 241–252
Regulatory considerations, 299–301
  advisory committee discussions and
    recommendations, 309–311
    catheter testing, 310
    large animal models, 310–311
    small animal models, 309
    study duration, 311
    in vitro data, 309–310
  clinical trial requirements, 299–300
  preclinical studies, 307–308
  product manufacturing and testing,
    300–306
    product considerations for cellular
      therapies, 300
    sources and collection of cellular
      products, 301–303
  swine model, 220
  testing cells for cardiac repair,
    303–306
    cell dose and viability, 305
    infectious disease, 304
    microbiological, 304–305
    product characterization, 305–306
  testing during clinical development,
    306–307
  U.S. government agencies, 299

Rejection, immunological: *see* Immune reaction
Remodeling in ischemic cardiomyopathy, 3–18
  bone marrow-derived stem cell tracking, 143–145
  canine model, 5, 7, 8
  cell therapy, 15–16
  contractile performance in, 12–14
  molecular and cellular remodeling, 11–12, 13
  pathophysiology, 3–7, 8
  reverse remodeling, pharmacological therapies and other devices inducing, 14–15
  structural remodeling, 8–11
Repair process, cellular components, 85
Resident stem cells, 122, 123
Restenosis, 127
Resynchronization therapy, 15
Reversed perfusion-metabolism mismatch, 261, 262
Reverse remodeling, 5, 11–12, 14–15, 17
Right ventricular assist device (RVAD), 11
Risk/benefit analysis, 308
Risk-benefit assessment, bone-marrow derived stem cell transplantation, 192–193
Risk stratification, PET, preoperative use of, 264
Routes of administration: *see* Delivery modes/routes
Ryanodine-sensitive calcium release channel, 11, 12, 13, 14

Safety
  bone marrow-derived stem cell transplantation, 180
  regulatory considerations, 300, 307; *see also* Regulatory considerations
  skeletal myoblast transplantation, 113, 115, 223–228
Sarcomere length, fiber shortening, 281
Sarcomere number, 276
Sarcomere stretch, 275, 276
Sarcomeric organization, bone marrow-derived stem cells, 146–147

Sarcoplasmic endoreticular calcium-ATPase subtype 2a (SERCA2a), 11, 12
  remodeling process, 13
Satellite cells (myoblasts), 27–28
Scar tissue
  bone marrow-derived stem cells, effects on regeneration, 160–162
  cell delivery to, 224
  porcine model of MI, 237
Sequential perfusion-FDG approach, PET, 261, 262
Shortening, fiber, velocity of (VCF), 280, 281
Shortening fraction, derivation of, 278–279
Signal average electrocardiogram (SAECG), 293
Sinus node cells, 292
Skeletal myoblasts, 17, 27–28, 28–29, 177
  clinical trials, 128
  electrophysiology, 292
  European experience, 95–102
  history of transplantation of, 61–71
  percutaneous transplantation, steps in research
    bioretention and distribution of cells, 221, 223
    catheter-cell biocompatibility, 217
    cell types, 213
    delivery modes/routes, 213–215
    feasibility of cell delivery, 221–222
    flow chart, 227
    instrumentation, 214, 215–217, 218, 219
    porcine animal model, 219–220, 221
    safety and efficacy, 223–228
  preclinical studies, 81–90
    comparisons of cell types, 87–88
    early experiments, 82–85
    future directions, 88–89
    present role, 85–87
  U.S. experience, 105–117
    cell culture, primary, 108, 109
    cell culture, propagation, 110–111
    demographics, 110–111
    efficacy and potential complications, 115–116, 117

Skeletal myoblasts (*cont.*)
  evaluation, 107
  evaluation, imaging methods for,
    112–113, 114
  feasibility, 111–113
  limitations, 116–117
  muscle excision, 107–108
  patient selection, 106
  safety, 113, 115
  transplantation, 108, 111
Slow twitch protein, 115–116
Small animal models, regulatory
  considerations, 309, 310–311
Smooth muscle cells (SMC), 27, 29–30
Sodium/calcium exchanger, 11, 12
Spain, bone-marrow derived stem cell
    transplantation experience, 187–198
  acute phase treatment prospects,
    196–197
  algorithm, 194
  clinical studies, 194–196
  extraction and management of cells,
    189
  follow-up, 190–194
  infusion procedure, 190, 191
  pathophysiology of heart failure,
    187–188
  risk-benefit assessment, 192–193
Spanish experience, 96
SPECT imaging, 263–264, 265, 266, 267
  bone marrow-derived stem cell
    transplantation, 176, 180
  patient selection, 107
SR200 MyoCath™ Percutaneous
  Catheter Delivery System, 318,
  319
STEMI, 188–197
Stiletto™ Endocardial Direct Injection
  Catheter, 320
Strain rate imaging, 281–282
Stretch, 17
  left ventricular dilatation and, 291
  sarcomere, 275, 276
Structural remodeling, 8–11
ST-segment elevation acute MI
  (STEMI), 188–197
Surface markers/antigens, 302
  cardiac stem cells, 44–45, 123
  embryonic stem cells, 124

Surface markers/antigens (*cont.*)
  hematopoietic stem cells, 301
  mesenchymal stem cells, 141
Surgical delivery
  bone marrow-derived stem cells,
    159–165
  cell types, identification of,
    162–163
  delivery modes/routes, 163–164
  mechanisms of action, 164–165
  scarred myocardium, effects on,
    160–162
  clinical trials, 127
Sustained ventricular tachycardia
  (SVT), 225
Symptom improvement
  angina, 180, 181
  PET prediction of, 263–264
Systolic function assessment,
    posttransplantation, 273–285
  bone marrow-derived stem cells,
    146–147
  contractility metrics, 277–285
    ejection phase indexes, 278–282
    end systolic volume and dimensions,
      282–285
    isovolumic indexes, 277–278
  definitions, 274–276
    afterload, 274–275
    preload, 275–276

Tachycardias, 116, 225, 292, 293, 294
Targeting, cardiac stem cells, 48
Technetium labeling, bone marrow-
  derived stem cells, 147–148
Teratomas, 123–124
Testing, regulatory requirements
  cells, product quality, 303–306
    cell dose and viability, 305
    infectious disease issues, 304
    microbiological issues, 304–305
    product characterization,
      305–306
  manufacturing process, 300–306
    product considerations for cellular
      therapies, 300
    sources and collection of cellular
      products, 301–303
Therapeutic cloning, 31

Three-dimensional cell culture, cardioid tissue engineering, 249–251
Three-dimensional guidance catheter delivery system, 214, 215, 216, 226
Three-dimensional map, 222
Time of treatment, bone marrow-derived stem cells, 148–149
Time to peak tension (TPT), cardioid tissue engineering, 248
Time varying elastance, 282–283, 284
Tissue Doppler imaging, 281–282
Tissue engineering, 241–252
    cardioid formation method, 244–246
    contractility metrics, 248–249
    delamination process, 246–247
    histological studies, 247–248
    physiological metrics, 249–251
    strategies for, 242–244
Tissue stem cells, 303
TOPCARE-AMI trial, 293
Total peripheral resistance (TPR), 275
Totipotent cells, 121
Toxicology
    catheter testing, 310
    product quality, regulatory requirements, 307–308
Tracking cells
    bone marrow-derived stem cells, 176–177
    mesenchymal stem cell markers, 142–145
    skeletal myoblasts, 221, 223
TransAccess® MicroLume™, 214, 321, 322
Transdifferentiation, 128
    bone marrow-derived stem cells, 142–143, 162–163
    defined, 122
    versus fusion, 125–126
Transplantation, U.S. experience with skeletal myoblasts, 108, 111
Tropisms, cardiac stem cells, 48
Two-dimensional fluoroscopy catheter guidance system, 214, 215

Umbilical cord blood, 128, 182
    harvesting and processing, 302
    regulatory considerations, 304
United States, experience with skeletal myoblasts, 116

United States, skeletal myoblast transplantation, 105–117
United States regulatory agencies, 299

Vascular endothelial growth factor (VEGF), 30, 90, 164, 303
Vascular infusion, 308
Vascularization, 16; see also Angiogenesis
Velocity of fiber shortening (VCF), 280, 281
Ventricular function
    bone marrow-derived stem cell transplantation and, 146–147
    German studies, 178–179, 180
    Spanish studies, 194–196
    surgical delivery, 160–162
    myocardial stretch secondary to left ventricular dilatation, 291
    patient evaluation, 107
    patient selection, 106
    PET studies, 258–261, 263
    porcine model of MI, 232
    posttransplantation assessment, 273–285
        contractility metrics, 277–285
        definitions, 274–276
    steps in research, 220, 228
Ventricular remodeling: see Remodeling in ischemic cardiomyopathy
Ventricular tachycardia, 116, 225, 292, 293, 294
Ventriculography, porcine model of MI, 233, 235
Viability of cells, regulatory considerations, 305
Voltage map, ventricle, 216, 222
    steps in research, 227, 228

Wall motion, porcine model of MI, 232
Wall stress
    afterload measures, 275
    bone marrow-derived stem cells and, 146
Wall thickness
    bone marrow-derived stem cell transplantation and, 180
    steps in research, 224–225
    swine model, 225